T0257744

Hematopoietic Stem Cell Research

Hematopoietic Stem Cell Research

Edited by **Rex Turner**

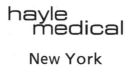

New York

Published by Hayle Medical,
30 West, 37th Street, Suite 612,
New York, NY 10018, USA
www.haylemedical.com

Hematopoietic Stem Cell Research
Edited by Rex Turner

International Standard Book Number: 978-1-63241-249-2 (Hardback)

Contents

Permissions

List of Contributors

Preface

This book was inspired by the evolution of our times; to answer the curiosity of inquisitive minds. Many developments have occurred across the globe in the recent past which has transformed the progress in the field.

Researches are being conducted around the globe for a better understanding of hematopoietic stem cells. This book provides a complete analysis of the biology and healing possibilities of hematopoietic stem cells, and is meant for those involved in stem cell study. Beginning from primary principles in hematopoiesis, this book assembles a wealth of information related to central devices that may control separation and growth of hematopoietic stem cells in usual conditions and throughout disease. It discusses the properties and regulation factors of hematopoietic stem cells. The book compiles researches from renowned experts involved in this field.

This book was developed from a mere concept to drafts to chapters and finally compiled together as a complete text to benefit the readers across all nations. To ensure the quality of the content we instilled two significant steps in our procedure. The first was to appoint an editorial team that would verify the data and statistics provided in the book and also select the most appropriate and valuable contributions from the plentiful contributions we received from authors worldwide. The next step was to appoint an expert of the topic as the Editor-in-Chief, who would head the project and finally make the necessary amendments and modifications to make the text reader-friendly. I was then commissioned to examine all the material to present the topics in the most comprehensible and productive format.

I would like to take this opportunity to thank all the contributing authors who were supportive enough to contribute their time and knowledge to this project. I also wish to convey my regards to my family who have been extremely supportive during the entire project.

Editor

Part 1

Hematopoietic Stem Cell Properties

Markers for Hematopoietic Stem Cells: Histories and Recent Achievements

Takafumi Yokota[1], Kenji Oritani[1], Stefan Butz[2],
Stephan Ewers[2], Dietmar Vestweber[2] and Yuzuru Kanakura[1]
[1]Department of Hematology and Oncology,
Osaka University Graduate School of Medicine, Suita
[2]Department of Vascular Cell Biology,
Max-Planck-Institute for Molecular Biomedicine, Münster,
[1]Japan
[2]Germany

1. Introduction

Hematopoietic stem cells (HSC) are characterized with the capacity for self-renewal as well as multi-lineage differentiation, maintaining the immune system and blood cell formation throughout life. Although studies for the HSC biology have been in the forefront of the stem cell research field, many questions still remain with regard to the origin, development, and aging of HSC. Furthermore, needless to say, HSC are very useful for clinical medicine, particularly in the transplantation and/or regeneration therapy for hematological malignancies. Success of those therapies depends on how effectively HSC are purified and transplanted to the patients. In order to address those important issues in both basic and clinical science, information of cell surface molecules that selectively mark HSC is essential.

Since the frequency of HSC in bone marrow or peripheral blood is extremely low, many studies have attempted to identify unique markers associated with those rare cells. As a result, it is now possible to purify long-term reconstituting HSC from mouse bone marrow with very high efficiency. However, many of these parameters change dramatically during ontogeny or inflammation, and what is worse still, they differ between mouse and man. Efficient HSC-based therapies and the emerging field of tissue-regenerative medicine will benefit from more precise information about what defines HSC.

In this chapter, we summarize a large body of information with respect to the HSC-related markers and introduce Endothelial cell-selective adhesion molecule (ESAM) as a novel marker for HSC (Yokota et al., 2009). Indeed, ESAM is expressed throughout the ontogeny in mouse and can be used as a gating parameter for sorting long-term repopulating HSC. In addition, the marker appears to be useful for the purification of human HSC.

2. Development of methodology for HSC purification from mouse bone marrow

In 1988, Spangrude et al tried to find a set of cell surface proteins that were associated with multi-lineage reconstitution ability, and succeeded to enrich such multipotential progenitors in the Lineage marker (Lin; generally including TER119, Mac1, Gr1, CD45R/B220, CD3, CD4, CD8)- Thy-1^{Low} Sca-1$^+$ fraction of mouse bone marrow (Spangrude et al, 1988). Indeed, they showed that only 30 Lin- Thy-1^{Low} Sca-1$^+$ cells injected via a tail vein could rescue 50% of lethally irradiated mice. Three years later, in 1991, Ogawa et al reported that hematopoietic progenitor activity of mouse bone marrow was excusive to the cells expressing c-kit, which is a receptor for stem cell factor (Ogawa et al., 1991). Since then, Lin- Sca-1$^+$ c-kit$^+$ (LSK) has been generally used as a canonical marker set for HSC enrichment.

It has been gradually recognized that the LSK fraction is heterogeneous, including long-term self-renewing HSC, short-term non-self-renewing HSC and lineage-committed progenitors. In 1996, Osawa et al reported that long-term HSC in adult bone marrow exist in the CD34 low to negative fraction among LSK cells (Osawa et al., 1996). Injection of a single CD34$^{-/Low}$ LSK cell resulted in multi-lineage long-term reconstitution in 21% of lethally irradiated mice whereas CD34$^+$ LSK cells revealed early but only short-term reconstitution. Transplantation of graded numbers of CD34$^{-/Low}$ LSK cells showed that the CD34$^{-/Low}$ LSK fraction contains long-term HSC at the frequency of 1 out of 5 cells. In 2001, Christensen and Weissman also showed that the LSK fraction is heterogeneous and long-term HSC are highly enriched in the Flk2/Flt3 receptor tyrosine kinase negative cells (Christensen & Weissman, 2001).

In addition to the cell surface markers, another approach has been developed to enrich long-term HSC activity by focusing on their high efflux activity. Using the fluorescent DNA-binding dye Hoechst33342, in 1996, Goodell et al found that cells in a small Hoechst^{low}-stained population (termed "Side population") can protect recipients from lethal irradiation at low cell doses (Goodell et al., 1996). A following study by Matsuzaki et al showed that, in combination with the CD34$^{-/Low}$ LSK phenotype, the strongest Hoechst33342 efflux activity (Tip-side population) can purify long-term multi-lineage HSC with almost absolute efficiency (Matsuzaki et al., 2004).

Recently, Morrison and colleagues reported an alternative method for HSC purification based on the expression pattern of the signaling lymphocytic activation molecule (SLAM) family proteins, i.e. CD150, CD244, and CD48 (Kiel et al., 2005). They showed that CD150$^+$ CD48$^-$ cells were uniformly CD244$^-$ and a simple gating for CD150$^+$ CD48$^-$ could enrich long-term HSC at approximately 1 in 5 cells. Moreover, combined with the canonical HSC marker LSK, the SLAM code could purify the HSC at 1 in 2 cells (Kiel et al., 2005).

Representative achievements during these 2 decades are summarized in Table 1. With surface markers, we can now purify the long-term multi-lineage HSC from adult mouse bone marrow with extremely high efficiency as Lin- Sca-1$^+$ c-kit$^+$ Thy1^{Low} CD34$^{-/low}$ CD150$^+$ CD48$^-$ cells. In fact, recent studies have demonstrated that the Lin- Sca-1$^+$ c-kit$^+$ CD34$^-$ CD150$^+$ CD48$^-$ fraction in adult mouse bone marrow contains truly dormant HSC, which divide only 5-6 times during the life span (Wilson et al., 2008; Foudi et al., 2009).

Markers	references
Lin⁻ Thy-1^{Low} Sca-1$^+$	Spangrude et al., 1988
CD34$^{-/Low}$ Lin⁻ Sca-1$^+$ c-kit$^+$	Osawa et al., 1996
Side Population (high Hoechst-efflux ability)	Goodell et al., 1996
*Tip-SP Lin⁻ Sca-1$^+$ c-kit$^+$	Matsuzaki et al., 2004
CD150$^+$ CD244 CD48⁻	Kiel et al., 2005
BrdU or Histone 2B-GFP-retaining, CD150$^+$ CD48⁻ CD34⁻ Lin⁻ Sca-1$^+$ c-kit$^+$	Wilson et al., 2008 Foudi et al., 2009

*Tip-SP: The highest Hoechst-efflux fraction in the Side Population

Table 1. Markers for hematopoietic stem cells in adult mouse bone marrow

3. Fickleness of HSC surface markers

It is important to stress here that none of the surface markers shown above is entirely specific to the long-term HSC. In addition, many of these parameters differ between strains of mice and change dramatically during developmental age. For example, Sca1, which has been a center in the canonical HSC marker "LSK", is not detectable on the emerging HSC in the aorta-gonad-mesonephros (AGM) area and only appears after day 11.5 of gestation on HSC in fetal liver (Matsubara et al., 2005; Our unpublished observation). Furthermore, the expression level of Sca1 on HSC differs between strains and is not very effective to enrich HSC from Balb/c mice (Spangrude & Brooks, 1993). Likewise, the SLAM family CD150 is not useful for the emerging and developing HSC in embryos (McKinney-Freeman et al., 2009). On the contrary, CD41, CD11b/Mac1, vascular endothelial (VE)-cadherin, and CD34 are known to mark the emerging and developing HSC during the fetal period, but gradually disappear along the ontogeny (Mikkola & Orkin, 2006).

It is also a well-recognized fact that cell surface markers on HSC in adult bone marrow do fluctuate according to the cell-cycle status and the differentiating behavior, which change depending on the physiological requirement. Bone marrow suppression by irradiation and/or chemotherapy revives several disappeared markers including CD11b/Mac1 and CD34 whereas it significantly down-regulates the expression level of c-kit on long-term HSC (Randall & Weissman, 1997; Ogawa 2002). Molecular crosstalk between HSC and bone marrow microenvironment is thought to control the status of HSC and influence their surface phenotypes, but precise mechanisms remain largely unknown. Therefore, researchers in the HSC field need to carefully choose an appropriate marker set and a sorting gate depending on the HSC characteristics, otherwise they would miss important target cells even in the lineage depletion step.

4. Difference between mouse and man

Another very critical issue on the topic of the HSC markers is their diversity between species. Although essential difference has not been observed between mouse and man regarding either the organs producing HSC or the transcription factors regulating their differentiation, completely different markers have been used to sort HSC in the two species. Human HSC do not express Sca1 or the SLAM family CD150 (Larochelle et al., 2011). While the CD34+ CD38- phenotype has been regarded as the canonical marker set for human HSC, it has been repeatedly reported that murine adult HSC locate in the CD34- CD38+ fraction (Randall et al., 1996; Matsuoka et al., 2001; Tajima et al., 2001). There is no reasonable explanation so far for the change along evolution, and such phenotypic differences between murine and human HSC have been an obstacle to apply achievement in mouse studies to human.

Early studies by Berenson et al demonstrated that autologous CD34+ cells enriched from bone marrow effectively radioprotected baboons and promoted hematopoietic recovery in human patients after marrow ablative therapy (Berenson et al, 1988, 1991). Over the past 2 decades, the use of CD34 as a marker for hematopoietic stem/progenitor cells has been a strong tool in the field of clinical hematology. Since the CD34+ fraction of human bone marrow contains lineage-committed progenitors as well as long-term multi-lineage HSC, many laboratories have sought additional markers to further enrich the CD34+ population for long-term HSC. CD90/Thy1, Tie, CD117/c-kit, and CD133/AC133 have been found as positive markers to enrich long-term-HSC whereas several negative markers including CD38 have been reported (Baum et al., 1992; Hasiyama et al., 1996; Gunji et al., 1993; Yin et al., 1997; Terstappen et al., 1991).

Recent advances of xenotransplantation models and techniques have enabled the assessment of pluripotency as well as self-renewal of human hematopoietic progenitors in vivo (Shultz et al., 2007). A series of studies by John Dick's laboratory have successfully enriched human long-term HSC within the Lin- CD34+ CD38- population (McKenzie et al., 2007; Doulatov et al., 2010). In a very recent report, they have purified human HSC from cord blood with a maker set of Lin- CD34+ CD38- CD45RA- CD90/Thy1+ Rhodamin123Low CD49f+. Indeed, those cells were capable of long-term multilineage engraftment in NOD/SCID/IL2 receptor common-γ chain null mice at a single-cell level (Notta et al., 2011). The information regarding human HSC markers is summarized in Table 2.

While CD34 has been playing an important role as a reliable marker for human hematopoietic stem/progenitor cells in the practical medicine, several studies have demonstrated that long-term reconstituting activity is also detectable in the CD34- Lin- population (Bhatia et al., 1998; Gallacher et al., 2000; Wang et al., 2003). A prior study using Hoechst 33342 by Goodell et al also identified CD34- cells in the side-population of human and rhesus bone marrow, and actually rhesus CD34- side-population cells acquired the ability to form hematopoietic colonies after long-term cultivation on bone marrow stromal cells (Goodell et al., 1997). It should be interesting to examine molecular signatures associated with those CD34- HSC in primates, and compare their features with murine CD34- LSK cells.

Markers	references
CD34$^+$	Berenson et al., 1988, 1991
CD34$^+$ CD38$^-$	Terstappen et al., 1991
CD34$^+$ Lin$^-$ Thy1$^+$	Baum et al., 1992
CD34$^+$ c-kit$^+$	Gunji et al., 1993
CD34$^+$ Tie$^+$	Hashiyama et al., 1996
CD34$^+$ CD133/AC133$^+$	Yin et al., 1997
CD34$^-$ Lin$^-$ CD133/AC133$^+$ CD7$^-$	Gallacher et al., 2000
CD34$^+$ CD38$^-$ Lin$^-$ Rhodamine123^{Low}	McKenzie et al., 2007
CD34$^+$ CD38$^-$ Lin$^-$ CD45RA$^-$ Rhodamine123^{Low} CD49f$^+$	Notta et al., 2011

Table 2. Markers for human hematopoietic stem cells

5. Endothelial-related markers

Hematopoietic cells are thought to originate from the hemangioblast and/or the hemogenic endothelium, which can produce hematopoietic cells and endothelial cells. Therefore, it seems quite natural that HSC share some surface molecules with the endothelial lineage. CD34, PECAM-1/CD31, endoglin, Tie2 and VE-cadherin are well-known endothelial antigens that also mark HSC particularly at early developmental stages (Mikkola & Orkin 2006; Takakura et al., 1998; Yokota et al, 2006). In addition, recent studies have identified endomucin, endothelial protein-C receptor/CD201, and junctional adhesion molecule-A that are common to HSC and endothelial cells (Matsubara et al., 2005; Balazs et al., 2006; Sugano et al., 2008). Although, as discussed above, the expression level of some of these antigens declines or even diminishes at later stages of development (Mikkola & Orkin 2006), each of these advances offered the promise of learning more about how HSC arise de novo and function throughout life. It is crucial to define the means to identify the authentic HSC at all developmental stages so that we can ultimately understand the precise molecular mechanisms of the HSC development.

6. Identification of ESAM as a novel HSC marker

We previously reported that Rag1/GFP- Lin- c-kit^{High} Sca1$^+$ cells derived from bone marrow or fetal liver of the Rag1/GFP reporter mice reconstituted lympho-hematopoiesis in lethally irradiated recipients, while Rag1/GFP$^+$ Lin- c-kit^{High} Sca1$^+$ cells only transiently contributed to T and B lymphopoiesis (Igarashi et al., 2002; Yokota et al., 2003). Those data demonstrated that Rag1 expression is useful to distinguish early lymphoid progenitors (ELP) from the long-term HSC. To learn more about the first step of HSC differentiation to the lymphoid lineage, microarray analyses were conducted to search for genes that characterize the initial transition of HSC to ELP. The search brought us a large body of information about genes potentially related to early lymphopoiesis whereas it also identified genes whose expression seemed to correlate with HSC. Among the HSC-related genes, ESAM strongly drew our attention because of its conspicuous expression in the HSC fraction and sharp down-regulation on differentiation to ELP.

ESAM was originally identified as an endothelial cell-specific protein (Hirata et al., 2001; Nasdala et al., 2002). Flow cytometry analyses with anti-ESAM antibodies showed that the HSC-enriched Rag1- c-kit^{High} Sca1$^+$ fraction of E14.5 fetal liver could be subdivided into two on the basis of ESAM level (Figure 1A). The subpopulation with the high density of ESAM was enriched for c-kit^{High} Sca1^{High} cells, while ones with negative or low levels of ESAM were found in the c-kit^{High} Sca1^{Low} subset. In addition, ESAM expression well correlated with hematopoietic stem/progenitor activity (Figure 1B). Cells in the ESAM^{High} Rag1- c-kit^{High} Sca1$^+$ fraction formed more and larger colonies than those in the ESAM$^{-/Low}$ Rag1- c-kit^{High} Sca1$^+$ fraction. Particularly, majority of CFU-Mix, multi-potent primitive progenitors, were found in the ESAM^{High} fraction (Figure 1B and 1C). In limiting dilution stromal cell co-cultures, we found that 1 in 2.1 ESAM^{High} Rag1- c-kit^{High} Sca1$^+$ cells and 1 in 3.5 ESAM$^{-/Low}$ Rag1- c-kit^{High} Sca1$^+$ cells gave rise to blood cells. However, 1 in 8 ESAM^{High} Rag1- c-kit^{High} Sca1$^+$ cells produced CD19$^+$ B lineage cells whereas only 1 in 125 ESAM$^{-/Low}$ Rag1- c-kit^{High} Sca1$^+$ cells were lymphopoietic under these conditions. Furthermore, in long-term reconstituting assays, ESAM^{High} Rag1- c-kit^{High} Sca1$^+$ cells contributed highly to the multi-lineage recovery of lympho-hematopoiesis in recipients, but no chimerism was detected in mice transplanted with ESAM$^{-/Low}$ Rag1- c-kit^{High} Sca1$^+$ cells. These results suggested that the long-term multi-lineage HSC in E14.5 fetal liver are exclusively present in the ESAM^{High} fraction.

7. ESAM marks HSC in different developmental stages and in different species

Hematopoietic cells arise from mesoderm precursors at different sites and stages of development (de Bruijn et al., 2000; Oberlin et al., 2002). We previously determined that, while myelo-erythroid progenitors emerge from the yolk sac, hematopoietic progenitors with lymphopoietic potential first develop in the paraaortic splanchnopleura (pSp) / AGM region (Yokota et al., 2006). ESAM$^+$ cells in the AGM were found to co-express c-kit and endothelial antigens, Tie2, CD34 and CD31/PECAM-1 that are known as a marker set for emerging HSC. However, the earlier hematopoietic progenitors in the yolk sac that have limited life span and little lymphopoietic activity were harbored in the ESAM^{Low} Tie2^{Low} c-kit^{High} fraction (Figure 2).

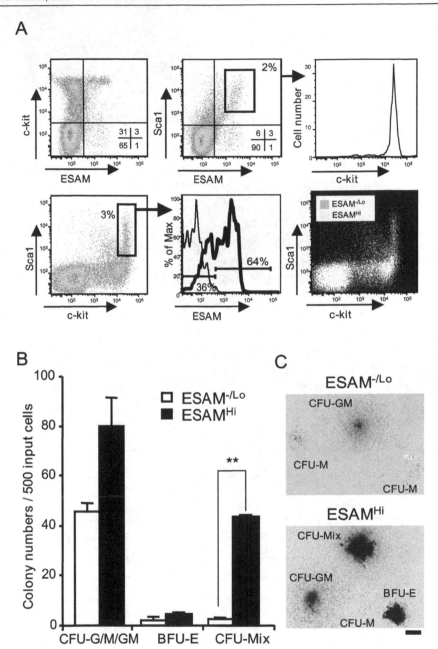

(A) Flow cytometry analysis was performed for mouse E14.5 fetal liver cells using anti-c-kit, anti- Sca1, and anti-ESAM Abs. ESAM$^{-/Lo}$ or ESAM^{Hi} cells of the Rag1/GFP$^-$ ckit^{Hi} Sca1$^+$ fraction were sorted and subjected to methylcellulose colony formation assay. Numbers of CFUs (B) and morphology of the colonies (C) are shown. (Modified from reference Yokota et al., 2009)

Fig. 1. ESAM expression on the HSC-enriched population of mouse fetal liver

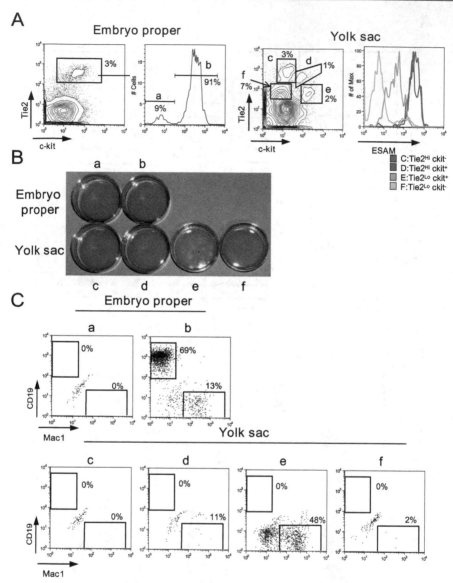

Yolk sac or the caudal half of embryo proper were obtained and pooled from E9.5 embryos of wild type C57B6 mice. The obtained cells were stained with the anti-ESAM Ab followed by goat anti-rat IgG-FITC, anti-c-kit-APC, anti-Tie2-PE, and 7AAD. (A) The profiles of Tie2 and c-kit expression are shown in the left panels. In the right panels, ESAM expression in each gate is shown in histograms. The sorted fractions were labeled with "a" to "f". The sorted cells were subjected to methylcellulose colony formation assay (B) and tested in the MS5 co-culture system (C). (Modified from reference Yokota et al., 2009)

Fig. 2. Yolk sac hematopoietic cells differ from those in the embryo proper with respect to ESAM expression and lymphopoietic activity.

ESAM expression was also detected on HSC within the Lin- c-kit^{High} Sca1$^+$ fraction in adult bone marrow. Interestingly, while the expression level was slightly decreased in the adolescent period, it was up-regulated again in aged mice. In addition, Ooi et al showed that the ESAM$^+$ Lin$^-$ Sca1$^+$ gating could more effectively enrich adult bone marrow for the long-term reconstituting HSC than the conventional LSK gating, and that ESAM expression in HSC is conserved between different mouse strains (Ooi et al., 2009). Based on these observations, we conclude that ESAM serves as an effective and durable marker for HSC throughout life in mice.

The importance of ESAM as a HSC marker has been further enhanced by the findings that its expression in HSC is conserved between mouse and man. Ooi et al detected abundant ESAM transcripts in human cord blood CD34$^+$ CD38$^-$ Lin$^-$ Thy1/CD90$^+$ cells (Ooi et al., 2009). Furthermore, by using a rabbit anti-human polyclonal ESAM antibody and flow cytometry, we also detected ESAM expression on human cord blood CD34$^+$ cells (Figure 3). The intensity of ESAM expression, however, was similar between CD34$^+$ CD38$^-$ and CD34$^+$ CD38$^+$ cells, suggesting that the ESAM$^+$ gate covers committed as well as non-committed hematopoietic progenitors. ESAM expression might serve as an alternative marker to CD34 for the selection of hematopoietic stem/progenitor cells in human. It is noteworthy that, although majority of human cord blood CD34$^-$ CD38$^+$ fraction were negative for the ESAM staining, the fraction contains a small ESAM$^+$ population. Further study is necessary to characterize those ESAM$^+$ CD34$^-$ cells.

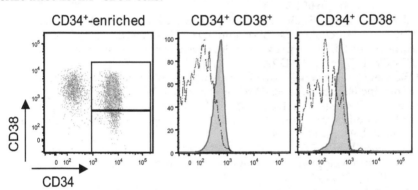

CD34$^+$ cells were firstly enriched from cord blood mononuclear cells by magnetic beads conjugated with an anti-human CD34 antibody, and then stained with anti-CD34, anti-CD38, and anti-ESAM antibodies. The left panel shows CD34 and CD38 expression profile of the CD34$^+$ enriched population. The middle and right panels indicate ESAM expression (red tinted) on CD34$^+$ CD38$^+$ or CD34$^+$ CD38$^-$ cells, respectively. Dot lines show background staining levels with control IgG for an anti-ESAM antibody.

Fig. 3. ESAM expression on human cord blood CD34$^+$ cells

8. Conclusion

In this chapter, we summarized 2 decades achievements for the identification of HSC and introduced our recent discovery of human ESAM as a new HSC marker. Although it is possible in mouse to purify the long-term multi-lineage HSC with high efficiency, characterization of human HSC has lagged behind partly due to insufficient information about their cell surface antigens. As a new tool, ESAM expression might contribute to improve the purification strategy of human HSC, not only from human hematopoietic tissues but also from cultures of embryonic stem cells or induced-pluripotent stem cells, for therapeutic application. In addition, our findings will be beneficial to basic studies of HSC themselves. Since ESAM is expressed on mesoderm precursors for HSC in the pSp/AGM region as well as expanding HSC in fetal liver, its expression will be potentially useful to trace developing HSC back to their origin and localize them in distinct hematopoietic organs. In addition, up-regulation of ESAM expression on aged HSC may provide some insights regarding molecular mechanisms of HSC senescence. We are expecting that a new HSC marker ESAM could help future studies regarding HSC in many directions.

9. References

Balazs AB, Fabian AJ, Esmon CT, & Mulligan RC. (2006). Endothelial protein C receptor (CD201) explicitly identifies hematopoietic stem cells in murine bone marrow. *Blood* Vol.107, pp 317-2321.

Baum CM, Weissman IL, Tsukamoto AS, Buckle AM, & Peault B. (1992). Isolation of a candidate human hematopoietic stem-cell population. *Proc Natl Acad Sci USA*. Vol. 89, pp 2804-2808.

Berenson RJ, Andrews RG, Bensinger WI, Kalamasz D, Knitter G, Buckner CD, & Bernstein ID. (1988). Antigen CD34+ marrow cells engraft lethally irradiated baboons. *J Clin Invest*. Vol. 81, pp 951-955.

Berenson RJ, Bensinger WI, Hill RS, Andrews RG, Garcia-Lopez J, Kalamasz DF, Still BJ, Spitzer G, Buckner CD, Bernstein ID, & Thomas ED. (1991). Engraftment after infusion of CD34+ marrow cells in patients with breast cancer or neuroblastoma. *Blood* Vol. 77, pp 1717-1722.

Bhatia M, Bonnet D, Murdoch B, Gan OI, & Dick JE. (1998). A newly discovered class of human hematopoietic cells with SCID-repopulating activity. *Nat Med*. Vol. 4, pp 1038-1045.

Christensen JL, & Weissman IL. (2001). Flk-2 is a marker in hematopoietic stem cell differentiation: a simple method to isolate long-term stem cells. *Proc Natl Acad Sci USA*. Vol. 98, pp 14541-14546.

de Bruijn MF, Speck NA, Peeters MC, & Dzierzak E. (2000). Definitive hematopoietic stem cells first develop within the major arterial regions of the mouse embryo. *EMBO J*. Vol. 19. pp 2465-2474.

Doulatov S, Notta F, Eppert K, Nguyen LT, Ohashi PS, & Dick JE. (2010). Revised map of the human progenitor hierarchy shows the origin of macrophages and dendritic cells in early lymphoid development. *Nat Immunol*. Vol. 11, pp 585-593.

Foudi A, Hochedlinger K, Van Buren D, Schindler JW, Jaenisch R, Carey V, & Hock H. (2009). Analysis of histone 2B-GFP retention reveals slowly cycling hematopoietic stem cells. *Nat Biotechnol*. Vol. 27, pp 84-90.

Gallacher L, Murdoch B, Wu DM, Karanu FN, Keeney M, & Bhatia M. (2000). Isolation and characterization of human CD34-Lin- and CD34+Lin- hematopoietic stem cells using cell surface markers AC133 and CD7. *Blood* Vol. 95, pp 2813-2820.

Goodell MA, Brose K, Paradis G, Conner AS, & Mulligan RC. (1996). Isolation and functional properties of murine hematopoietic stem cells that are replicating in vivo. *J Exp Med*. Vol. 183, pp 1797-1806.

Goodell MA, Rosenzweig M, Kim H, Marks DF, DeMaria M, Paradis G, Grupp SA, Sieff CA, Mulligan RC, & Johnson RP. (1997). Dye efflux studies suggest that hematopoietic stem cells expressing low or undetectable levels of CD34 antigen exist in multiple species. *Nat Med*. Vol. 3, pp 1337-1345.

Gunji Y, Nakamura M, Osawa H, Nagayoshi K, Nakauchi H, Miura Y, Yanagisawa M, & Suda T. (1993). Human primitive hematopoietic progenitor cells are more enriched in KIT^{low} cells than in KIT^{high} cells. *Blood* Vol. 82, pp 3283-3289.

Hashiyama M, Iwama A, Ohshiro K, Kurozumi K, Yasunaga K, Shimizu Y, Masuho Y, Matsuda I, Yamaguchi N, & Suda T. (1996). Predominant expression of a receptor tyrosine kinase, TIE, in hematopoietic stem cells and B cells. *Blood* Vol. 87, pp 93-101.

Hirata K, Ishida T, Penta K, Rezaee M, Yang E, Wohlgemuth J, & Quertermous T. (2001). Cloning of an immunoglobulin family adhesion molecule selectively expressed by endothelial cells. *J Biol Chem.* Vol. 276, pp 16223-16231.

Igarashi H, Gregory SC, Yokota T, Sakaguchi N, & Kincade PW. (2002). Transcription from the RAG1 locus marks the earliest lymphocyte progenitors in bone marrow. *Immunity* Vol. 17, pp 117-130.

Kiel MJ, Yilmaz OH, Iwashita T, Yilmaz OH, Terhorst C, & Morrison SJ. (2005). SLAM family receptors distinguish hematopoietic stem and progenitor cells and reveal endothelial niches for stem cells. *Cell* Vol. 121, pp 1109-1121.

Larochelle A, Savona M, Wiggins M, Anderson S, Ichwan B, Keyvanfar K, Morrison SJ, & Dunbar CE. (2011). Human and rhesus macaque hematopoietic stem cells cannot be purified based only on SLAM family markers. *Blood* Vol. 117, pp1550-1554.

Matsubara A, Iwama A, Yamazaki S, Furuta C, Hirasawa R, Morita Y, Osawa M, Motohashi T, Eto K, Ema H, Kitamura T, Vestweber D, & Nakauchi H. (2005). Endomucin, a CD34-like sialomucin, marks hematopoietic stem cells throughout development. *J Exp Med.* Vol. 202, pp 1483-1492.

Matsuoka S, Ebihara Y, Xu M, Ishii T, Sugiyama D, Yoshino H, Ueda T, Manabe A, Tanaka R, Ikeda Y, Nakahata T, & Tsuji K. (2001). CD34 expression on long-term repopulating hematopoietic stem cells changes during developmental stages. *Blood* Vol. 97, pp 419-425.

Matsuzaki Y, Kinjo K, Mulligan RC, & Okano H. (2004). Unexpectedly efficient homing capacity of purified murine hematopoietic stem cells. *Immunity* Vol. 20, pp 87-93.

McKenzie JL, Takenaka K, Gan OI, Doedens M, & Dick JE. (2007). Low rhodamine 123 retention identifies long-term human hematopoietic stem cells within the Lin⁻CD34$^+$CD38$^-$ population. *Blood* Vol. 109, pp 543-545.

McKinney-Freeman SL, Naveiras O, Yates F, Loewer S, Philitas M, Curran M, Park PJ, & Daley GQ. (2009). Surface antigen phenotypes of hematopoietic stem cells from embryos and murine embryonic stem cells. *Blood* Vol. 114, pp 268-278

Mikkola HKA, & Orkin SH. (2006). The journey of developing hematopoietic stem cells. *Development* Vol. 133, pp 3733-3744.

Nasdala I, Wolburg-Buchholz K, Wolburg H, Kuhn A, Ebnet K, Brachtendorf G, Samulowitz U, Kuster B, Engelhardt B, Vestweber D, & Butz S. (2002). A transmembrane tight junction protein selectively expressed on endothelial cells and platelets. *J Biol Chem.* Vol. 277, pp 16294-16303.

Notta F, Doulatov S, Laurenti E, Poeppl A, Jurisica I, & Dick JE. (2011). Isolation of single human hematopoietic stem cells capable of long-term multilineage engraftment. *Science* Vol. 333, pp 218-221.

Oberlin E., Tavian M., Blazsek I., & Péault B. (2002). Blood-forming potential of vascular endothelium in the human embryo. *Development* Vol. 129, pp 4147-4157.

Ogawa M, Matsuzaki Y, Nishikawa S, Hayashi S, Kunisada T, Sudo T, Kina T, Nakauchi H, & Nishikawa S-I. (1991). Expression and function of c-kit in hemopoietic progenitor cells. *J Exp Med.* Vol. 174, pp 63-71.

Ogawa M. (2002). Changing phenotypes of hematopoietic stem cells. *Exp Hematol.* Vol. 30, pp 3-6.

Ooi AG, Karsunky H, Majeti R, Butz S, Vestweber D, Ishida T, Quertermous T, Weissman IL, & Forsberg EC. (2009). The adhesion molecule esam1 is a novel hematopoietic stem cell marker. *Stem Cells* Vol. 27, pp 653-661.

Osawa M, Hanada K, Hamada H, & Nakauchi H. (1996). Long-term lymphohematopoietic reconstitution by a single CD34-low/negative hematopoietic stem cell. *Science* Vol. 273, pp 242-245.

Randall TD, Lund FE, Howard MC, & Weissman IL. (1996). Expression of murine CD38 defines a population of long-term reconstituting hematopoietic stem cells. *Blood* Vol. 87, pp 4057-4067.

Randall TD, & Weissman IL. (1997). Phenotypic and functional changes induced at the clonal level in hematopoietic stem cells after 5-fluorouracil treatment. *Blood* Vol. 89, pp 3596-3606.

Shultz LD, Ishikawa F, & Greiner DL. (2007). Humanized mice in translational biomedical research. *Nat Rev Immunol.* Vol. 7, pp 118-130.

Spangrude GJ, Heimfeld S, & Weissman IL. (1988). Purification and characterization of mouse hematopoietic stem cells. *Science* Vol. 241, pp 58-62.

Spangrude GJ, & Brooks DM. (1993). Mouse strain variability in the expression of the hematopoietic stem cell antigen Ly-6A/E by bone marrow cells. *Blood* Vol. 82, pp 3327-3332.

Sugano Y, Takeuchi M, Hirata A, Matsushita H, Kitamura T, Tanaka M, & Miyajima A. (2008). Junctional adhesion molecule-A, JAM-A, is a novel cell-surface marker for long-term repopulating hematopoietic stem cells. *Blood* Vol. 111, pp 1167-1172.

Tajima F, Deguchi T, Laver JH, Zeng H, & Ogawa M. (2001). Reciprocal expression of CD38 and CD34 by adult murine hematopoietic stem cells. *Blood* Vol. 97, pp 2618-2624.

Takakura N, Huang XL, Naruse T, Hamaguchi I, Dumont DJ, Yancopoulos GD, & Suda T. (1998). Critical role of the TIE2 endothelial cell receptor in the development of definitive hematopoiesis. *Immunity* Vol. 9, pp 677-686.

Terstappen LW, Huang S, Safford M, Lansdorp PM, & Loken MR. (1991). Sequential generations of hematopoietic colonies derived from single nonlineage-committed CD34+CD38- progenitor cells. *Blood* Vol. 77, pp 1218-1227.

Wang J, Kimura T, Asada R, Harada S, Yokota S, Kawamoto Y, Fujimura Y, Tsuji T, Ikehara S, & Sonoda Y. (2003). SCID-repopulating cell activity of human cord blood-derived CD34- cells assured by intra-bone marrow injection. *Blood* Vol. 101, pp 2924-2931.

Wilson A, Laurenti E, Oser G, van der Wath RC, Blanco-Bose W, Jaworski M, Offner S, Dunant CF, Eshkind L, Bockamp E, Lió P, Macdonald HR, & Trumpp A. (2008). Hematopoietic stem cells reversibly switch from dormancy to self-renewal during homeostasis and repair. *Cell* Vol. 135, pp1118-1129.

Yin AH, Miraglia S, Zanjani ED, Almeida-Porada G, Ogawa M, Leary AG, Olweus J, Kearney J, & Buck DW. (1997). AC133, a novel marker for human hematopoietic stem and progenitor cells. *Blood* Vol. 90, pp 5002-5012.

Yokota T, Kouro T, Hirose J, Igarashi H, Garrett KP, Gregory SC, Sakaguchi N, Owen JJ, & Kincade PW. (2003). Unique properties of fetal lymphoid progenitors identified according to RAG1 gene expression. *Immunity* Vol. 19, pp 365-375.

Yokota T, Huang J, Tavian M, Nagai Y, Hirose J, Zúñiga-Pflücker JC, Péault B, & Kincade PW. (2006). Tracing the first waves of lymphopoiesis in mice. *Development* Vol. 133, pp 2041-2051.

Yokota T, Oritani K, Butz S, Kokame K, Kincade PW, Miyata T, Vestweber D, & Kanakura Y. (2009). The endothelial antigen ESAM marks primitive hematopoietic progenitors throughout life in mice. *Blood* Vol. 113, pp 2914-2923.

2

Transcriptional Quiescence of Hematopoietic Stem Cells

Rasmus Freter

Ludwig Institute for Cancer Research, University of Oxford
United Kingdom

1. Introduction

Haematopoietic stem cells (HSC) have the exceptional capacity to undergo continuous self-renewal and differentiation into multiple lineages, which is essential for haematopoietic homeostasis and response to injury. To achieve this life long function, these cells have to be protected from cytotoxic and genetic damage. On the other hand, rapid activation of haematopoietic stem cell proliferation in response to stimuli must be ensured. While cellular quiescence is thought to be the key mechanism underlying this paradoxical nature of HSC, the molecular basis of induction and maintenance of quiescence remains unresolved.

Quiescence is commonly defined as a reversible cell cycle exit. Induction and maintenance of stem cell quiescence has been studied at the level of cell cycle regulation (Orford & Scadden, 2008), cellular metabolism (Tothova & Gilliland, 2007) or interaction with the specific niche (Fuchs et al., 2004). Genome-wide association studies have been performed on a variety of quiescent model systems, such as serum starvation of fibroblasts (Coller et al., 2006), primary lymphocytes (Garriga et al., 1998) or yeast in stationary phase (Patturajan et al., 1998, Radonjic et al., 2005). All of these studies revealed a significant decrease of productive mRNA transcription in these model systems. However, if quiescent adult stem cells share this down regulation of mRNA transcription has never been examined.

Due to their relative ease of isolation, cells of the haematopoietic lineage have been extensively studied. Importantly, several assays for hematopoietic stem cell function have been developed, such as colony forming ability and rescue of lethally irradiated mice. These functional tests are lacking in most other adult stem cell models, with the exception of spermatogonia and mammary gland stem cells (Brinster & Nagano, 1998, Shackleton et al., 2006). Functional assays for HSC ability have provided us with the notion that most defined populations of long term repopulating HSC still contain progenitor cells, which can only transiently contribute to repopulation of the haematopoietic system. This heterogeneity is not only evident in defined cell populations, but also in the in vivo niche for HSC, the bone marrow. HSC in the bone marrow are interspersed with transient amplifying cells and differentiated cells, complicating stem cell identification by spatial organization of the tissue. Other stem cell systems, such as spermatogonia, keratinocyte or crypt stem cells have a clearly defined niche architecture, enabling stem cell identification by location only (Fuchs et al., 2004). In this case, resting stem cells and activated progenitors can be separated by location and molecular markers can be easily identified. If all adult stem cells share a repertoire of molecular markers, findings from other adult stem cells can be transferred to HSC and should lead to characterization of haematopoietic stem cell subpopulations.

In our previous work, we found that adult melanocyte stem cells exhibit a 10 to 100fold lower level of housekeeping gene mRNA compared to differentiated cells, suggesting a global repression of mRNA transcription (Osawa et al., 2005). We could then show that the largest subunit of RNA polymerase II (RNApII), which is responsible for all mRNA transcription, exhibits a partly phosphorylated C-terminal domain (CTD), characteristic of initiated, but paused mRNA transcription (Freter et al., 2010). In line with this, we found the RNApII kinase CDK9 absent in adult melanocyte stem cells. Inhibition of CDK9 resulted in cellular resistance to withdrawal of essential growth factors, conferring a stem cell-like phenotype to progenitor cells. Interestingly, various other adult stem cells, including keratinocyte, muscle, spermatogonia and also HSC exhibited a similar partial phosphorylation of RNApII (Freter et al., 2010). We concluded that transcriptional quiescence is an early, specific and conserved marker for adult stem cells. This feature can be used to isolate and characterize pure populations of stem cell-like cells from any tissue, enabling a deeper understanding of stem cell biology and recapitulation of the stem cell niche, in order to expand immature stem cells in vitro.

In this chapter I would like to summarize our findings that HSC exhibit a reduction in productive mRNA transcription. I would like to elaborate on the implications arising from transcriptional quiescence of a subset of HSC, both in development and disease. Technical challenges and resulting applications of identifying and isolating transcriptionally quiescent HSC in vitro will be discussed.

2. The mRNA transcription cycle

Regulation of gene expression is essential for all single- and multi cellular organisms. This fundamental process is executed at the level of mRNA transcription by RNApII, typically in distinct transcription steps. The different stages of mRNA transcription, initiation, promoter clearance, elongation, mRNA processing and release of RNApII from DNA are tightly regulated by modifications of the CTD of RNApII (Sims et al., 2004, Fig1). This characteristic domain is in mammalian cells composed of 52 repeats of the consensus sequence YS_2PTS_5PS. During mRNA transcription several posttranslational modifications of the CTD are occurring, most prominently phosphorylation of Serine 5 (Ser5) and Serine 2 (Ser2). These phosphorylation events are requisite for binding of proteins essential for RNA processing, splicing and polyadenylation. Using antibodies specifically detecting these phosphorylation events enables determination of global mRNA transcription activity in single cells in vivo.

Gene expression in mammalian cells has been comprehensively studied at the transcription initiation step that is controlled by cell-specific transcription factors. In fact, it has been thought for long time that assembly of the preinitiation complex and subsequent recruitment on RNApII is the rate-limiting step for gene transcription. However, early results indicated that RNApII is initiated, but paused at Drosophila heat shock genes (Boehm et al., 2003, Ni et al., 2004). More recently, it was observed using genome-wide association studies that initiated but stalled polymerase is not only present on immediate-response or developmentally regulated genes, but also many non-expressed genes, suggesting transcription elongation as the critical step in gene expression (Guenther *et al.*, 2007, Muse *et al.*, 2007, Zeitlinger *et al.*, 2007).

Transcription initiation requires phosphorylation of Ser5 of the CTD by TFIIH, a heterodimeric kinase consisting of CDK7 and Cyclin H. These phosphorylation events enable binding of the mRNA capping machinery (Ho & Shuman, 1999) and promoter clearance. Typically, a short (~40nt) nascent RNA is then produced by RNApII. However, mRNA transcription is paused at many genes due to the action of negative elongation factor (NELF) and DRB-sensitivity inducing factor (DSIF) (Wu *et al.*, 2003, Yamaguchi *et al.*, 2002).

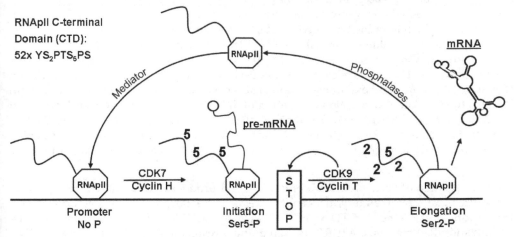

Fig. 1. The mRNA transcription cycle is characterized by phosphorylation of the RNA polymerase (RNApII) CTD. Phosphorylation of Ser5 (5) by CDK7/Cyclin H induces promoter clearance and pre-mRNA capping. RNApII is then halted (STOP), until activation of CDK9/Cyclin T. Phosphorylation of the inhibitory complex and RNA polymerase II CTD Ser2 (2) leads to productive elongation and release of mature mRNA.

Recruitment of positive transcription elongation factor b (P-TEFb), a heterodimeric protein consisting of the kinase CDK9 and one of the regulatory subunits Cyclin T1, T2 or K, to stalled polymerases is required for alleviation of the transcriptional block by NELF and DSIF (Peterlin & Price, 2006, Rahl *et al.*, 2010). P-TEFb phosphorylates RNA recognition motif-containing protein RD, a component of NELF, and Spt5, a subunit of DSIF (Aida *et al.*, 2006, Fujinaga *et al.*, 2004). NELF then dissociates from RNApII, while DSIF remains associated with RNApII and becomes a positive transcription elongation factor (Chen *et al.*, 2009). Importantly, phosphorylation of Ser2 of the CTD by P-TEFb triggers transcription elongation, mRNA processing, and release of mature mRNA (Kohoutek, 2009, Ni *et al.*, 2004).

CDK9 has first been identified as a CDC2-related kinase with a PITALRE motif (Grana *et al.*, 1994). The cyclin partner of CDK9 is Cyclin T1, T2 or K. Unlike other CDK/Cyclin heterodimers, neither P-TEFb levels nor kinase activity is fluctuating during the cell cycle (Garriga *et al.*, 2003, Grana *et al.*, 1994). CDK9 exists in two isoforms, a major 42kD sized peptide and an N-terminal extended peptide, whose transcription starts from an alternative

TATA box upstream of the housekeeping-type promoter of the 42kD isoform (Shore *et al.*, 2003). The expression of both isoforms varies between developmental stages and organs (Shore *et al.*, 2005). For example, the expressed isoform shifts from the longer 55kD form to the shorter 42kD isoform during lymphocyte activation (Liu & Herrmann, 2005). However, the target gene specificity is very similar between the two isoforms (Liu & Herrmann, 2005).

P-TEFb is present in the cell as either a large or small multiprotein complex. The inactive, large complex consists of 7SK non-coding RNA, Hexim1, LARP7 and MEPCE (Li *et al.*, 2005), while the small, active complex is formed by binding of Brd4 to P-TEFb (Yang *et al.*, 2005). Brd4 binds to acetylated histones and may therefore target P-TEFb to actively transcribed genes, when no specific transcription factor is present (Jang *et al.*, 2005) but can also recruit P-TEFb to inducibly acetylated histones (Hargreaves *et al.*, 2009). However, even the large complex contains primarily active P-TEFb, which is sequestered away from the kinase targets. Cellular stresses, such as UV irradiation, cytokines or changes in the microenvironment result in release of active P-TEFb to support quick mRNA transcription to respond to stimuli. Several transcription factors have been shown to interact directly with P-TEFb to stimulate transcription elongation of RNApII. These include NF-kB (Barboric *et al.*, 2001), c-Myc (Eberhardy & Farnham, 2001), CIITA (Kanazawa *et al.*, 2000), GATA1 (Elagib *et al.*, 2008) and Runx1 (Jiang *et al.*, 2005), amongst others. Thus, P-TEFb can be either recruited directly to promoters by specific transcription factors or to acetylated histones by Brd4.

Phosphorylation of Ser2 in the CTD of RNApII and productive transcription elongation is the critical target for eukaryotic gene expression (Bentley, 1995, Chao & Price, 2001). Inhibition of the CTD Ser2 kinase CDK9 by 5,6-Dichloro-1-β-D-ribofuranosylbenzimidazole (DRB) or Flavopiridol results in degradation of most mRNA (Chao & Price, 2001, Sehgal & Darnell, 1976) and induces apoptosis (Chen *et al.*, 2005, Gojo *et al.*, 2002). Similarly, knockdown of CDK9 in vivo results in complete absence of mRNA synthesis and embryonic lethality (Eissenberg *et al.*, 2007, Shim *et al.*, 2002). Cyclin T1 KO mice exhibit minor immunological defects (Oven *et al.*, 2007), while the Cyclin T2 KO mouse is embryonic lethal (Kohoutek *et al.*, 2009) with an extremely early phenotype before implantation of the blastocyst. This difference in phenotype of CDK9 Cyclin partners can partly be explained by a limited overlap in target genes of these isoforms (Ramakrishnan *et al.*, 2011).

On the other hand, ectopic activation of P-TEFb by ablation of Hexim1 results in embryonic lethality as well, due to hypertrophy of the heart (Huang *et al.*, 2004). Similarly, inactivation of the inhibitory large complex member LARP7 results in aberrant splicing and embryonic death in zebrafish, highlighting the essential role of P-TEFb for pre-mRNA splicing (Barboric *et al.*, 2009). However, overexpression of CDK9 from the endogenous Rosa26 promoter did not result in any phenotype in mice, mainly due to a low level of expression of CDK9 from this promoter (Freter *et al.*, 2010). Limiting P-TEFb activity is necessary for development of germ line cells in both D. melanogaster and C. elegance (Batchelder *et al.*, 1999, Hanyu-Nakamura *et al.*, 2008, Zhang *et al.*, 2003). Ectopic activation of P-TEFb by overexpression or knock down of inhibitors results in misexpression of somatic genes in germ line cells and their subsequent degeneration, resulting in sterile offspring. In summary, levels of P-TEFb and thus the global activity of RNApII need to be maintained within a certain limits, not exceeding and not below a basal threshold.

Most cells, including proliferating, terminally differentiated and senescent cells, actively synthesize mRNA. In these cells, RNApII is phosphorylated on CTD Ser2 and Ser5 independent of the cell cycle (Garriga *et al.*, 2003, Marshall *et al.*, 2005). However, some cells do not display this active phosphorylation pattern. For example, deeply dormant cells, such as primary T and B lymphocytes, exhibit an almost complete absence of RNApII phosphorylation (Garriga *et al.*, 1998, Marshall *et al.*, 2005). Activation of these cells by antigen encounter results in upregulation of Ccnt1 both on mRNA and protein level and subsequent phosphorylation of CTD Ser2 (Marshall *et al.*, 2005).

On the other hand, RNApII in yeast cells in the stationary phase (Patturajan *et al.*, 1998, Radonjic *et al.*, 2005) or on Drosophila heat shock genes (Boehm *et al.*, 2003, Ni *et al.*, 2004) is phosphorylated on Ser5, but not on Ser2. Stimulation of these cells, such as the addition of nutrients or heat shock, ensures rapid activation of gene transcription. Thus, analysis of the specific phosphorylated sites in RNApII can distinguish cells featuring phases of productive mRNA elongation or paused mRNA transcription initiation.

3. mRNA transcription in the hematopoietic lineage

Most of our knowledge of P-TEFb function derived from studies involving HIV replication (Barboric & Peterlin, 2005). Human Cyclin T1 is an essential co-factor of the immediate-early HIV gene product Tat, which recruits P-TEFb to the tar RNA located 5' on HIV genes to activate gene expression (Mancebo *et al.*, 1997, Zhu *et al.*, 1997). In resting lymphocytes, P-TEFb activity is low and thus HIV replication is blocked. Upon stimulation, upregulation of Cyclin T1 results in activation of P-TEFb and transcription of viral genes (Garriga *et al.*, 1998). Human Cyclin T1 (Ccnt1), the major Cyclin associated with CDK9, is characterized by a TAR recognition motif, which is essential for the formation of a ternary complex between tar RNA/Tat and P-TEFb to activate HIV gene transcription in cells (Wei *et al.*, 1998). This motif contains an essential Cysteine, which is required for complex formation with HIV Tat. Mutagenesis of mouse Ccnt1 at this position, which normally contains a Tyrosine in mouse, activates HIV transcription in murine cells (Fujinaga *et al.*, 2002).

P-TEFb is also required for normal hematopoietic development and function. Knock down of CDK9 in zebrafish embryos results in severe defects in definitive erythropoiesis, but no gross developmental defects despite a smaller body size (Meier *et al.*, 2006). Given the ubiquitous requirement of CDK9 for mRNA transcription this surprising observation may be explained by incomplete knockdown using morpholino DNA. Similarly, partial depletion of Ccnt1 in mice results in modest immunological phenotypes, such as appearance of autoimmunity due to impaired negative selection of autoreactive T cells in thymus (Oven *et al.*, 2007). Together, these results suggest that the hematopoietic lineage may be very susceptible for small changes in P-TEFb activity.

Recruitment of P-TEFb by transcription factors to heterochromatin converts this general elongation factor to a repressor of transcription. Runx1 binds the CD4 silencer in thymocytes and leads to active suppression of CD4 transcription during development. Interestingly, despite an engaged RNApII on the CD4 promoter and in the presence of an active CD4 enhancer in these cells, CD4 transcription is silenced (Jiang *et al.*, 2005). This is achieved by binding of Cyclin T1 to Runx1 and sequestering of P-TEFb into inactive chromatin loops (Jiang & Peterlin, 2008). Thus, inactive genes can be loaded with a poised polymerase and induction of chromatin remodelling complexes result in rapid activation of gene transcription by release of active P-TEFb from adjacent loci (Jiang & Peterlin, 2008). In this sense, assembly of the transcriptional machinery on inactive promoters can be seen as a transcription bookmark, to facilitate future expression.

Activation of hematopoietic gene transcription can also be achieved via binding of P-TEFb to actively acetylated chromatin. Studies on LPS-induced inflammatory gene expression in macrophages revealed that primary response genes have a stalled polymerase at their promoters, already phosphorylated at Ser5 of the CTD (Hargreaves et al., 2009). In response to LPS stimulation, acetylation of H4K5/8/12 recruits Brd4, this in turn engages P-TEFb leading to CTD Ser2 phosphorylation and mRNA transcription (Hargreaves et al., 2009).

Hematopoietic lineages are very susceptible for inhibition of P-TEFb activity and require specific co-factors for their respective differentiation. For example, differentiating macrophages and murine erythroleukemic cells down regulate the 42kD isoform, and up regulate the 55 kD isoform of CDK9 (Liu & Herrmann, 2005). Megakaryocyte differentiation depends on activation of P-TEFb and can be blocked by CDK9 inhibitors or dominant negative CDK9 (Elagib et al., 2008). Erythroid differentiation depends on stabilization of a GATA-1/SCL/LMO2 complex on β-globin chromatin, subsequent association of P-TEFb and RNApII Ser2 phosphorylation in the locus by the ubiquitous enhancer facilitator/chromatin factor Ldb1 (Song et al., 2010). Interestingly, deletion of Ldb1 in vivo results in defects in adult haematopoietic stem cell maintenance and diminished long-term reconstitution potential upon transplantation (Li et al., 2011). However, the authors did not examine activity of P-TEFb in their knock-out mice, which may be reduced and thus result in defects in HSC specification. Certainly, many other genes and cells depend on P-TEFb activity during development and differentiation. Using the hematopoietic lineage as a model system for the basal mRNA transcription machinery will shed light onto many aspects of eukaryotic mechanisms of transcription control.

Conversely, some leukemic cancers are characterized by dysregulation of P-TEFb activity. Several fusion genes of the histone methytransferase MLL1 involved in chromosomal rearrangements leading to myeloid and lymphoblastic leukaemia associate with mRNA transcription elongation factor encoded by ELL or P-TEFb (Benedikt et al., 2011, Lin et al., 2010), suggesting that one major mechanism for leukomogenesis is deregulated transcription elongation (Shilatifard et al., 1996). Indeed, targeting P-TEFb with the specific CDK9 inhibitor Flavopiridol induces apoptosis in chronic lymphocytic leukemic cells by suppression of short-lived anti-apoptotic genes, such as Mcl-1 (Chen et al., 2005). Dysregulation of P-TEFb activity is involved in several other cancer types. For example Hexim1, a negative regulator of P-TEFb activity, was found down regulated in invasive breast cancer samples compared to normal breast tissue (Wittmann et al., 2003). Exploiting the susceptibility of the hematopoietic lineage for disturbance of their mRNA transcription may result in novel targets of cancer therapy.

4. Transcriptional quiescence of hematopoietic stem cells

Hematopoietic stem cells (HSC) have been in the focus of basic and applied research since many decades. Definition of subsets of transplantable HSC and their in vitro culture have advanced considerably in recent years. However, so far no reliable marker for the isolation of pure HSC exists and our use of transplants is limited by the inability to expand these cells ex vivo. A sensitive marker of HSC quiescence and activation could be useful to isolate unadulterated long-term repopulating HSC and screen for factors that enable stem cell expansion while maintaining their undifferentiated state. It has been known for three decades that HSC down regulate productive mRNA transcription. Low retention of Pyronin Y, an RNA binding dye, can be used to isolate HSC (Shapiro, 1981), suggesting that global suppression of mRNA transcription is a feature of quiescent HSC. However, this observation has not been followed up by analysis of the global status of RNApII activity, which is responsible for all mRNA transcription.

We have previously observed that adult melanocyte stem cells (MelSC) down regulate many housekeeping genes, including ActB, ActG and GapDH, suggesting a global repression of mRNA synthesis in these cells (Osawa et al., 2005). Melanocytes are pigmented cells in the hair follicle and skin, providing melanin granules to differentiating keratinocytes. The MelSC system in mouse hair follicles can serve as a model system for adult stem cell systems. It has the advantage of spatial separation of stem and differentiated cells and a non-lethal but obvious hair graying phenotype if this system is perturbed (Nishimura et al., 2002). We observed that adult MelSC show a complete absence of RNApII CTD Ser2 phosphorylation, while Ser5 was phosphorylated (Freter et al., 2010), suggesting a global down regulation of productive mRNA transcription. In line with this, CDK9 protein and mRNA was down regulated in MelSC as well. This suggests that RNApII is present at many genes in quiescent MelSC, but P-TEFb levels are not sufficient to induce active transcription elongation. Importantly, inhibition of CDK9 in vitro protected melanocyte precursors from stress-induced apoptosis and converted them to a stem cell-like state (Freter et al., 2010).

We then expanded our observation to other stem cell systems, and found CTD Ser2-negative cells in all stem cell systems tested, including keratinocyte, muscle, spermatogonia and hematopoietic stem cells. This suggests that global suppression of mRNA transcription elongation is a conserved feature of adult stem cells. Interestingly, some stem cell systems showed heterogeneity of CTD Ser2 staining. For example, we observed that spermatogonia stem cells attached to the basal lamina are negative for CTD Ser2 phosphorylation, while those detaching up-regulate Ser2 phosphorylation, even though they are still positive for the spermatogonia stem cell marker CD9 (Freter et al., 2010). Attachment to the basal lamina is often a requirement for stem cell function by directing planes of division or maintenance of the undifferentiated state. Thus, the CTD Ser2 negative population seems to be the more stem cell-like population in CD9 positive spermatogonia.

Similarly, murine CD34- c-Kit+Sca1+Lin- (KSL) long-term repopulating hematopoietic stem cells clearly showed two different populations. One population exhibited CTD Ser2 phosphorylation levels as high as short-term repopulating CD34+ KSL cells, while ~27% of all CD34- KSL cells were negative for CTD Ser2 phosphorylation (Freter et al., 2010). Heterogeneity of the HSC pool has been described previously, with a transplantable fraction of 15-25% of CD34- KSL HSC population, also using additional markers (Ema et al., 2005, Foudi et al., 2009, Wilson et al., 2008). Importantly, analysis of transcriptionally quiescent HSC requires isolation of pure subpopulations of cells. We found that adult MelSC exhibit up to 100fold lower levels of total RNA per cell (Osawa et al., 2005), suggesting that one activated stem cell may be sufficient to mask the RNA signal of 100 quiescent stem cells.

In order to identify the transcriptionally quiescent subpopulation of CD34- KSL cells, we performed sorting of bone marrow cells and antibody staining of sorted populations. Unfortunately, this procedure always includes fixation of cells, so they can not be used for assessment of in vivo repopulation ability. In order to validate stem cell function in vivo, it is necessary to convert the negative CTD Ser2 phosphorylation event into a readout which can be measured in living cells. Kinase activity can be measured using fusion proteins of Cyan and Yellow fluorescent proteins (CFP and YFP respectively), separated by a kinase target, a flexible linker and a phosphoprotein binding domain. Phosphorylation events result in binding of the phosphoacceptor to the kinase target and folding of the fusion protein resulting in Foerster resonance energy transfer (FRET) between CFP and YFP (Sato *et al.*, 2007). However, autofluorescence of cellular organelles in low energetic wavelengths, such as CFP, results in low signal to noise ratios, which is particularly difficult for cell sorting of multiparametric cell suspensions, such as bone marrow cells. Furthermore, even a complete lack of FRET by spatial separation results in FRET signal due to high concentration of expressed fluorescent proteins (Nguyen & Daugherty, 2005). Thus, a FRET-based approach can be useful for single-cell based imaging approaches, such as time lapse imaging of individual cells in vitro, but rather not for FACS sorting of heterogenic cell populations.

Recently, the development of circular permuted green fluorescent proteins (cpGFP) has enabled researchers to measure phosphorylation events in living cells using a single wavelength (Kawai *et al.*, 2004). However, the increase in fluorescence was only around 10-15%, which would be too little for separation by FACS. Novel mutations of circular GFP and ratiometric measurement of absorbance at different wavelengths increased the dynamic range up to 16fold between free and saturated forms of cpGFP, at least for measurement of pH or Ca^{2+} in living cells (Bizzarri *et al.*, 2006, Souslova *et al.*, 2007). Yet, if a kinase reporter can be constructed using these advanced cpGFP mutants has still to be shown.

We could observe a specific down regulation of CDK9, the RNApII CTD Ser2 kinase, in adult melanocyte stem cells both on the mRNA and protein levels (Freter *et al.*, 2010). The CDK9 promoter has many features of a housekeeping gene promoter (Bagella *et al.*, 2000, Liu & Rice, 2000), thus down regulation of this promoter may be due to a similar mechanism as other down regulated housekeeping genes in MelSC. Reporters for promoter function, for example GFP, Luciferase or LacZ have been used extensively to isolate or trace specific cells in vivo. However, isolating CDK9 promoter negative cells as transcriptionally quiescent stem cells could be biased by secondary effects on the reporter, such as silencing of reporter constructs or heterogeneity of expression between cells. One solution would be to label all cells with a constitutive reporter, and isolate constitutive promoter positive, CDK9 promoter reporter negative cells. The constitutive promoter has to be carefully chosen, as for example expression from the CMV promoter highly depends on CDK9 (Peng *et al.*, 1998). Given our observation of low activity of CDK9 in HSC, it is not surprising that HSC show limited CMV promoter activity (Salmon *et al.*, 2000). Constitutive promoters, but also promoters used for overexpression of genes in quiescent stem cells thus need to be validated for activity in vivo.

In vitro culture and expansion of immature hematopoietic stem cells could help to achieve better transplantation response in patients, but has not been achieved yet. So far culture of immature HSC leads to almost immediate differentiation and loss of multi-lineage repopulation ability. It has been shown recently that the xenobiotic Aryl receptor is present on HSC (Singh *et al.*, 2009). Activation by ligands results in nuclear translocation, recruitment of Ccnt1 and activation of hematopoietic gene transcription (Tian *et al.*, 2003). Interestingly, antagonists of the Aryl receptor prevent differentiation of HSC in vitro (Boitano *et al.*, 2010), suggesting that transcriptional quiescence may be beneficial for in vitro stem cell expansion. It would be very interesting to determine if inhibitors of P-TEFb activity have an effect on maintenance of undifferentiated HSC.

Transcriptional quiescence could also be used as a read-out of stem cell function in vitro. Screens of small molecular compounds in in vitro culture of primary HSC for maintenance of the human HSC markers CD34 and CD133 have led to some promising results (Boitano *et al.*, 2010). However, surface proteins may be unstable or unreliable, and may not be an immediate read-out of stem cell function. Transcriptional quiescence could serve as an alternative marker for stem cell identity. The development of fluorescent reporters for this screening is required to evaluate the impact of cytokines or small molecules on maintenance and expansion of HSC in vitro.

We and others have shown that inhibition of P-TEFb activity can be favourable for cell survival during cellular stresses, such as serum or growth factor starvation (Freter *et al.*, 2010, Kanazawa *et al.*, 2003). Down regulation of P-TEFb activity could thus also be advantageous for cancer cell survival during metastasis or therapy. Flavopiridol, a very specific CDK9 inhibitor has been used in BLL with some success (Chen *et al.*, 2005), but failed in most cases as a single agent in cancer chemotherapy (Blagosklonny, 2004). If transcriptionally quiescent cancer cells are present in primary or metastatic tumours, further inhibition of CDK9 activity may not be required. Rather, activation of mRNA transcription in these cells may render them susceptible to therapy and prevent metastasis and relapse. The first step towards this goal would be to identify and isolate transcriptionally quiescent cancer cells from a given tumour using a kinase activity reporter or CDK9 promoter reporter. Next, it would be necessary to determine if transcriptionally quiescent tumour cells have an enhanced tumour forming capacity in vivo or survive treatment with chemotherapeutic agents better than transcriptionally activated cells. Finally, high throughput screens for small molecular compounds which activate transcriptional quiescent cancer cells using the same reporter systems will enable us to activate dormant cancer stem cell-like cells in vivo and improve treatment of metastasis and prevent relapse of cancer in patients.

5. Conclusion

Adult stem cells have the unique capacity to self-renew and give rise to differentiated cells. To fulfil their lifelong function, these cells must be protected from cellular and genetic damage. Most adult stem cells are thought to enter a state of reversible cell cycle quiescence to preserve their role (Orford & Scadden, 2008). Indeed, activation of the cell cycle leads to premature stem cell exhaustion (Cheng *et al.*, 2000, Kippin *et al.*, 2005, Park *et al.*, 2003). However, most cells in the adult body have withdrawn from the cell cycle and can be induced to proliferate again, resulting in their eventual depletion (Bond *et al.*, 2004, Pajalunga *et al.*, 2007). Some somatic cells are able to resume proliferation and even self-renew, for example differentiated T and B lymphocytes (Fearon *et al.*, 2001). It has thus been proposed that adult stem cells are distinguished by other mechanisms rather than cell cycle quiescence (Mikkers & Frisen, 2005). Yet, what kind of defining mechanisms or marker this property integrates, and if it is shared by various adult stem cells, is unclear at the moment.

It has been long known that adult HSC can be isolated by their low retention of Pyronin Y, an RNA binding dye (Shapiro, 1981), suggesting that global mRNA transcriptional quiescence is a hallmark of quiescent stem cells. This observation however, has never been addressed further in terms of the precise molecular mechanism underlying global transcriptional quiescence. Analysis of the distinct phosphorylation patterns of the CTD of RNApII during the different stages of mRNA transcription can reveal initiation, paused transcription or productive elongation. Our analysis of various adult stem cell systems showed that down regulation of productive mRNA transcription elongation is a conserved, specific and early feature of adult stem cells (Freter *et al.*, 2010). In line with this, the CTD kinase CDK9 was absent and its inhibition improved cell survival during cellular stresses, suggesting a beneficial function of transcriptional quiescence for stem cell maintenance and survival. However, we could not induce activation of mRNA transcription by overexpression of CDK9 in vivo. It is thus not clear what the in vivo function of this down regulation is. New animal models with a constitutively active RNApII have to be developed to elucidate if transcriptional quiescence is necessary for adult stem cell maintenance or just a symptom of their quiescence.

Interestingly, we could observe some heterogeneity in terms of mRNA transcription elongation in the HSC pool, where only 27% of cells showed a clear absence of mRNA transcription elongation. Yet, identification and isolation of these transcriptionally quiescent cells depends on the availability of genetically encoded reporters of mRNA transcription. CDK9 activity reporters need to be specific for this kinase, and a large dynamic range has to be provided to clearly separate cell populations. A particular challenge will be to convert the negative observation of CTD Ser2 dephosphorylation into a signal-positive output, in order to avoid false-positive events by untransfected cells.

Taken together, we defined a novel molecular mechanism for adult stem cell quiescence, which may lead to the identification of pure stem cell-like cell populations from various sources, including heterogeneous adult stem cell populations or cancerous tissue. Even though some technical questions and functional tests are still to be answered, transcriptional quiescence is a novel and exciting mechanism to detect, isolate and characterize adult stem cells in an unprecedented purity from various sources.

6. References

Aida, M., Chen, Y., Nakajima, K., Yamaguchi, Y., Wada, T. & Handa, H. (2006) Transcriptional pausing caused by NELF plays a dual role in regulating immediate-early expression of the junB gene. *Mol Cell Biol*, 26, 6094-6104.

Bagella, L., Stiegler, P., De Luca, A., Siracusa, L.D. & Giordano, A. (2000) Genomic organization, promoter analysis, and chromosomal mapping of the mouse gene encoding Cdk9. *J Cell Biochem*, 78, 170-178.

Barboric, M., Lenasi, T., Chen, H., Johansen, E.B., Guo, S. & Peterlin, B.M. (2009) 7SK snRNP/P-TEFb couples transcription elongation with alternative splicing and is essential for vertebrate development. *Proc Natl Acad Sci U S A*, 106, 7798-7803.

Barboric, M., Nissen, R.M., Kanazawa, S., Jabrane-Ferrat, N. & Peterlin, B.M. (2001) NF-kappaB binds P-TEFb to stimulate transcriptional elongation by RNA polymerase II. *Mol Cell*, 8, 327-337.

Barboric, M. & Peterlin, B.M. (2005) A new paradigm in eukaryotic biology: HIV Tat and the control of transcriptional elongation. *PLoS Biol*, 3, e76.

Batchelder, C., Dunn, M.A., Choy, B., Suh, Y., Cassie, C., Shim, E.Y., Shin, T.H., Mello, C., Seydoux, G. & Blackwell, T.K. (1999) Transcriptional repression by the Caenorhabditis elegans germ-line protein PIE-1. *Genes Dev*, 13, 202-212.

Benedikt, A., Baltruschat, S., Scholz, B., Bursen, A., Arrey, T.N., Meyer, B., Varagnolo, L., Muller, A.M., Karas, M., Dingermann, T. & Marschalek, R. (2011) The leukemogenic AF4-MLL fusion protein causes P-TEFb kinase activation and altered epigenetic signatures. *Leukemia*, 25, 135-144.

Bentley, D.L. (1995) Regulation of transcriptional elongation by RNA polymerase II. *Curr Opin Genet Dev*, 5, 210-216.

Bizzarri, R., Arcangeli, C., Arosio, D., Ricci, F., Faraci, P., Cardarelli, F. & Beltram, F. (2006) Development of a novel GFP-based ratiometric excitation and emission pH indicator for intracellular studies. *Biophys J*, 90, 3300-3314.

Blagosklonny, M.V. (2004) Flavopiridol, an inhibitor of transcription: implications, problems and solutions. *Cell Cycle*, 3, 1537-1542.

Boehm, A.K., Saunders, A., Werner, J. & Lis, J.T. (2003) Transcription factor and polymerase recruitment, modification, and movement on dhsp70 in vivo in the minutes following heat shock. *Mol Cell Biol*, 23, 7628-7637.

Boitano, A.E., Wang, J., Romeo, R., Bouchez, L.C., Parker, A.E., Sutton, S.E., Walker, J.R., Flaveny, C.A., Perdew, G.H., Denison, M.S., Schultz, P.G. & Cooke, M.P. (2010) Aryl hydrocarbon receptor antagonists promote the expansion of human hematopoietic stem cells. *Science*, 329, 1345-1348.

Bond, J., Jones, C., Haughton, M., DeMicco, C., Kipling, D. & Wynford-Thomas, D. (2004) Direct evidence from siRNA-directed "knock down" that p16(INK4a) is required for human fibroblast senescence and for limiting ras-induced epithelial cell proliferation. *Exp Cell Res*, 292, 151-156.

Brinster, R.L. & Nagano, M. (1998) Spermatogonial stem cell transplantation, cryopreservation and culture. *Semin Cell Dev Biol*, 9, 401-409.

Chao, S.H. & Price, D.H. (2001) Flavopiridol inactivates P-TEFb and blocks most RNA polymerase II transcription in vivo. *J Biol Chem*, 276, 31793-31799.

Chen, R., Keating, M.J., Gandhi, V. & Plunkett, W. (2005) Transcription inhibition by flavopiridol: mechanism of chronic lymphocytic leukemia cell death. *Blood*, 106, 2513-2519.

Chen, Y., Yamaguchi, Y., Tsugeno, Y., Yamamoto, J., Yamada, T., Nakamura, M., Hisatake, K. & Handa, H. (2009) DSIF, the Paf1 complex, and Tat-SF1 have nonredundant, cooperative roles in RNA polymerase II elongation. *Genes Dev*, 23, 2765-2777.

Cheng, T., Rodrigues, N., Shen, H., Yang, Y., Dombkowski, D., Sykes, M. & Scadden, D.T. (2000) Hematopoietic stem cell quiescence maintained by p21cip1/waf1. *Science*, 287, 1804-1808.

Coller, H.A., Sang, L. & Roberts, J.M. (2006) A new description of cellular quiescence. *PLoS Biol*, 4, e83.

Eberhardy, S.R. & Farnham, P.J. (2001) c-Myc mediates activation of the cad promoter via a post-RNA polymerase II recruitment mechanism. *J Biol Chem*, 276, 48562-48571.

Eissenberg, J.C., Shilatifard, A., Dorokhov, N. & Michener, D.E. (2007) Cdk9 is an essential kinase in Drosophila that is required for heat shock gene expression, histone methylation and elongation factor recruitment. *Mol Genet Genomics*, 277, 101-114.

Elagib, K.E., Mihaylov, I.S., Delehanty, L.L., Bullock, G.C., Ouma, K.D., Caronia, J.F., Gonias, S.L. & Goldfarb, A.N. (2008) Cross-talk of GATA-1 and P-TEFb in megakaryocyte differentiation. *Blood*, 112, 4884-4894.

Ema, H., Sudo, K., Seita, J., Matsubara, A., Morita, Y., Osawa, M., Takatsu, K., Takaki, S. & Nakauchi, H. (2005) Quantification of self-renewal capacity in single hematopoietic stem cells from normal and Lnk-deficient mice. *Dev Cell*, 8, 907-914.

Fearon, D.T., Manders, P. & Wagner, S.D. (2001) Arrested differentiation, the self-renewing memory lymphocyte, and vaccination. *Science*, 293, 248-250.

Foudi, A., Hochedlinger, K., Van Buren, D., Schindler, J.W., Jaenisch, R., Carey, V. & Hock, H. (2009) Analysis of histone 2B-GFP retention reveals slowly cycling hematopoietic stem cells. *Nat Biotechnol*, 27, 84-90.

Freter, R., Osawa, M. & Nishikawa, S. (2010) Adult stem cells exhibit global suppression of RNA polymerase II serine-2 phosphorylation. *Stem Cells*, 28, 1571-1580.

Fuchs, E., Tumbar, T. & Guasch, G. (2004) Socializing with the neighbors: stem cells and their niche. *Cell*, 116, 769-778.

Fujinaga, K., Irwin, D., Huang, Y., Taube, R., Kurosu, T. & Peterlin, B.M. (2004) Dynamics of human immunodeficiency virus transcription: P-TEFb phosphorylates RD and dissociates negative effectors from the transactivation response element. *Mol Cell Biol*, 24, 787-795.

Fujinaga, K., Irwin, D., Taube, R., Zhang, F., Geyer, M. & Peterlin, B.M. (2002) A minimal chimera of human cyclin T1 and tat binds TAR and activates human immunodeficiency virus transcription in murine cells. *J Virol*, 76, 12934-12939.

Garriga, J., Bhattacharya, S., Calbo, J., Marshall, R.M., Truongcao, M., Haines, D.S. & Grana, X. (2003) CDK9 is constitutively expressed throughout the cell cycle, and its steady-state expression is independent of SKP2. *Mol Cell Biol*, 23, 5165-5173.

Garriga, J., Peng, J., Parreno, M., Price, D.H., Henderson, E.E. & Grana, X. (1998) Upregulation of cyclin T1/CDK9 complexes during T cell activation. *Oncogene*, 17, 3093-3102.

Gojo, I., Zhang, B. & Fenton, R.G. (2002) The cyclin-dependent kinase inhibitor flavopiridol induces apoptosis in multiple myeloma cells through transcriptional repression and down-regulation of Mcl-1. *Clin Cancer Res*, 8, 3527-3538.

Grana, X., De Luca, A., Sang, N., Fu, Y., Claudio, P.P., Rosenblatt, J., Morgan, D.O. & Giordano, A. (1994) PITALRE, a nuclear CDC2-related protein kinase that phosphorylates the retinoblastoma protein in vitro. *Proc Natl Acad Sci U S A*, 91, 3834-3838.

Guenther, M.G., Levine, S.S., Boyer, L.A., Jaenisch, R. & Young, R.A. (2007) A chromatin landmark and transcription initiation at most promoters in human cells. *Cell*, 130, 77-88.

Hanyu-Nakamura, K., Sonobe-Nojima, H., Tanigawa, A., Lasko, P. & Nakamura, A. (2008) Drosophila Pgc protein inhibits P-TEFb recruitment to chromatin in primordial germ cells. *Nature*, 451, 730-733.

Hargreaves, D.C., Horng, T. & Medzhitov, R. (2009) Control of inducible gene expression by signal-dependent transcriptional elongation. *Cell*, 138, 129-145.

Ho, C.K. & Shuman, S. (1999) Distinct roles for CTD Ser-2 and Ser-5 phosphorylation in the recruitment and allosteric activation of mammalian mRNA capping enzyme. *Mol Cell*, 3, 405-411.

Huang, F., Wagner, M. & Siddiqui, M.A. (2004) Ablation of the CLP-1 gene leads to down-regulation of the HAND1 gene and abnormality of the left ventricle of the heart and fetal death. *Mech Dev*, 121, 559-572.

Jang, M.K., Mochizuki, K., Zhou, M., Jeong, H.S., Brady, J.N. & Ozato, K. (2005) The bromodomain protein Brd4 is a positive regulatory component of P-TEFb and stimulates RNA polymerase II-dependent transcription. *Mol Cell*, 19, 523-534.

Jiang, H. & Peterlin, B.M. (2008) Differential chromatin looping regulates CD4 expression in immature thymocytes. *Mol Cell Biol*, 28, 907-912.

Jiang, H., Zhang, F., Kurosu, T. & Peterlin, B.M. (2005) Runx1 binds positive transcription elongation factor b and represses transcriptional elongation by RNA polymerase II: possible mechanism of CD4 silencing. *Mol Cell Biol*, 25, 10675-10683.

Kanazawa, S., Okamoto, T. & Peterlin, B.M. (2000) Tat competes with CIITA for the binding to P-TEFb and blocks the expression of MHC class II genes in HIV infection. *Immunity*, 12, 61-70.

Kanazawa, S., Soucek, L., Evan, G., Okamoto, T. & Peterlin, B.M. (2003) c-Myc recruits P-TEFb for transcription, cellular proliferation and apoptosis. *Oncogene*, 22, 5707-5711.

Kawai, Y., Sato, M. & Umezawa, Y. (2004) Single color fluorescent indicators of protein phosphorylation for multicolor imaging of intracellular signal flow dynamics. *Anal Chem*, 76, 6144-6149.

Kippin, T.E., Martens, D.J. & van der Kooy, D. (2005) p21 loss compromises the relative quiescence of forebrain stem cell proliferation leading to exhaustion of their proliferation capacity. *Genes Dev*, 19, 756-767.

Kohoutek, J. (2009) P-TEFb- the final frontier. *Cell Div*, 4, 19.

Kohoutek, J., Li, Q., Blazek, D., Luo, Z., Jiang, H. & Peterlin, B.M. (2009) Cyclin T2 is essential for mouse embryogenesis. *Mol Cell Biol*, 29, 3280-3285.

Li, L., Jothi, R., Cui, K., Lee, J.Y., Cohen, T., Gorivodsky, M., Tzchori, I., Zhao, Y., Hayes, S.M., Bresnick, E.H., Zhao, K., Westphal, H. & Love, P.E. (2011) Nuclear adaptor Ldb1 regulates a transcriptional program essential for the maintenance of hematopoietic stem cells. *Nat Immunol*, 12, 129-136.

Li, Q., Price, J.P., Byers, S.A., Cheng, D., Peng, J. & Price, D.H. (2005) Analysis of the large inactive P-TEFb complex indicates that it contains one 7SK molecule, a dimer of HEXIM1 or HEXIM2, and two P-TEFb molecules containing Cdk9 phosphorylated at threonine 186. *J Biol Chem*, 280, 28819-28826.

Lin, C., Smith, E.R., Takahashi, H., Lai, K.C., Martin-Brown, S., Florens, L., Washburn, M.P., Conaway, J.W., Conaway, R.C. & Shilatifard, A. (2010) AFF4, a component of the ELL/P-TEFb elongation complex and a shared subunit of MLL chimeras, can link transcription elongation to leukemia. *Mol Cell*, 37, 429-437.

Liu, H. & Herrmann, C.H. (2005) Differential localization and expression of the Cdk9 42k and 55k isoforms. *J Cell Physiol*, 203, 251-260.

Liu, H. & Rice, A.P. (2000) Genomic organization and characterization of promoter function of the human CDK9 gene. *Gene*, 252, 51-59.

Mancebo, H.S., Lee, G., Flygare, J., Tomassini, J., Luu, P., Zhu, Y., Peng, J., Blau, C., Hazuda, D., Price, D. & Flores, O. (1997) P-TEFb kinase is required for HIV Tat transcriptional activation in vivo and in vitro. *Genes Dev*, 11, 2633-2644.

Marshall, R.M., Salerno, D., Garriga, J. & Gra√ ±a, X. (2005) Cyclin T1 expression is regulated by multiple signaling pathways and mechanisms during activation of human peripheral blood lymphocytes. *J Immunol*, 175, 6402-6411.

Meier, N., Krpic, S., Rodriguez, P., Strouboulis, J., Monti, M., Krijgsveld, J., Gering, M., Patient, R., Hostert, A. & Grosveld, F. (2006) Novel binding partners of Ldb1 are required for haematopoietic development. *Development*, 133, 4913-4923.

Mikkers, H. & Frisen, J. (2005) Deconstructing stemness. *EMBO J*, 24, 2715-2719.

Muse, G.W., Gilchrist, D.A., Nechaev, S., Shah, R., Parker, J.S., Grissom, S.F., Zeitlinger, J. & Adelman, K. (2007) RNA polymerase is poised for activation across the genome. *Nat Genet*, 39, 1507-1511.

Nguyen, A.W. & Daugherty, P.S. (2005) Evolutionary optimization of fluorescent proteins for intracellular FRET. *Nat Biotechnol*, 23, 355-360.

Ni, Z., Schwartz, B.E., Werner, J., Suarez, J.R. & Lis, J.T. (2004) Coordination of transcription, RNA processing, and surveillance by P-TEFb kinase on heat shock genes. *Mol Cell*, 13, 55-65.

Nishimura, E.K., Jordan, S.A., Oshima, H., Yoshida, H., Osawa, M., Moriyama, M., Jackson, I.J., Barrandon, Y., Miyachi, Y. & Nishikawa, S. (2002) Dominant role of the niche in melanocyte stem-cell fate determination. *Nature*, 416, 854-860.

Orford, K.W. & Scadden, D.T. (2008) Deconstructing stem cell self-renewal: genetic insights into cell-cycle regulation. *Nat Rev Genet*, 9, 115-128.

Osawa, M., Egawa, G., Mak, S.S., Moriyama, M., Fretcr, R., Yonetani, S., Beermann, F. & Nishikawa, S. (2005) Molecular characterization of melanocyte stem cells in their niche. *Development*, 132, 5589-5599.

Oven, I., Brdickova, N., Kohoutek, J., Vaupotic, T., Narat, M. & Peterlin, B.M. (2007) AIRE recruits P-TEFb for transcriptional elongation of target genes in medullary thymic epithelial cells. *Mol Cell Biol*, 27, 8815-8823.

Pajalunga, D., Mazzola, A., Salzano, A.M., Biferi, M.G., De Luca, G. & Crescenzi, M. (2007) Critical requirement for cell cycle inhibitors in sustaining nonproliferative states. *J Cell Biol*, 176, 807-818.

Park, I.K., Qian, D., Kiel, M., Becker, M.W., Pihalja, M., Weissman, I.L., Morrison, S.J. & Clarke, M.F. (2003) Bmi-1 is required for maintenance of adult self-renewing haematopoietic stem cells. *Nature*, 423, 302-305.

Patturajan, M., Schulte, R.J., Sefton, B.M., Berezney, R., Vincent, M., Bensaude, O., Warren, S.L. & Corden, J.L. (1998) Growth-related changes in phosphorylation of yeast RNA polymerase II. *J Biol Chem*, 273, 4689-4694.

Peng, J., Zhu, Y., Milton, J.T. & Price, D.H. (1998) Identification of multiple cyclin subunits of human P-TEFb. *Genes Dev*, 12, 755-762.

Peterlin, B.M. & Price, D.H. (2006) Controlling the elongation phase of transcription with P-TEFb. *Mol Cell*, 23, 297-305.

Radonjic, M., Andrau, J.C., Lijnzaad, P., Kemmeren, P., Kockelkorn, T.T., van Leenen, D., van Berkum, N.L. & Holstege, F.C. (2005) Genome-wide analyses reveal RNA polymerase II located upstream of genes poised for rapid response upon S. cerevisiae stationary phase exit. *Mol Cell*, 18, 171-183.

Rahl, P.B., Lin, C.Y., Seila, A.C., Flynn, R.A., McCuine, S., Burge, C.B., Sharp, P.A. & Young, R.A. (2010) c-Myc regulates transcriptional pause release. *Cell*, 141, 432-445.

Ramakrishnan, R., Yu, W. & Rice, A.P. (2011) Limited redundancy in genes regulated by Cyclin T2 and Cyclin T1. *BMC Res Notes*, 4, 260.

Salmon, P., Kindler, V., Ducrey, O., Chapuis, B., Zubler, R.H. & Trono, D. (2000) High-level transgene expression in human hematopoietic progenitors and differentiated blood lineages after transduction with improved lentiviral vectors. *Blood*, 96, 3392-3398.

Sato, M., Kawai, Y. & Umezawa, Y. (2007) Genetically encoded fluorescent indicators to visualize protein phosphorylation by extracellular signal-regulated kinase in single living cells. *Anal Chem*, 79, 2570-2575.

Sehgal, P.B. & Darnell, T. (1976) The inhibition by DRB (5,6-dichloro-1-beta-D-ribofuranosylbenzimidazole) of hnRNA and mRNA production in HeLa cells. *Cell*, 9, 473-480.

Shackleton, M., Vaillant, F., Simpson, K.J., Stingl, J., Smyth, G.K., Asselin-Labat, M.L., Wu, L., Lindeman, G.J. & Visvader, J.E. (2006) Generation of a functional mammary gland from a single stem cell. *Nature*, 439, 84-88.

Shapiro, H.M. (1981) Flow cytometric estimation of DNA and RNA content in intact cells stained with Hoechst 33342 and pyronin Y. *Cytometry*, 2, 143-150.

Shilatifard, A., Lane, W.S., Jackson, K.W., Conaway, R.C. & Conaway, J.W. (1996) An RNA polymerase II elongation factor encoded by the human ELL gene. *Science*, 271, 1873-1876.

Shim, E.Y., Walker, A.K., Shi, Y. & Blackwell, T.K. (2002) CDK-9/cyclin T (P-TEFb) is required in two postinitiation pathways for transcription in the C. elegans embryo. *Genes Dev*, 16, 2135-2146.

Shore, S.M., Byers, S.A., Dent, P. & Price, D.H. (2005) Characterization of Cdk9(55) and differential regulation of two Cdk9 isoforms. *Gene*, 350, 51-58.

Shore, S.M., Byers, S.A., Maury, W. & Price, D.H. (2003) Identification of a novel isoform of Cdk9. *Gene*, 307, 175-182.

Sims, R.J., 3rd, Belotserkovskaya, R. & Reinberg, D. (2004) Elongation by RNA polymerase II: the short and long of it. *Genes Dev*, 18, 2437-2468.

Singh, K.P., Casado, F.L., Opanashuk, L.A. & Gasiewicz, T.A. (2009) The aryl hydrocarbon receptor has a normal function in the regulation of hematopoietic and other stem/progenitor cell populations. *Biochem Pharmacol*, 77, 577-587.

Song, S.H., Kim, A., Ragoczy, T., Bender, M.A., Groudine, M. & Dean, A. (2010) Multiple functions of Ldb1 required for beta-globin activation during erythroid differentiation. *Blood*, 116, 2356-2364.

Souslova, E.A., Belousov, V.V., Lock, J.G., Stromblad, S., Kasparov, S., Bolshakov, A.P., Pinelis, V.G., Labas, Y.A., Lukyanov, S., Mayr, L.M. & Chudakov, D.M. (2007) Single fluorescent protein-based Ca2+ sensors with increased dynamic range. *BMC Biotechnol*, 7, 37.

Tian, Y., Ke, S., Chen, M. & Sheng, T. (2003) Interactions between the aryl hydrocarbon receptor and P-TEFb. Sequential recruitment of transcription factors and differential phosphorylation of C-terminal domain of RNA polymerase II at cyp1a1 promoter. *J Biol Chem*, 278, 44041-44048.

Tothova, Z. & Gilliland, D.G. (2007) FoxO transcription factors and stem cell homeostasis: insights from the hematopoietic system. *Cell Stem Cell*, 1, 140-152.

Wei, P., Garber, M.E., Fang, S.M., Fischer, W.H. & Jones, K.A. (1998) A novel CDK9-associated C-type cyclin interacts directly with HIV-1 Tat and mediates its high-affinity, loop-specific binding to TAR RNA. *Cell*, 92, 451-462.

Wilson, A., Laurenti, E., Oser, G., van der Wath, R.C., Blanco-Bose, W., Jaworski, M., Offner, S., Dunant, C.F., Eshkind, L., Bockamp, E., Li$\sqrt{\geq}$, P., Macdonald, H.R. & Trumpp, A. (2008) Hematopoietic stem cells reversibly switch from dormancy to self-renewal during homeostasis and repair. *Cell*, 135, 1118-1129.

Wittmann, B.M., Wang, N. & Montano, M.M. (2003) Identification of a novel inhibitor of breast cell growth that is down-regulated by estrogens and decreased in breast tumors. *Cancer Res*, 63, 5151-5158.

Wu, C.H., Yamaguchi, Y., Benjamin, L.R., Horvat-Gordon, M., Washinsky, J., Enerly, E., Larsson, J., Lambertsson, A., Handa, H. & Gilmour, D. (2003) NELF and DSIF cause promoter proximal pausing on the hsp70 promoter in Drosophila. *Genes Dev*, 17, 1402-1414.

Yamaguchi, Y., Inukai, N., Narita, T., Wada, T. & Handa, H. (2002) Evidence that negative elongation factor represses transcription elongation through binding to a DRB sensitivity-inducing factor/RNA polymerase II complex and RNA. *Mol Cell Biol*, 22, 2918-2927.

Yang, Z., Yik, J.H., Chen, R., He, N., Jang, M.K., Ozato, K. & Zhou, Q. (2005) Recruitment of P-TEFb for stimulation of transcriptional elongation by the bromodomain protein Brd4. *Mol Cell*, 19, 535-545.

Zeitlinger, J., Stark, A., Kellis, M., Hong, J.W., Nechaev, S., Adelman, K., Levine, M. & Young, R.A. (2007) RNA polymerase stalling at developmental control genes in the Drosophila melanogaster embryo. *Nat Genet*, 39, 1512-1516.

Zhang, F., Barboric, M., Blackwell, T.K. & Peterlin, B.M. (2003) A model of repression: CTD analogs and PIE-1 inhibit transcriptional elongation by P-TEFb. *Genes Dev*, 17, 748-758.

Zhu, Y., Pe'ery, T., Peng, J., Ramanathan, Y., Marshall, N., Marshall, T., Amendt, B., Mathews, M.B. & Price, D.H. (1997) Transcription elongation factor P-TEFb is required for HIV-1 tat transactivation in vitro. *Genes Dev*, 11, 2622-2632.

3

Networks Establishing Hematopoietic Stem Cell Multipotency and Self-Renewal

Eliana Abdelhay, Luciana Pizzatti and Renata Binato
Instituto Nacional de Câncer, Rio de Janeiro,
Brazil

1. Introduction

Hematopoiesis is a tightly regulated process maintained by a small pool of hematopoietic stem cells (HSC) capable of undergoing self-renewal and generating mature progeny of all of the hematopoietic cell lineages. To sustain the proper levels of blood cells, HSCs must continuously monitor and regulate the balance between self-renewal and lineage differentiation. To produce all hematopoietic cells, hematopoiesis proceeds in a step-wise manner from the primordial long-term (LT)-HSCs. LT-HSCs possess the ability to self-renew and the capacity for long-term reconstitution of lethally irradiated hosts. After a first step of differentiation, LT-HSCs lose their capacity for self-renewal and give rise to a population of short-term (ST)-HSCs. The ST-HSCs has a limited ability to self-renew and reconstitute lethally irradiated hosts, but differentiate into a multipotent progenitor (MPP) population. The MPPs lack the capacity to undergo self-renewal, but retain multipotency. From these multipotent progenitors develops a series of intermediate progenitors that give rise to the assorted hematopoietic lineages. In the classical pathway of hematopoiesis, these intermediates include the common lymphoid progenitors (CLPs) that differentiate into lymphoid, but not myeloid progeny, and the common myeloid progenitors (CMPs), which retain full erythromyeloid potential. The CMPs further differentiate to form the granulocyte/macrophage progenitors (GMPs) that differentiate to the myelomonocytic lineage and the megakaryocytic/erythrocyte progenitors (MEPs) that eventually differentiate to form red blood cells and platelets. All these blood cells produced daily in high numbers (1×10^{12} cells/day) are derived from a relatively small but rare fraction of multipotent cells, the HSCs (Weissman, 2000).

Transcriptional regulation is a key mechanism controlling HSC homeostasis, development, and lineage commitment.

2. Transcription factors in hematopoietic development

Hematopoiesis is regulated at the level of pluripotent HSCs and committed progenitors through growth and/or differentiation inducing factors (like EPO, G-CSF, GM-CSF, IL-1, IL-3) that interact with receptors and initiate signal transduction processes that culminate in the activation of new genetic programs. These external stimuli trigger intrinsic determinants of cell fate, the transcription factors which contribute to the reprogramming of HSCs into cell-lineage restricted pathways of maturation (Zon, 2008). Although the transcription factors involved in hematopoietic development belong to all classes of DNA-binding proteins some of them are involved in the regulation of self-renewal function primarily on HSCs while the others act on MPPs and/or early committed progenitors entering the cell-lineage restricted pathways of differentiation. While transcription factors as MLL, RUNX1, TEL/ETV6, SCL/TAL1 and LMO2 are required for HSC formation and function, others are necessary as key lineage restricted factors acting at the level of early pre-committed progenitors, using key partners that act synergistically or competing to restrict cell-lineage hematopoietic differentiation. GATA-1 and PU-1, for example, physically interact and antagonize with each other to promote either myeloid or erythroid maturation (Rekhtman et al., 1999; Zhang et al., 1999), which means that suppression of GATA-1 expression favors myeloid differentiation while inhibition of PU-1 promotes erythroid maturation. Additional, antagonistic interactions with other transcription factors have also been reported as C/EBPα that antagonizes FOG-1 in eosinophilic differentiation, EKLF antagonizes Fli-1 for erythroid versus megakaryocytic differentiation. Finally, repression of the *Pax-5* gene prevented Pro-B cell maturation to B cells, while promoting multi-potentiality into macrophage, T-NKs and dendritic cells (Huntly & Gilliland, 2005).

Transcription factors also interact with other proteins associated with chromatin modification and form active or repressive transcriptional complexes. Knockout of *Scl/Tal1* or *Lmo2* abrogates hematopoietic development. The precise mechanism through which such transcription activator or repressor complexes regulate the expression of several genes is critical, since the gene expression pattern regulates cell fate decision via cell-lineage restricted maturation. A critical point, however, for all these transcriptional complexes is the concentration of the transcription factor itself and its affinity to other interactive proteins.

Under normal hematopoiesis, several groups of hematopoietic and mature blood cells are generated. Hematopoiesis occurs unidirectionally and commitment from one step to the next occurs irreversibly, suggesting that transcription factors regulate cell fate along the specific cell-lineage pathways irreversibly. This occurs in such a way because intrinsic transcription factor network is coordinated with inputs resulting from external stimuli initiated within the hematopoietic cell niche. The question, however, whether one cell type of progenitors can be reprogrammed into another phenotype at the level of manipulation of transcription factor activation, is a potentially interesting one. Indeed, evidence now indicates that transfection of *Gata-1* into CMPs and/or CLPs redirects their commitment to another cell-lineage restricted pathway as megakaryocytic/erythroid. Similarly, pre-T cells can be reprogrammed to myeloid dendritic cells upon *PU-1* overexpression (Laiosa et al., 2006; Orkin & Zon, 2008).

3. Ontogeny of HSCs

In vertebrates, the production of blood stem cells is accomplished by the allocation and specification of distinct embryonic cells in a variety of sites that change during development. In mammals, the sequential sites of hematopoiesis include the yolk sac; an area surrounding the dorsal aorta termed the aorta-gonad mesonephros (AGM) region, the fetal liver, and finally the bone marrow. Recently, the placenta has been recognized as an additional site that participates during the AGM to fetal liver period. The properties of HSCs in each site differ, presumably reflecting diverse niches that support HSC expansion and/or differentiation and intrinsic characteristics of HSCs at each stage. For instance, HSCs present in the fetal liver are in cycle, whereas adult bone marrow HSCs are largely quiescent.

The initial wave of blood production in the mammalian yolk sac is termed "primitive." The primary function for primitive hematopoiesis is the production of red blood cells that facilitate tissue oxygenation as the embryo undergoes rapid growth. The hallmark of primitive erythroid cells is expression of embryonic globin proteins. The primitive hematopoietic system is transient and rapidly replaced by adult-type hematopoiesis that is termed "definitive". In mammals, the next site of hematopoietic potential is the AGM region. Hematopoietic cells were first detected in the aorta of the developing pig more than 80 years ago. Morphological examination revealed that a sheet of lateral mesoderm migrates medially, touches endoderm, and then forms a single aorta tube. Clusters of hematopoietic cells subsequently appear in the ventral wall. Similarly, an intraembryonic source of adult HSCs in mice capable of long-term reconstitution of irradiated hosts resides in the AGM region (Muller et al., 1994). At embryonic day 10.5, little HSC activity is detectable, whereas by day 11 engrafting activity is present. Additional hematopoietic activity in the mouse embryo was detected subsequently in other sites, including the umbilical arteries and the allantois in which hematopoietic and endothelial cells are co-localized (Inman & Downs, 2007). Umbilical veins lack hematopoietic potential, suggesting that a hierarchy exists during definitive hematopoiesis in which HSCs arise predominantly during artery specification. In addition, significant numbers of HSCs are found in the mouse placenta (Gekas et al., 2005; Ottersbach & Dzierzak, 2005), nearly coincident with the appearance of HSCs in the AGM region and for several days thereafter. Placental HSCs could arise through de novo generation or colonization upon circulation, or both. The relative contribution of each of the above sites to the final pool of adult HSCs remains largely unknown.

Subsequent definitive hematopoiesis involves the colonization of the fetal liver, thymus, spleen, and ultimately the bone marrow. It is believed that none of these sites is accompanied by de novo HSC generation. Rather, their niches support expansion of populations of HSCs that migrate to these new sites. However, until very recently, there has been no evidence by fate mapping or direct visualization that HSCs from one site colonize subsequent sites.

4. Pathways involved in the emergence of HSCs

The AGM has been characterized largely by morphology and functional assays, but the pathways involved in HSC generation remain incompletely defined. Studies of chick embryos demonstrate that endoderm has a prominent role and secretes inducing factors. Somitic mesoderm also contributes to the dorsal aspect of the aorta, and the addition of factors such as VEGF, TGF-β, and FGF to the somitic mesoderm leads to induction of hematopoietic tissue. In contrast, TGF-α and EGF suppressed formation of hematopoietic cells (Pardanaud & Dieterlen-Lievre, 1999).

Signaling pathways that regulate the induction of the AGM have been uncovered in mouse and zebrafish, *Notch 1* is required for artery identity and aortic HSC production (Kumano et al., 2003). The fate decisions imposed on mesodermal progenitors within the AGM are clearly influenced by the *Notch* pathway (Burns et al., 2005). For instance, mice deficient in *RBPj* (a downstream component of the *Notch* pathway) show expanded *VE-Cadherin* and *CD31/PECAM* endothelial cell expression with concomitant loss of definitive HSCs (Robert-Moreno et al., 2005). Ablation of the COUP-TFII transcription factor in endothelial cells enabled veins to acquire arterial characteristics, including the expression of *Notch1* and the formation of ectopic HSCs (You et al., 2005). This result would favor *Notch* acting to induce HSCs from a hemogenic endothelial cell. The model in which the *Notch* pathway regulates arterial and HSC fate choice either from distinct mesodermal populations or over different developmental windows since each decision can be uncoupled *in vivo* is very attractive. The finding that both aorta and vein express HSC markers in the *Notch*-activated state with minimal change in *ephrinB2a* expression indicates that *Notch* independently regulates mesoderm–HSC and artery–vein cell fate decisions.Lateral inhibition has been proposed in the central nervous system whereby *Notch* signaling promotes non-neural fates while inhibiting neural development (Lewis, 1998). HSC fate may be established by a similar mechanism whereby *Notch* activation in an endothelial or mesenchymal cell causes down-regulation of ligand production. Consequently, a cell that produces more ligand will force its neighbor to produce less, thus generating a salt-and-pepper pattern of cells containing elevated *Notch* activity. In this model, cells containing high levels of Notch Intra Cytoplasmatic Domain (NICD) would become HSCs, while those with low NICD activity would remain endothelial or mesenchymal.

5. Hematopoietic niches

Stem cells depend on their microenvironment, the niche, for regulation of self-renewal and differentiation. As the site of hematopoiesis changes during vertebrate development, the nature of the stem cell niche must also change. Mutant mice in which the *BMP* pathway is disrupted have increased numbers of osteoblasts and HSCs (Calvi et al., 2003; Zhang et al., 2003). These findings suggest that osteoblasts may represent a critical component of the bone marrow niche for HSCs. Microscopical examination revealed that HSCs appear to reside in the periosteal area of calvarium marrow, where osteoblasts represent an essential component of the bone marrow niche (Papadimitriou et al., 1994). Most recent live animal tracking experiments by using real-time imaging of individual HSCs have indicated that endosteum forms a special zone where HSCs reside (Lo Celso et al., 2009; Xie et al., 2009). The bone marrow HSC niche is constituted of mesenchymal cells type osteoblasts, extracellular matrix components and minerals (high density calcium salts), all of which contribute to the unique micro-environment (niche) (Moore & Lemischka, 2006; Wilson & Trumpp, 2006). At least two distinct hematopoietic progenitor cell supportive niches in bone marrow have been identified thus far: the osteoblastic, which is regulated by *BMP*, *osteopontin, angiopoietin-1, notch* and maybe others (Adams & Scadden, 2006; Wilson & Trumpp, 2006) and the other one, the vascular niche. The vascular niche is thought to be the site where actively dividing stem or progenitor cells is located, and osteoblastic niche is an environment promoting maintenance of quiescent HSCs (Calvi et al., 2003). Currently, how these two different niches communicate with each other is largely unknown.

The number of HSCs in the bone marrow niche is highly controlled through physical interactions among different cell types, in a way that maintains stem cell state. HSCs remain in a quiescent state through close interaction with osteoblasts where this interaction is not only crucial to attach HSCs to niche osteoblasts, but is also essential to maintain HSC dormancy and function. Many factors, including ligands for Notch receptors and N-cadherin, are liberated by osteoblasts, although the contribution of these to adult hematopoiesis remains to be established. The role of N-cadherin as a mediator of interactions with osteoblasts (Zhang et al., 2003), as well as the prominence of osteoblasts for HSC adherence, has been challenged (Kiel et al., 2007). Recent findings suggest that HSCs are maintained in a quiescent state through interaction with thrombopoietin-producing osteoblasts (Yoshihara et al., 2007). Thrombopoietin (TPO) is the primary cytokine that regulates megakaryocyte and platelet development. Thrombopoietin and its receptor Mpl also exert profound effects on primitive hematopoietic cells. All HSCs express Mpl; $TPO-/-$ or $Mpl-/-$ mice have a decreased number of repopulating HSCs (Solar et al., 1998). *In vitro* culture studies (Matsunaga et al., 1998) also indicate a role of TPO in promoting the survival of repopulating HSCs. Through study of AGM and fetal liver $Mpl-/-$ HSCs, Petit-Cocault et al. (2007) showed that TPO contributes to both generation and expansion of HSCs during definitive hematopoiesis. An intracellular adaptor, Lnk, induces a negative signaling pathway downstream of TPO in HSCs (Buza-Vidas et al., 2006; Seita et al., 2007). Another study (Tong et al., 2007) on mice that express Mpl lacking the C-terminal 60 amino acids revealed a pivotal role of an unknown signal emanating from the membrane proximal region of the Mpl receptor or from JAK2 that is critical for maintenance of HSC activity.

The association of HSCs with osteoblasts is countered by other studies that place HSCs adjacent to vascular cells. The chemokine CXCL12 regulates the migration of HSCs to the vascular cells (Kiel & Morrison, 2006). Taken together, these findings suggest that HSCs reside in various sites within the marrow and that their function might depend on their precise localization. Much of the existing debate may be semantic, however, if the osteoblastic and vascular niches are intertwined and not physically separate. Alternatively, HSCs may truly reside in distinct sub-regions, which may endow them with different activities. Cellular dynamics within the niche are relevant to clinical marrow transplantation. For example, recent findings suggest that antibody-mediated clearance of host HSCs facilitates occupancy of the niche and transplantation by exogenous HSCs (Czechowicz et al., 2007).

The physical interactions between individual HSCs and osteoblasts may be effective in determining the stem cell number by facilitating asymmetric or symmetric divisions, which in turn enable HSCs to either self-renew themselves or give birth to early progenitors for blood cells production (Moore & Lemischka, 2006; Wilson and Trumpp, 2006). HSCs are not of static nature, but exist in a dynamic state, since they migrate from the bone marrow into the peripheral blood (frequent trafficking). Whether, or not, HSCs contribute into the repair of the vascular system, is still not known (Janzen & Scadden, 2006).

5.1 Signaling in the niche

Many cell culture experiments have shown that HSCs respond to multiple cytokines and that the fate of a HSC self renewal, apoptosis, mobilization from the niche, formation of differentiated progeny cells depends on multiple cytokines, adhesion proteins, and other signals produced by stromal cells and likely other cells in the body. Since osteoblast (a cell derived from mesenchymal stem cells) is a key component in the HSC niche for the regulation of HSC number via self-renewal (Adams & Scadden, 2006; Huang et al., 2007), modifications of osteoblast functions in co-orchestration with other niche components, would be pivotal for HSCs survival, self-renewal, differentiation and apoptosis under certain circumstances.

HSCs fate decisions is activated by external environmental stimuli and coordinated by intrinsic factors. External stimuli include hematopoietic growth factors such as SCF, BMP/TGF-β, FGF, TPO, WNT proteins (WNT3A), Angiopoietin-1, IL-3, IL-6, Flt3-ligand, as well as Ca2+, hypoxia, PGE2 and retinoic acid (Wilson & Trumpp, 2006) while intrinsic factors are essentially genes controlling cell cycle, apoptosis and chromatin remodeling.

5.2 How some extrinsic factors act in the niche

Stem cell factor receptor, also known as *c-kit* and its ligand *SCF* play a central role in hematopoiesis, melanogenesis and gametogenesis (Edling & Hallberg, 2007; Kent et al., 2008). *C-kit* is a member of the type-III subfamily of receptor tyrosine kinases that also includes the receptor for *M-CSF*, *Flt-3* and *PDGF*. It is expressed in HSCs (LT-HSCs, ST-HSCs and MPPs) (Zayas et al., 2008), normal B- and T-cell progenitors, mast cells, germ cells, melanocytes, neurons, glial cells, placenta, kidney, lung and gut cells. Deficiency and/or deregulation in *SCF* or *c-kit* produce defects in hematopoiesis leading to Acute Myeloid Leukemia (AML) (Scholl et al., 2008). Sporadic mutations of *c-kit* and autocrine/paracrine activation pathways of the *SCF/c-kit* pathway have been implicated in a variety of malignancies. Gain of function mutations of *c-kit* are associated with malignancies such AML, gastrointestinal tumors and mastocytomas. Moreover, expression of a defective *c-kit* leads to a decrease in repopulating HSCs (Ikuta & Weissman, 1992).

Binding of SCF to c-kit promotes dimerization and activation of protein kinase that auto-phosphorylates the receptor. Although SCF may not be essential for the generation of HSCs, numerous studies have shown that it prevents HSC apoptosis. Almost all cytokine combinations used to date for culturing HSCs include SCF. SCF potentiates the greater ability of fetal liver HSCs than adult HSCs to undergo symmetric self-renewal in culture this activity likely needs the cooperation of other factors. The membrane-bound form of SCF is also an adhesive molecule for HSCs to the bone marrow environment (Heissig et al., 2002) as interruption of the interaction between the membrane-bound stem cell factor on osteoblasts with the c-kit receptor on HSCs by blocking antibodies has demonstrated that *c-kit* signaling is essential to maintain HSC dormancy and function (Suzuki et al., 2006), and an increased number of osteoclasts was associated with HSC mobilization. Receptor activator of nuclear factor (NF)-κB (RANK) ligand and cathepsin K mediate the cleavage of membrane-bound SCF; this decreases the abundance of SCF and, therefore, increases HSC mobilization (Kollet et al., 2006). The involvement of SCF in survival, mobility and possibly self-renewal of HSCs in culture and in the HSC niche likely reflects the complex relationship of different cell fates of HSCs.

Transforming growth factor (TGF)-β potently inhibits HSC activity *in vitro* (Blank et al., 2008). However, a *TGF-β* signaling deficiency *in vivo* does not affect proliferation of HSCs. TGF-β and BMP are secreted ligands that are recognized by different receptors that dimerizes and activates downstream cytosolic targets, culminating with the translocation of these activated transcription factors to the nucleus. BMPs, members of the TGF-β superfamily, play important roles in HSC specification during development. A negative role of *BMP* signaling in maintenance of mouse HSCs was shown by its control of the size of the HSC endosteal niche (Ross & Li, 2006). BMP4 supports HSC expansion in culture and partially mediates the effects of Sonic hedgehog on cultured human HSCs (Bhardwaj et al., 2001). Recently, expression characterization of TGF-β superfamily ligands, receptors, and Smads in mouse HSCs was published; primary HSCs and the Lhx2-HPC cell line express most of the proteins required to transmit signals from several TGF-β family ligands (Utsugisawa et al., 2006). In addition, Pimanda et al. (2007) demonstrated the integration of *BMP4/Smad* pathway and *Scl* and *Runx1* activity in HSC development.

All long-term repopulating bone marrow HSCs express a fibroblast growth factor (FGF) receptor (Yeoh et al., 2006); both FGF-1 and FGF-2 support HSC expansion when unfractionated mouse bone marrow cells are cultured in serum-free medium. Crcareva et al. (2005) confirmed that FGF-1 stimulates *ex vivo* expansion of HSCs and showed that the expanded cells were efficiently transduced by retrovirus vectors. Conditional derivatives of FGF receptor-1 have also been used to support short-term HSC expansion and long-term HSC survival in culture (Schiedlmeier et al, 2007). However, the role of the *FGF* pathway in regulating adult HSCs or embryonic hematopoietic development is controversial as the same authors showed that the treatment of purified mouse HSCs that ectopically express *HoxB4* with the fibroblast growth factor receptor (FGFR) inhibitor SU5402 enhanced HSC repopulating activity. Similar results were obtained using primitive hematopoietic colonies derived from embryonic stem cells. These inconsistent results were obtained from different starting cell populations and under different culture conditions, suggesting that the crosstalk of FGF signaling with other pathways is complex.

The WNT protein binds to a receptor complex consisting of a member of the Frizzled family of seven transmembrane proteins and the LDL receptor-related proteins LRP5 or LRP6 (Clevers, 2006). In the canonical *Wnt* pathway, receptor activation leads to stabilization of β-catenin, which accumulates and translocates to the nucleus where it activates target gene expression in concert with transcription factors such as TCF and LEF. Fleming et al. (2008) analyzed the role of *Wnt* signaling on HSC activity, including its effects on cell-cycle quiescence and the capacity of HSCs to reconstitute the hematopoietic system of recipient mice (whose bone marrow has been ablated by radiation). In contrast to previous studies that genetically manipulated the HSCs themselves, they analyzed the effects of blocking *Wnt* signaling in the mouse bone marrow microenvironment by overexpression of dickkopf1 (*Dkk1*), an antagonist of *Wnt/ β-catenin* signaling. Dkk1 is a soluble secreted protein that interacts with the Wnt co-receptors LRP5 and LRP6 (Kawano & Kypta, 2003). It is known that the number of osteoblasts directly affects the number of long-term repopulating HSCs (Calvi et al., 2003; Zhang et al., 2003). The overexpression of *Dkk1* in the osteoblastic lineage under the control of a 2.3 kb fragment of the *collagen 1α* promoter reduced activation of the *Tcf/Lef* transcription factors in HSCs in a non-cell-autonomous manner.

The transgenic mice showed no significant alteration in the proportion of HSCs and common lymphoid progenitor cells under steady-state conditions. Although HSCs from the *Dkk1* transgenic mice could reconstitute the hematopoietic system of irradiated recipient mice, they lost their reconstituting capacity after repeated bone marrow transplantation, indicating that the inhibition of *Wnt* signaling in the niche results in the premature loss of self-renewal activity. These findings show that *Wnt/β-catenin* activity is crucial for the maintenance of HSC quiescence in the bone marrow niche.

The angiopoietin (*Ang*) family of growth factors is composed of four members that bind to the Tie-2 tyrosine kinase receptor; Ang growth factors are important modulators of angiogenesis. Members of the angiopoietin family of proteins contain an N-terminal coiled–coil domain that mediates homo-oligomerization and a C-terminal fibrinogen-like domain that binds Tie-2. To identify the HSCs in situ, Arai et al. (2004) analyzed the receptor tyrosine kinase Tie-2 expression in bone marrow and found that 5-FU-resistant Tie-2 expressing HSCs adhere to osteoblasts at the endosteal surface, in agreement with previous findings of Calvi et al. (2003) and Zhang et al (2003). They also demonstrated that angiopoietin-1 (*Ang-1*), a Tie-2 receptor ligand, is produced primarily by osteoblasts, indicating that Tie-2 and Ang-1 are expressed complementarily in the niche. Tie-2 together with Tie-1 was also found required for homing of HSCs to bone marrow. Taken together, Tie receptors seem one group of the likely candidates for localizing stem cells to the stem cell niche.

Mineral content of bone contributes to compose a unique extracellular matrix in bone marrow and distinguishes it from other mesenchymal tissues. The extracellular calcium concentrations are recognized by the seven-transmembrane calcium-sensing receptors and therefore can initiate an intracellular G protein–coupled response. Those receptors are found on hematopoietic cells and have also been identified on the surface of HSCs (Adams et al., 2006). Local calcium gradient is involved in retaining HSCs in close physical proximity to the endosteal surface of bone. Extracellular calcium ion concentrations in the endosteum are likely higher than in the central marrow region (Silver et al., 1988). In receptor deficient mice models, HSCs were found not to engraft in the bone marrow (Adams et al., 2006) suggesting that the ability of stem cells to sense and respond to the increased calcium concentrations at the endosteal surface participates in creating the unique stem cell-niche interaction that enables bone marrow hematopoiesis.

Most slow-cycling hematopoietic cells are found in the hypoxic zones close to bone surface and distant from capillaries (Kubota et al., 2008), raising the possibility that these hypoxic niches are important for diminished HSC proliferation. Evidence for quiescent HSCs situated in a hypoxic environment has lately been confirmed by analyzing bone marrow cells from mice injected with a Hoechst dye. Transplantation results showed that the bone marrow fraction with the lowest Hoechst-dye uptake, inferred to be hypoxic, had the highest amount of long-term repopulating cells (Parmar et al., 2007). Consistently, HSCs were found to be the most positive for binding of the hypoxic probe pimonidazole. The molecular mechanisms involve the hypoxia-inducible factor-1a regulated gene expressions in stromal cells, such as c-Kit, stromal cell derived factor–1, and others (Ceradini et al., 2004).

Other molecules were recently identified to have role in signaling pathways inside the niche. DNA array experiments showed that, among other proteins, IGF-2 is specifically expressed in cells that do support HSC expansion in culture. Moreover, it was showed that all fetal liver and bone marrow HSCs express receptors for IGF-2. The inclusion of IGF-2 with SCF, TPO, and FGF-1 supports an eight-fold increase of highly enriched HSCs in culture (Zhang & Lodish, 2004). Whether IGF-2 acts on self-renewal, apoptosis, differentiation, or homing of HSCs is unclear. Interestingly, IGF-2 was found to bind and stimulate self-renewal of human embryonic stem cells (Bendall et al., 2007). Angiopoietin-like proteins (Angptls) were also implicated in HSC expansion. Angptls are a family of seven secreted glycoproteins that share sequence homology with the angiopoietins (Morisada et al., 2006). Similar to the angiopoietins, each Angptl contains an N-terminal coiledcoil domain and a C-terminal fibrinogen-like domain. However, unlike angiopoietins, Angptls do not bind to Tie-2 or Tie-1 and their receptors are unknown. This suggests that Angptls may have different functions from the angiopoietins. Angptl7 was suggested to be a target of the *Wnt/β-catenin* signaling pathway. However, most of the physiological activities of the Angptls remain unknown. Recently Angptl2 and Angptl3 were identified as growth factors that stimulate *ex vivo* expansion of bone marrow HSCs. Other analogues, including Angptl5, Angptl7, and Mfap4, also support *ex vivo* expansion of HSCs.

5.3 Signaling through cell adhesion molecules

In addition to signaling pathways as described above, extracellular matrix components of the niche have also been shown to play role in regulating the HSC dynamics. A matrix glycoprotein, osteopontin (OPN), as a constraining factor on HSCs within the bone marrow microenvironment is produced by osteoblasts in response to stimulation (Stier et al., 2005). Using studies that combine OPN-deficient mice and exogenous OPN, Stier et al. (2005) demonstrated that OPN modifies primitive hematopoietic cell number and function in a stem cell non-autonomous manner. The OPN-null microenvironment is sufficient to increase the number of stem cells associated with increased stromal *Jagged-1* and *Ang-1* expression and reduced primitive hematopoietic cell apoptosis. The activation of the stem cell microenvironment with PTH was shown to induce a super-physiologic increase in stem cells in the absence of OPN. Therefore, OPN seems to be a negative regulatory element of the stem cell niche that limits the size of the stem cell pool and may provide a mechanism for restricting excess stem cell expansion under conditions of niche stimulation.

The production of OPN by osteoblasts is likely to be an essential requirement as shown by Karahuseyinoglu et al. (2007). Osteogenically induced umbilical cord stromal cells express OPN during the first week of induction followed by a third week expression of another matricellular protein, bone sialoprotein-2 (BSP-2). In the following weeks, in conditioned media differentiating osteoblasts express osteonectin and osteocalcin that led us to suggest that all those proteins have roles in autocrine regulation of osteoblast maturation and thus might serve to determine the conditional status of the partner cell(s) in hematopoietic niche microenvironment.

Previous studies showed that cell adhesion molecules, such as cadherins and integrins, are crucial for the interactions between HSCs and the osteoblastic niche. N-cadherin–mediated adhesion mediates slowing cell cycling of HSCs and may keep HSCs quiescent. Some studies showed that specialized spindle-shaped N-cadherin+ osteoblasts are a key component of the bone marrow stem cell niche. HSCs are thought to be anchored to spindle-shaped N-cadherin+ osteoblast cells via a homotypic N-cadherin interaction. Also, N-cadherin and β1-integrin are identified as the downstream targets in *Tie-2/Ang-1* signaling and *TPO/MPL* signaling (Yoshihara et al., 2007) in HSCs, respectively, suggesting a link between adhesion molecules and cell-cycle regulators in modulating the HSC–niche interaction. These data suggest cell-adhesion molecules not only contribute to the anchoring of HSCs to the niche, but also regulate cell-cycle quiescence of HSCs in the niche. However, the studies by conditional deletion of N-cadherin fail to support the effects of N-cadherin on hematopoiesis (Kiel et al., 2007).

The members of the *Notch* family are developmental morphogens shown to be expressed in self-renewing tissues, enhance the self-renewal capacity of HSCs and promote T-cell differentiation. *Notch* signaling is initiated by the involvement of the extracellular portion of Notch with its ligands Jagged/Delta. Activation of the *Notch* signaling pathway has been shown to potentiate self-renewal of HSCs. It is initiated by the binding of Jagged ligand to Notch protein followed by metalloproteinase (γ-secretase) cleavage in the extracellular receptor portion leading to the intracellular release of Notch (NICD). Then Notch translocate into the nucleus, where it forms a multimeric transcriptional complex with other transcription factors (Huntly & Gilliland, 2005). Inhibitors of γ-secretase abrogate the Notch signaling activation (Rizzo et al., 2008; Shih & Wang, 2007).

Calvi et al. (2003) and Duncan et al. (2005) demonstrated that the *Notch* signaling pathway plays a role in the osteoblast bone marrow HSCs niche. Notch ligands have positive effects on *ex vivo* expansion of HSCs: activated *Notch* is able to immortalize primitive mouse hematopoietic progenitors and Notch ligands support HSC expansion in culture (Chiba, 2006). Recently, by culturing human cord blood cells in serum-free medium supplemented with SCF, TPO, Flt3L, IL-3, IL-6/sIL-6R, and Delta 1, Suzuki et al. (Suzuki et al., 2006) reported an approximate six-fold increase in SCID-repopulating cell (SRC) number. It is noteworthy that there exists a dose effect for Notch ligands in HSC culture. Whereas a low amount of Delta 1 supports human cord blood SRC expansion, high amounts of the cytokine induce apoptosis (Chiba, 2006).

This emphasizes the complicated relationship among the different fates of HSCs. As conditional knockouts of *Notch1* and *Jagged1* have normal *in vivo* HSC activities (Mancini et al., 2005), there likely is functional redundancy of different *Notch* isoforms and their ligands.

Endothelial cells in the vascular niche environment contacting HSCs also provide maintenance signals on the HSC behaviour (Coultas et al., 2005 ; Li & Li, 2006). The main components of vascular niche – hematopoietic cells and endothelial cells – are closely related during development since they are both derived from haemangioblasts (Kopp et al., 2005). Previous studies have suggested that the vascular niche is the place for HSC differentiation and mobilization (Avencilla et al., 2004). Endothelial cells expressing vascular cell-adhesion molecule-1 (VCAM-1) associate closely with megakaryocytes and their progenitors through VLA-4 in response to chemotactic factors, stromal cell-derived factor- 1 (SDF1) and fibroblast growth factor-4 (FGF4), and thus provide a niche for megakaryocyte maturation and platelet production. The immediate juxtaposition of HSCs to endothelial cells also facilitates their rapid mobilization and entry into circulation in response to stress and, in the case of megakaryocytes, release of platelets directly into the blood. Endothelial cells promote survival of HSCs in culture, but this seems to be limited to certain populations of endothelial cells (Li et al., 2004). Fractions of HSCs in both adult bone marrow and spleen were found in close association with endothelial sinusoids (Kiel et al., 2005), suggesting that endothelial cells provide support to HSCs *in vivo*. Depending on these data, it is now plausible to note that while the osteoblastic niche provides a quiescent environment for HSC maintenance, the vascular niche offers an alternative niche for mobilized stem cells and promotes proliferation and further differentiation or maturation into the circulatory system. It would be interesting to further define the respective contributions of endothelial and endosteal niches to HSC behaviour.

5.4 Cell intrinsic responses

Recent studies have shown that Polycomb group (PcG) proteins and their interaction are important in the regulation of HSC self-renewal and lineage restriction. In particular, members of the PRC1 (Polycomb repression complex 1), such as *Bmi1*, *Mel18* and *Rae28*, have been implicated. *Bmi1* plays an important role in regulating the proliferative activity of stem and progenitor cells. It is required for the self-renewal of both adult HSCs and neural stem cells (Molofsky et al., 2005; Park et al, 2003). *Bmi1* enhances symmetrical expansion of the stem cell pool through self-renewal, induces a marked *ex vivo* expansion of multipotent progenitors, and increases the ability of HSCs to repopulate bone marrow *in vivo* (Iwama et al., 2004). Leukemic cells lacking *Bmi1* undergo proliferation arrest, differentiation and apoptosis, leading to failure of leukemia in a mouse transplant model (Lessard & Sauvageau, 2003). In *Bmi1*-deficient bone marrow there is an up-regulation of cell cycle inhibitors *p16* and *p19*, and the *p53*-induced gene *Wig1*, and a down-regulation of the apoptosis inhibitor *AI-6*. This suggests that a mechanism exists whereby *Bmi1* functions by modulating proliferation and preventing apoptosis (Park et al., 2004). *Bmi1* has also been shown to regulate the expression of *Hox* genes that are required for differentiation during hematopoiesis (van der Lugt et al., 1996).Loss or knockdown of another Polycomb gene, *Mel18*, leads to increased expression of *Hoxb4* (Kajiume et al., 2004), and transplanted *Mel18*-deficient bone marrow showed an increase in overall HSC numbers but a decrease in their activity owing to arrest in G_0 phase of the cell cycle. *Rae28*-deficient HSCs were defective in their long-term repopulating ability in serial transplantation experiments (Kim et al., 2004; Ohta et al., 2002). Taken together, these studies show the importance of the Polycomb proteins in HSC self-renewal and maintenance of the blood system.

Transcriptional repression by PcG proteins is essential for maintenance of HSC identity. Part of the mechanism by which it functions is by repression of genes that promote lineage specification, cell death and cell cycle arrest. More recently, PcG complexes have been shown to be essential for maintenance of the undifferentiated state in murine embryonic stem (ES) cells and human ES cells by directly repressing a large number of developmental regulators (Boyer et al., 2006; Lee et al., 2006). PcG complexes bind to and presumably repress the expression of a subset of these genes linked to differentiation. This represents a dynamic repression of genes required for differentiation, and a scenario in which PcG proteins act as transcription repressors by cooperating with a specific set of transcription factors in stem cells. Some target genes include *Hox* family members important for induction of differentiation. Expression of *Hox* genes that are involved in differentiation is repressed in the ES cells by PcG proteins. Thus, PcG complex repression is also necessary for ES cell identity. Taken together, these studies suggest that differentiation is the default state during stem cell replication, and self-renewal requires active repression of transcription factors that prevent self-renewal

The transcription factor *Tel* (Translocation Ets leukemia; also known as Etv6 [Ets variant gene 6]), an *Ets* (E-26 transforming-specific)-related transcriptional repressor, is also required for HSC maintenance. Conditional inactivation of *Tel/Etv6* in HSCs rapidly leads to the depletion of *Tel/Etv6*-deficient bone marrow. However, *Tel/Etv6* is not required for the maintenance of committed precursors. When it is conditionally inactivated in most hematopoietic lineages, it does not affect their differentiation or survival (Hock et al., 2004). At the moment, the mechanism by which *Tel/Etv6* modulates adult HSCs renewal is not known. Study of the downstream targets it represses should shed light on other players essential for HSC maintenance.

Pbx1 (pre–B-cell acute lymphoblastic leukemia) is a TALE class homeodomain transcription factor that critically regulates numerous embryonic processes, including hematopoiesis. *Pbx1* is preferentially expressed in LT-HSCs compared to more mature short-term HSCs and multipotent progenitor cells (Ficara et al., 2008). By using *Pbx1*-conditional knockout mice, it was revealed that *Pbx1* positively regulates HSC quiescence. Transcriptional profiling showed that a significant proportion of *Pbx1*-dependent genes are associated with the *TGF-β* pathway.

The homeobox (*Hox*) genes encode transcription factors that regulate embryonic body patterning and organogenesis. They play a role in the regulation of hematopoiesis. Overexpression of *HoxB4* in bone marrow leads to expansion of HSCs *in vivo* and *in vitro*, therefore appearing to be a positive regulator of HSC self-renewal (Antonchuck et al., 2002; Krosl et al., 2003; Miyake et al., 2006; Sauvageau et al., 1995). It therefore came as a surprise when *HoxB4*-deficient mice had normal hematopoietic development but exhibited only mild proliferative HSC defects (Brun et al., 2004). In an attempt to determine if this was due to compensatory mechanisms, the entire *HoxB* cluster was deleted. However, this did not lead to major defects in hematopoiesis (Bijl et al., 2006), possibly owing to compensation by *HoxA4* and/or *HoxC4*.

Gfi1 (Growth factor independence 1), a zinc-finger repressor, has been recently implicated as a regulator of HSC self-renewal. Two groups working independently determined that *Gfi1* controls self-renewal of HSCs by restraining their proliferative potential (Hock et al 2004; Zeng et al., 2004). They showed that *Gfi1*-deficient HSCs display increased proliferation rates and are also functionally compromised in competitive repopulation and serial transplantation assays. *Gfi1* might exert its effects on HSC proliferation by regulating the cell cycle inhibitor p21.

Gfi1 is originally recognized for its role in T-cell differentiation and lymphoma. *Gfi1* gene knockout is one of the first targeted mutants to exhibit the combination of an increase in cycling HSCs at the expense of HSC function. Both *Gfi1* knockout models displayed an increase in cycling cells within the HSC pool, a large decrease in HSC function in transplantation experiments. Profoundly reduced expression of *p21*, the cyclin-dependent kinase inhibitor, in *Gfi1* null HSCs may account for the mechanism. Thus, under normal homeostasis, *Gfi1* is thought to suppress the proliferation of HSCs, thereby keeping HSCs in quiescence.

Numerous studies have identified roles for *p53* in the proliferation, differentiation, apoptosis, and aging of hematopoietic cells. LT-HSCs express high levels of *p53* transcripts, which is an indication of roles of *p53* in HSC physiology (Dumble et al., 2007). Recently, *p53* has been identified as a positive regulator of HSC quiescence through analysis of $p53^{-/-}$ mice (Liu et al., 2009). Furthermore, in the same study, it was demonstrated that the increased quiescence of HSCs from MEF null mice, in which both $p53$ and $p21$ are up-regulated, is dependent on $p53$, but not $p21$, further confirming the positive role of $p53$ in maintaining HSC in quiescence. $Gfi1$ was identified as $p53$ target gene, which is both shown important in regulating HSC quiescence by up-regulation or knockdown experiments.

Stem cell leukemia/T-cell acute lymphoblastic leukemia 1 ($SCL/TAL1$) plays a key role in controlling development of primitive and definitive hematopoiesis during mouse development. In adult HSCs, it is highly expressed in LT-HSCs compared with short-term HSCs and progenitors (Lacombe et al., 2010). SCL impedes G_0-G_1 transition in HSCs. The function of HSCs from $Scl^{+/-}$ mice or with decreased dosage of SCL protein by $in\ vitro$ interference was shown decreased in various transplantation assays. At the molecular level, SCL maintains HSC quiescence by regulating gene expression of $Cdkn1a$ and $Id1$.

Recently, many other transcriptional factors, such as interferon regulatory factor−2, a transcriptional suppressor of interferon signaling (Sato et al., 2009); $Nurr1$, a nuclear receptor transcription factor (Sirin et al., 2010); and thioredoxin-interacting protein, a transcriptional repressor (Shao et al., 2010), have been identified as positive regulators of HSC quiescence. Loss of HSC quiescence was observed in mice with deletion of each of these factors.

Individual member of Retinoblastoma (Rb) tumor suppressor gene family serves critical roles in the control of cellular proliferation and differentiation with functional redundancy for each other. The mice with conditional triple knockout of Rb family genes including Rb, $p107$, and $p130$ display a cell-intrinsic myeloproliferation that originates from hyperproliferative early hematopoietic progenitors due to the loss of quiescence, and the mutant HSCs show strong short-term repopulation capacity but impaired long-term repopulation ability on transplantation. Thus, Rb family members collectively maintain HSC quiescence (Viatour et al., 2008).

It has been shown that the conditional inactivation of c-Myc induces excessive expression of $integrins$ and N-$cadherin$ in HSCs, leading to the enhanced HSC interaction with the niche, which subsequently enable Myc-deficient HSCs stay in quiescence. Conversely, enforced c-Myc expression in HSCs downregulates N-$cadherin$ and $integrins$, leading to a loss of HSC function (Wilson et al., 2004).

$p21$ mRNA expression levels are dramatically lower in the $Gfi1$-deficient HSCs. $p21$ itself has been implicated in the regulation of HSCs (Cheng et al., 2000). In its absence, HSCs have an impaired serial transplantation capacity. Another cell cycle inhibitor, $p18$, has also been shown to affect HSC self-renewal. The absence of $p18$ leads to increased HSC self-renewal (Yuan et al., 2004; Yu et al., 2006). Therefore, intricate control of the cell cycle and proliferation machinery is required for self-renewal regulation.

In contrast to $p21$, little is known about the role of $p57$ in adult stem cell populations. Using primary human hematopoietic cells and microarray analysis, Scandura et al. (2004) identified $p57$ as the only cyclin-dependent kinase inhibitor induced by TGF-β. Up-regulation of $p57$ is essential for TGF-β−induced cell-cycle arrest in these cells, which may represent the mechanisms by which TGF-β affects cell-cycle arrest and stem cell quiescence.

Bone marrow is a very low oxygen tension environment that would protect cells from exposure to oxidative stress. Various intrinsic factors have also been identified to function in maintaining low oxidant levels in HSCs. ATM, a cell-cycle checkpoint regulator activated after DNA damage, is shown to regulate oxidant levels in HSCs (Ito et al., 2006). ATM deficiency-induced ROS elevation in HSCs specifically activates the p38 mitogen-activated protein kinase (MAPK) pathway, a signaling pathway responding to diverse cellular stresses, leading to a defect in the maintenance of HSC quiescence (Ito et al., 2004). $ATM^{-/-}$ mice over the age of 24 weeks show progressive bone marrow failure due to a defect in HSC function associated with elevated levels of ROS. Treatment with anti-oxidative reagents, N-acetyl cysteine or with a MAPK inhibitor restores reconstitutive capacity and quiescence of $ATM^{-/-}$ HSCs.

Members of the FoxO subfamily of forkhead transcription factors have been shown to protect HSCs from oxidative stress by up-regulating genes involved in their detoxification. Triple knockout mice of *FoxO1*, *FoxO3*, and *FoxO4* exhibited defective long-term repopulating activity of HSCs, which correlated with increased cycling and apoptosis of HSCs, as well as increased levels of ROS in HSCs (Tothova et al., 2007). Similarly, the HSC compartment in *FoxO3a* null mice suffers from augmented levels of ROS and subsequent bone marrow failure (Miyamoto et al., 2007). The HSC defect resulting from loss of *FoxOs* could also be rescued by administration of the antioxidant N-acetyl cysteine.

It is conceivable that both the hypoxic environment in which the HSCs reside and the intrinsic factors in HSCs serve to protect HSCs from oxygen radicals, keeping HSCs' quiescent status.

The *JAK–STAT* (Janus family kinase–signal transducer and activator of transcription) pathway is a common downstream pathway of cytokine signaling that promotes hematopoiesis. Constitutive activation of the transcription factors of the *Stat* family, particularly *Stat3* and *Stat5*, are frequently detected in leukemias, lymphomas and solid tumors. In order to evaluate their role in HSCs, constitutively active *Stat* mutants were used to activate signaling in HSCs. Activation of *Stat5* in HSCs led to the dramatic expansion of multipotent progenitors and promoted HSC self-renewal *ex vivo* (Kato et al., 2005). Deletion of *Stat5* resulted in profound defects in hematopoiesis and markedly reduced ability of the mutant cells to repopulate the bone marrow of lethally irradiated mice (Snow et al., 2002). In a mouse model of myeloproliferative disease (MPD), sustained *Stat5* activation in HSCs and not multipotent progenitors induced fatal MPD, suggesting that the capacity of *Stat5* to promote self-renewal of hematopoietic stem cells is crucial for MPD development. Another group showed that transduction of adult mouse bone marrow cells with a constitutively activated form of *Stat3* increased their regenerative activity in lethally irradiated recipients, whereas the transduction of these cells with a dominant negative form of *Stat3* suppressed their regenerative activity (Chung et al., 2006). These studies suggest that Stat proteins play a role in HSC self-renewal and potentially in other tissues; owing to the wide range of solid tissue and blood malignancies that harbor constitutively activated Stats.

Studies using transgenic mice constitutively expressing *BCL2* (*B-cell lymphoma* 2) in all hematopoietic tissues provide evidence directly supporting this theory. The forced expression of the oncogene *Bcl2* resulted in increased numbers of transgenic HSCs *in vivo* and gave these cells a competitive edge over wild type HSCs in competitive reconstitution experiments (Domen et al., 1998; Domen et al., 2000) suggesting that cell death plays a role in regulating the homeostasis of HSCs. Recently, *Mcl1* (Myeloid cell leukemia 1), another anti-apoptotic *Bcl2* family member, has been shown to be required for HSC survival (Opferman et al., 2005).

6. Quiescence or self-renewal

In order to both maintain a supply of mature blood cells and not exhaust HSCs throughout the lifetime of an individual, under steady state, most HSCs remain quiescent and only a small number enter the cell cycle. However, in response to hematopoietic stress such as blood loss, HSCs exit quiescence and rapidly expand and differentiate to repopulate the peripheral hematopoietic compartments. When quiescence is disrupted, HSCs displayed defective maintenance in G_0 phase of cell cycle, leading to premature exhaustion of the stem cell pool under conditions of hematopoietic stress, impaired self-renewal, and loss of competitive repopulating capacity, eventually causing hematological failure.

Quiescence of HSCs is not only critical for protecting the stem cell compartment and sustaining stem cell pools over long periods, but it is also critical for protecting stem cells by minimizing their accumulation of replication-associated mutations. The balance between quiescence and proliferation is tightly controlled by both HSC-intrinsic and -extrinsic mechanisms. Understanding quiescence regulation in HSC is of great importance not only for understanding the physiological foundation of HSCs, but also for understanding the pathophysiological origins of many related disorders.

In steady state conditions HSCs are in a slowly dividing state, termed relative quiescence, with a cell division cycle in the mouse in the range of 2–4 weeks, localized in close contact with stromal cells, including osteoblasts (Calvi et al., 2003; Zhang et al., 2003). This is in contrast to the rapidly cycling hematopoietic progenitor cells, which are more committed to differentiation than HSCs. The balance between quiescent and cycling stem cells was proposed to rely on the amount of soluble cytokines, which result in HSCs relocating from the osteoblastic to the vascular niche (Heissig et al., 2002). However new results indicate that it depends on a complex network of signals.

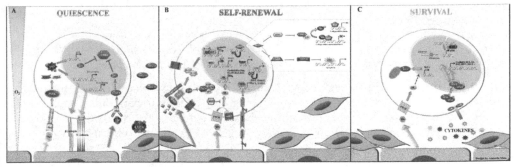

Fig. 1. Networks interaction model for: A) quiescence, B) self-renewal and C) survival.

In part, the dramatic contrast in cell cycle status between stem and progenitor cells has led to the hypothesis that cell cycle regulation plays a fundamentally important role in stem cell fate determination. This hypothesis is supported by recent data demonstrating a slower rate of division in Hoxb4hiPbx1lo cells, which extensively self-renewal *in vitro*, compared to control cells (Cellot et al., 2007). It is essential for an HSC to undergo cell division if it is to self-renew, but how the cell division cycle is integrated into the process of self-renewal is unclear. It is also unknown as to whether cell cycle regulation represents an intrinsic or extrinsic modifier of HSC fate.

6.1 How HSC maintain quiescence

Negative regulators of both $Cdk2$ and $Cdk4/6$ activity, and therefore Rb function, have been demonstrated to have roles in regulating HSCs (Cheng et al., 2000; Janzen et al., 2006; Stepanova & Sorrentino, 2005; Van Os et al., 2007; Walkley et al., 2005). For the most part however these phenotypes have been relatively subtle, particularly when compared to hematopoietic phenotypes apparent after disruption of transcription factors such as C/EBPα (Hock et al., 2004) and Tel (Zhang et al., 2004) amongst others, and are often apparent only after serial transplantation. The "Rb pathway" has also been implicated in phenotypes observed in both the $Bmi1-/-$ and $ATM-/-$ HSCs (Ito et al., 2004; Lessard & Sauvageau, 2003; Park et al., 2003). The interaction of cell cycle regulators with other factors such as Hoxb4 or telomerase deficiency has produced much more striking phenotypes than that observed for the cell cycle mutants in isolation (Choudhury et al., 2007; Miyake et al., 2006). While clearly demonstrating that cell cycle modifiers have roles in regulating stem cells, particularly HSCs, the aforementioned studies have not been able to clearly discriminate between intrinsic or extrinsic contributions to HSC fate as all studies to date had utilized non-hematopoietic restricted mutant alleles. A study demonstrating that the $p27Kip1-/-$ microenvironment mediates the myelo-lymphoid expansion observed in the $p27Kip1-/-$ animals raises the possibility that the HSC expansion observed in $p27Kip1-/-$ bone marrow is extrinsic in nature (Chien et al., 2006; Walkley et al, 2005). This result suggested that cell cycle regulators might play a role in regulating the competence of the hematopoietic niche, in addition to having potential intrinsic roles in HSC fate determination. Moreover Daria et al (2007) observed a requirement for Rb in the stress response of HSCs and this has also previously been suggested in the context of the role of Rb in erythropoiesis (Spike et al., 2004; Spike & Macleod, 2005).

Also of note is that the cell division dynamics of HSCs change during development, from rapidly cycling and dividing cells during the fetal liver and early stages of life to relatively quiescent and more slowly cycling in the adult context (Bowie et al., 2007; Bradford et al., 1997; Ito et al, 2000; Kiel et al., 2007; Sato et al., 1999). Thus the role for Rb may be context dependent, both in terms of stress response and developmentally in the regulation of HSC fate.

One important point that is becoming clearer recently is how some HSCs are maintained quiescent while others enter self-renewal program. Although bone–lining cells in the endosteal surface are often described as osteoblasts in the literature, they are heterogeneous in their degree of differentiation, and only a minority of these cells are actually bone synthesizing osteoblasts. So a good hypothesis is that in the endosteal niche some cells are in contact with true osteoblasts that expresses the necessary factors to maintain quiescence while others are not receiving the same signalization so will follow other fate.

Li (2008) proposed that HSC quiescence is maintained through several signaling pathways including positive and negative regulators from extrinsic and intrinsic factors already described. In this context the *Tie-2/Ang-1* signaling pathway plays a critical role in the maintenance of HSCs in a quiescent state in the bone marrow niche (Adams et al., 2006). HSCs express the receptor tyrosine kinase Tie-2 and osteoblasts are the source of the Ang-1 ligand for Tie-2. *Tie-2/Ang-1* signaling activates its key downstream targets, *β1-integrin* and *N-cadherin* in lineage-negative, *Sca-1*, *C-kit* double-positive (LSK), and *Tie-2*-positive cells, and promotes HSC interactions with extracellular matrix and cellular components of the niche. This interaction is sufficient to maintain the quiescence and enhanced survival of HSCs by preventing cell division (Arai et al., 2007). *Ang-1/Tie-2* signaling also activates the phosphatidylinositol 3-kinase/Akt signaling pathway (Visnjic et al., 2004). Phosphatidylinositol 3-kinase/Akt signaling regulates several cell-cycle regulators, such as the CDK inhibitor, p21, which in turn leads to HSC quiescence.

Other pathway that has been proven to enhance quiescence is TPO/MPL. TPO is secreted by osteoblast while MPL is expressed in the membrane of HSCs. Interaction of these two proteins maintain HSCs attached to osteoblasts by activation of a pathway that results in the expression of their adhesion molecules targets and at the same time activate genetic programs which will control entry in cell cycle and survival of HSC. How these positive regulators interact with other positive and negative regulators is not completely understood. Moreover, which signaling pathways are being activated and which genes have their expression changed waits to be clarified.

A recent study by Wang et al. (2009) recently identified STAT5, a downstream target of MPL, as a positive regulator of HSC quiescence by analyzing *STAT5-/-* mice. Expression of quiescence regulators including *Tie-2* and *p57* are decreased in *STAT5-/-* HSCs. This study demonstrated that *STAT5* might mediate *MPL* effects in maintaining HSC quiescence during steady state hematopoiesis and that the same pathway directly or indirectly regulates *Tie-2* and *p57*. Interestingly, up-regulation of *p57* is essential for TGF-β−induced cell-cycle arrest. How these pathways are connected awaits more investigation.

Two other signaling pathways that act as positive and negative regulators of quiescence deserve more discussion, the Hypoxia induced factor (HIF) and Osteopontina signaling pathway. Hypoxia microenvironment seems to be important for maintaining HSC quiescence The molecular mechanisms for this involve the hypoxia-inducible factor-1a (HIF-1a) regulated gene expressions in stromal cells. Two genes known to be targets of the HIF pathway are *c-Kit* and stromal cell derived factor−1 (*SDF-1* or *CXCL12*) that both have proven to be important to HSC maintenance.

Osteopontina (*OPN*) is a negative regulator of HSC quiescence as an OPN-null microenvironment is sufficient to increase the number of stem cells associated with increased stromal *Jagged-1* and *Ang-1* expression and reduced primitive hematopoietic cell apoptosis. OPN seems to function by preventing HSC cycling. It is interesting to note that the release of this inhibition occurs in parallel with the possible activation of the *Notch* pathway.

As we can see there is many connections between intrinsic factors and extrinsic cues and between different intrinsic factors or different extrinsic factors. Some intrinsic factors function through affecting extrinsic factors, such as *c-Myc*, which negatively regulates HSC quiescence by controlling *N-cadherin* expression level, reducing the *N-cadherin*–mediated interaction between HSCs and niche. Some extrinsic cues function through certain intrinsic factors, such as *STAT5*, which may serve as a component of *MPL*–induced signaling pathway, mediating MPL's effects in maintaining HSC quiescence.

Interestingly, among those HSC quiescence regulators that have been identified so far, the majority are positive regulators; few are negative for the maintenance of HSCs quiescence. This is consistent with the idea showing that the bias toward reduced gene expression that actively maintains HSC quiescence is an important mechanism of HSC proliferation, suggesting that various positive regulators of HSC quiescence are actively restricting proliferation of HSCs, and that there may exist signals in the environment to promote HSC proliferation.

6.2 Deciding for self-renewal

Many signaling pathways are thought to contribute to stem cell self-renewal in the marrow niche including *Notch* (Maillard et al., 2003), Wnt (Duncan et al. 2005; Reya et al., 2003; Willert et al., 2003) and *Hedgehog* (Baron, 2001 ; Bhardwaj et al., 2001; Gering & Patient 2005).

Activated *Notch* expands the stem and progenitor cell compartment by either influencing undifferentiated cells to adopt a HSC fate or by causing a G_0 HSC population to up-regulate *runx1*-dependent gene expression. Findings that the stem cell markers *runx1*, *scl*, and *lmo2* were transcriptionally increased in response to NICD (Notch Intra-Cytoplamatic Domain) indicate that stem and progenitor cells were expanded in the adult marrow, possibly by increasing stem cell self-renewal. A conditional allele of *runx1* was generated in the mouse to study the loss of *Runx1* function during adult hematopoiesis (Growney et al., 2005; Ichikawa et al., 2004). In transplantation studies, *Runx1*-excised marrow cells showed a reduced competitive repopulating ability in long-term engraftment assays (Growney et al., 2005), demonstrating that Runx1 is essential for normal stem cell function.

The *Wnt/β-catenin* signaling pathway also plays a crucial role during self-renewal of HSCs (Nemeth & Bodine, 2007). Deregulation of this pathway has been implicated in the formation of solid tumors, like lung epidermal adenocarcinomas, breast carcinomas and intestinal colorectal tumors just to mention a few (Reya & Clevers, 2005). Although several *Wnt* genes are expressed in bone marrow, the precise role of *Wnt* signaling pathway in HSCs and its mechanism(s) of action remained unclear until very recently.

There is a multitude of *Wnt* signaling cascades some of them regulating one another. Using different receptors, Wnt proteins can trigger at least three intracellular signaling pathways: the canonical b-catenin pathway, the non-canonical calcium pathway and the c-Jun N-terminal kinase pathway (Zeng et al., 2004). Several components of the *Wnt* signaling machinery have been shown to play a role in HSC self-renewal. Both canonical as well as non-canonical pathways seem to be involved, since the canonical ligand *Wnt3a* intrinsically promotes self-renewal (Luis et al., 2009). On the other hand, the non-canonical ligand *Wnt5a* has been shown to extrinsically promote self-renewal by inhibiting canonical signaling (Murdoch et al., 2003). The mechanistic basis for the balance between canonical and non-canonical pathways is not fully understood. It is likely that numerous *Wnt* inhibitors or antagonists are modulating *Wnt* signaling.

Taken together, the existing studies suggest that canonical Wnt signaling may not be strictly required for HSC function, but that canonical Wnt signaling may affect self-renewal and differentiation of HSCs depending on the extent of canonical Wnt signaling and on the context of expression of additional genes. Non-canonical Wnt signaling and/or other signaling pathways may also compensate for the absence of canonical Wnt signaling in maintaining the self-renewal of HSCs (Huang, 2007).

To exactly control the fine tune of *Wnt* in HSC it is likely that the numerous Wnt-signaling inhibitors (Dickkopf homolog (Dkk), Wnt inhibitory factor (Wif) or secreted frizzled-related protein (Sfrp), or other Wnt antagonists, such as Kremen, Ctgf, Cyr61, Sost and Sostdc1) have to be the correctly expressed. Interestingly, some of these molecules also directly stimulate certain Fzds independent of Wnt factors. For example, Sfrp1 directly activates Fzd2, as well as Fzd4, and Fzd7 but can also interact with Wnt5a (Rodriguez et al., 2005; Dufourc et al, 2008; Matsuyama et al, 2009 & Kirstetter et al., 2006). This balance and feedback mechanisms between canonical and non-canonical Wnt signaling, suggests that β-*catenin* is the primary regulatory target of Wnt signaling. However, overexpression or stabilization of β-*catenin* results in expansion of the HSC pool, but, at the same time, the loss of myelopoiesis is due to a differentiation block (Renstrom et al., 2010), suggesting that b-catenin promotes self-renewal and/or inhibits differentiation.

Conversely, Wnt signaling also induces increased expression of *HOXB4*, *Bmi1* and targets of *Notch-1*, genes that are implicated in self-renewal of HSCs . Transcription factors of homeodomain family (HOX family) have been found to regulate HSC self-renewal and downregulate differentiation. Disruption of HOX genes in mice led to abnormalities in multiple hematopoietic cell lineages. Moreover, overexpression of HOX genes (like HOXB4) has been associated with HSCs ex vivo expansion and HOX gene mutation with acute leukemia. *Bmi1*,a polycomb gene, seems to have a repressor role over *p16* inhibiting apoptosis of HSCs and thus contributing to its maintenance . So the correct Wnt signaling seems to be essential to integrate the intracellular response in the decision to self-renew or differentiate (Reya et al., 2003).

The investigation of the interactions between Bmi1 and Hoxb4, showed that Bmi1 is not required for the in vivo expansion of fetal HSCs but is essential for the long-term maintenance of adult HSCs. Moreover, Hoxb4 overexpression induces an expansion of Bmi1-/- STR-HSCs leading to a rescue of their repopulation defect. Together, these results support the emerging concept that fate and sustainability of this fate are two critical components of self-renewal in adult stem cells such as HSCs.

Moreover Polycomb group (PcG) proteins play a role in the transcriptional repression of genes through histone modifications. Recent studies have clearly demonstrated that PcG proteins are required for the maintenance of embryonic as well as a broad range of adult stem cells, including hematopoietic stem cells (HSCs). PcG proteins maintain the self-renewal capacity of HSCs by repressing tumor suppressor genes and keep differentiation programs poised for activation in HSCs by repressing a cohort of hematopoietic developmental regulator genes via bivalent chromatin domains. Enforced expression of one of the PcG genes, Bmi1, augments the self-renewal capacity of HSCs. PcG proteins also maintain redox homeostasis to prevent premature loss of HSCs. These findings established PcG proteins as essential regulators of HSCs and underscored epigenetics as a new field of HSC research (Li et al., 2010; Komuna, 2010).

Recently we demonstrated that another polycomb group member, Suz12 gene, is activated by the non canonical Wnt pathway and may epigenetically inhibit genes involved in hematopoietic differentiation. These data pointed to cell cycle changes, deregulation of early differentiation genes and regulation of PRC2 polycomb complex genes, due to Suz12 role in CML blast crisis. This observation indicates that the cross talk between Wnt and Polycomb pathways may promotes hematopoietic differentiation. (Pizzatti et al., 2010).

Taken together all these data fits in a model were HSCs fated to self renew are in contact in the endosteal niches with osteoblasts expressing *Notch* legends (*Jagged*) so the pathway that will be induced is *Notch* pathway.

The *Hedgehog* (*Hh*) is a ligand that binds and represses the *Patched* receptor and thereby releases the latent activity of the multipass membrane protein Smoothened, which is essential for transducing the *Hh* signal. Using *Patched*$^{+/-}$ mouse with increased *Hh* signaling activity, it was demonstrated that constitutive activation of the *Hh* signaling pathway results in the steady-state accumulation of phenotypically defined HSCs and an increase in the proportion of cycling cells within this population (Kuhn et al., 1995). However, HSC activity on secondary transplantation is reduced 3-fold, indicating the functional exhaustion of the HSC pool in this mutant. In vivo treatment with an inhibitor of the *Hh* pathway rescues these transcriptional and functional defects in HSCs. This study establishes *Hh* signaling as a negative regulator of the HSC quiescence. In contrast to the germline *Patched*$^{+/-}$ mode, the mode of conditional deletion of Smoothened in the adult hematopoietic compartment was used in other two studies. However, the negative effects of the Hh pathway on HSC quiescence were shown in one study (Walkley & Orkin, 2006) and not in another (Stead et al., 2002). The discrepancy is possibly due to a distinct mode of deletion. How this pathway collaborate with the two others is not clear although interaction through GSK3 have been already proposed.

The outcome of *Hh* signaling varies according to the receiving cell type. GLI, the cytoplasmic effector of *Hh* signaling activates the transcription of several target genes as *CyclinD1 and D2,N-Myc,Wnts, FoxM1,Hes 1,Bcl2,Osteopontin* and others. If these genes are activated in HSCs has not yet been defined but if they are, a clear interconnection between several important signaling pathways is visualized.

One important point when talking about self-renewal is how to prevent exhaustion of the HSC pool.

7. Role of telomerase in hematopoietic stem cell

Stem cells self renewal capacity is believed to be closely associated with tissue degeneration during aging. Studies of human genetic diseases and gene-targeted animal models have provided evidence that functional decline of telomeres and deregulation of cell cycle checkpoints contribute to the aging process of tissue stem cells. Telomere dysfunction can induce DNA damage response via key cell cycle checkpoints, leading to cellular senescence or apoptosis depending on the tissue type and developmental stage of a specific stem cell compartment (Ju Z et al., 2011).

Studies in hematopoietic stem cell (HSC) biology are often focused on "self-renewal" and differentiation. Implicit in the word self-renewal is that the two daughter cells generated by a self-renewal division are identical to the parental cell. Strictly speaking, this is not possible because DNA is continuously damaged and repaired by DNA-repair mechanisms that are not 100% efficient (Lansdorp et al., 2005).

It is important to note that the efficiency of DNA repair varies greatly among different stem cell types. For example, embryonic stem cells are quite resistant to DNA damage and maintain the length of telomere repeats on serial passage, whereas HSCs are quite sensitive to DNA damage and less able to maintain telomere length. This idea has given rise to the notion that many aspects of normal aging could primarily reflect limitations in DNA repair and telomere-maintenance pathways in the (stem) cells of the soma (Lansdorp et al., 2005).

The loss of telomere repeats in adult hematopoietic cells (including purified "candidate" HSCs) relative to fetal hematopoietic cells also fits a model that postulates a finite and limited replicative potential of HSCs (Vaziri et al., 1994; Lansdorp et al., 1995; Lansdorp et al., 1997). How this collaborates with the model of LT-HSCs given rise to ST-HSCs has not still been addressed.

Eukaryotic chromosomes are capped by special structures called telomeres, which are guanine-rich, simple repeat sequences. Telomeres act to guarantee chromosome integrity by preventing illegitimate recombination, degradation, and end fusions (Blackburn et al., 1991; Stain et al ., 2004).

Synthesis and maintenance of telomeric repeats are accomplished by a specialized ribonucleoprotein complex known as telomerase. Telomerase consists of an essential RNA template and protein components, one of which appears to resemble reverse transcriptase. In the absence of telomerase, the failure of DNA polymerase to fully synthesize DNA termini leads to chromosome shortening (Stain et al., 2004; Lee et al., 1998).

In contrast to mice were short telomeres maintain cell survival for some generations, a modest two fold reduction in telomerase levels in humans (resulting from haploinsufficiency for the telomerase RNA template gene) typically results in premature death from complications of aplastic anemia or immune deficiency. Recent studies indicate that short telomeres and eventual marrow failure may also result from haploinsufficiency for the telomerase reverse transcriptase(hTERT) gene (Yamaguchi et al., 2005).

Moreover the large number of HSCs typically used in clinical transplant settings may effectively prevent their replicative exhaustion. Variations in telomere length between cells and individuals have even made it difficult to reproducibly document a decline in telomere length following transplantation. Nevertheless, a significant shortening of telomeres was observed in the first year after allogeneic bone marrow transplantation (Landsdorp et al., 2005). Furthermore, marrow failure with pronounced telomere shortening has been described in a few long-term survivors of HSC transplants. Although there is little evidence to suggest that telomere shortening will result in an epidemic of marrow failure in HSC transplant recipients, caution remains warranted when the cell number available for transplantation is limited or when the telomere length in HSCs for transplantation is short, as in cells from old donors or patients with telomerase deficiencies. It is tempting to speculate that some of the advantages of cord blood HSC transplants are related to the longer telomeres in individual cord blood HSCs (Awaya et al ., 2002).

It has been proposed that telomeres can switch between an open state (in principle allowing elongation by telomerase) and a closed state (inaccessible to telomerase) with the likelihood of the open state inversely related to the length of the repeat track (Blackburn et al., 2001). In most human cells, telomerase appears to be present at limiting levels, allowing elongation of only a limited number of critically short telomeres. Accumulation of short telomeres before replicative senescence has been observed and replicative senescence or apoptosis could result when the number of critically short telomeres exceeds the telomere repair capacity in a cell (Ju Z et al., 2011). In this context the ability of HSCs to modulate telomerase activity may be crucial in maintaining the self-renewal process. In human BM cells, low telomerase activity levels were demonstrated in multipotent HSCs, whereas significant upregulation of enzyme activity was apparent in the presence of proliferation-inducing cytokines (Samper et al., 2002; Stein et al., 2004). So cytokines and JAK-STAT signaling pathway may contribute to self renewal by maintaining telomerase activity.

The role of DNA repair pathways and telomeres/telomerase in the biology of normal and malignant human HSCs cells as well as the biology of aging clearly needs further study. New insight in the role of telomerase in HSCs has been provided by recent studies of patients with inborn errors in telomerase activity. Therefore, a further understanding of the molecular mechanisms underlying HSC aging may help identity new therapeutic targets for stem cell-based regenerative medicine.

8. Asymmetric cell division – A mechanism to generate progenitors while maintaining HSC

In both invertebrates like the insect *Drosophila*, and mammals, the major characteristic of stem cells is their ability to self-renew. Using various modes of proliferation, stem cells maintain or expand the available stem cell pool, but they can also generate more specialized progeny that constitute the majority of cells in an adult individual. In multi-cellular organisms, totipotent zygotes generate pluripotent stem cells, which become increasingly restricted in their lineage potential during development, and subsequently give rise to mature tissue-specific, multipotent stem cells. Stem cells show either 'proliferative' symmetric divisions or 'differentiative' asymmetric divisions to regulate a balance between the maintenance of stem cell pool and the supply of mature cells. It is critical for stem cells to tightly control this balance between the two different modes of division, both during development and adulthood, because, failure in maintaining cellular homeostasis may lead to incomplete tissue or organ development, whereas uncontrolled proliferation can lead to tumorigenesis.

Symmetric cell divisions commonly occur during development of invertebrates and vertebrates, phenomena that can also be observed during wound healing and regeneration of tissues. This mode of division is defined by the generation of two daughter cells that acquire the same fate, thereby expanding the pool of stem cells required or generating two differentiating daughter cells. Asymmetric cell divisions play a key role in generating cellular diversity during development by generating two daughter cells that are committed to different fates in a single division, simultaneously self-renewing to generate a daughter cell with stem cell properties, as well as to give rise to a more differentiated progeny.

Asymmetric stem cell divisions can be controlled by intrinsic mechanisms or the asymmetric exposure to extrinsic cues. Intrinsic mechanisms use apical-basal or planar polarity along the mitotic spindle to asymmetrically segregate cell fate determinants into only one daughter cell. Extrinsic mechanisms rely on contact with the so called stem cell niche, a cellular microenvironment that provides external cues (Doe, 2008; Li & Xie, 2005; Morrison & Spradling, 2008). Orientation of its mitotic spindle perpendicular to the niche surface allows the asymmetric segregation of cell fate determinants relative to the external stimuli to maintain self-renewal potential.

Much progress has been made in understanding intercellular mechanisms, especially the identification of niches for various types of tissue stem cells and elucidation of the role of the niche in regulating asymmetric stem cell division.

Although the role of niche in the asymmetric division of mammalian stem cells has not been clearly illustrated, Fuchs (2008) have shown that embryonic basal epidermal cells use their polarity to divide asymmetrically with respect to the underlying basal lamina, generating a committed suprabasal cell and a proliferative basal cell. Because skin stem cells are a subpopulation of mitotically active basal epidermal cells, it is conceivable that these stem cells divide in an asymmetric fashion to self-renew and to produce differentiated keratinocytes. Moreover, integrins and cadherins in the basal lamina are essential for the proper localization of apical complexes containing atypical PKC (aPKC), the Par3 – LGN – Inscuteable protein, and NuMA (nuclear mitotic apparatus protein) – dynactin. This asymmetric localization may be functionally important because similar complexes in *Drosophila* neuroblasts are essential for asymmetric division (Chia et al., 2008).

In addition to basal epidermal cells, mouse neuroepithelial stem cells and hematopoietic precursor cells undergo both asymmetric and symmetric divisions. In the mammalian central nervous system, embryonic neuroepithelial cells first undergo symmetric division to expand their population and then switch to asymmetric divisions for neurogenesis. This switch involves a change in cleavage plane orientation from perpendicular to parallel to the plane of the apical lamina, leading to an asymmetric distribution to the daughter cells of the apical plasma membrane, which constitutes only a minute fraction (1 – 2%) of the entire neuroepithelial cell plasma membrane (Kosodo et al., 2004). Somewhat similarly, mouse hematopoietic progenitor cells are capable of both symmetric and asymmetric divisions in cultures supported by stromal cells (Wu et al., 2007). A pro-differentiation stromal cell line increased the frequency of asymmetric division, whereas a pro-proliferation stromal cell line promoted symmetric division. These observations indicate that niche signaling can also control the asymmetry of stem cell division at a populational level.

Although niche induction accounts for asymmetric division in some types of stem cells, it may not play a role in all types of stem cells. In some stem cells there is an intrinsic polarity where molecules are segregated along an axis and serves as determinant of cell fate after cell division. In these cases the orientation of mitotic spindle has to be coordinated with the asymmetric localization of the cell fate regulators. This is the case, for example of *Numb* homologue during hematopoietic precursor cell division. So looking for hematopoietic niche and signaling between microenviroment cells and the stem cell we could " envisage"(imagine; idealize, construct) a model for stem cell to decide between symmetric or asymmetric division.

A particularly exciting development in basic stem cell research in the past few years is the discovery of novel functions of cell cycle regulators in controlling the asymmetry of stem cell division, as timely reviewed by Chia et al (2008). For example, the *cdc2/cdk1* level controls whether a neural or muscle progenitor undergoes symmetric or asymmetric division. In neuroblasts, high levels of CDK1 during mitosis are required for the asymmetric localization of apical and basal protein complexes. In addition, Aurora and Polo kinases act as tumor suppressors in neuroblasts by preventing excess self-renewal, implicating the function of asymmetric division in restricting over-proliferation. The mutations of these two kinase genes affect the asymmetric localization of aPKC, Numb, Partner of Numb, and Notch, causing symmetric division to generate two daughter neuroblasts. In addition, anaphase-promoting complex/cyclosome is also required for the localization of Miranda and its cargo proteins (Prospero, Brain Tumor, and Staufen). More surprisingly, even cyclin E, a G1 cyclin, is involved in asymmetric neuroblast division.

Interestingly in epidermal progenitors the decision of choosing between symmetric cell division or asymmetric cell decision is tightly regulated. Two control points have been indentified: expression of Inscutable and recruitment of NuMA to the apical cell cortex. Moreover in embryonic lung distal epithelium Eya1 protein regulates cell polarity, spindle orientation and the localization of Numb, which inhibits Notch signaling with the participation of NuMa protein (El-Hashad et al , 2011).

9. Conclusion

In the last ten years a body of evidence has accumulated on the hematopoietic stem cell niches and the mechanisms by which they regulate HSCs homeostasis. However many questions remain to be addressed. What we can speculate with today data is that in the endosteal niche dissimilar stages of differentiating osteoblasts provides diverse signals. These signals induce a quiescent or a self-renewal fate. However after leaving quiescence HSCs are prone to accumulate mutations that will lead to senescence. To prevent HSCs exhaustion mechanisms to enhance survival are also induced. Several of these additional signals come from the osteoblasts but also from other cells from microenvironment as stromal cells and endothelial cells. This is specially visualized in the decision of a symmetric or asymmetric division. From the control of all these interconnected pathways depends a normal hematopoiesis.

10. Acknowledgements

We thank Amanda Maia and André Mencalha for the excellent figures design.

11. References

Adams, G.B. & Scadden, D.T.(2006). The hematopoietic stem cell in its place. *Nat Immunol.* Apr;7(4):333-7.
Antonchuk, J.; Sauvageau, G. & Humphries, R.K.(2002). HOXB4-induced expansion of adult hematopoietic stem cells ex vivo. *Cell.* Apr 5;109(1):39-45.

Arai, F.; Hirao, A.; Ohmura, M.; Sato, H.; Matsuoka, S.; Takubo, K.; Ito, K.; Koh, G.Y. & Suda,T.(2004). Tie2/angiopoietin-1 signaling regulates hematopoietic stem cell quiescence in the bone marrow niche. *Cell*. Jul 23;118(2):149-61.

Arai, F.& Suda T.(2007). Maintenance of quiescent hematopoietic stem cells in the osteoblastic niche. *Ann N Y Acad Sci*. Jun;1106:41-53.

Avecilla, S.T.; Hattori, K.; Heissig, B.; Tejada, R.; Liao, F.; Shido, K.; Jin, D.K.; Dias, S.; Zhang, F.; Hartman. T.E.; Hackett, N.R.; Crystal, R.G.; Witte, L.; Hicklin, D.J.; Bohlen, P.; Eaton, D.; Lyden, D.; de Sauvage, F.& Rafii, S.(2004). Chemokine-mediated interaction of hematopoietic progenitors with the bone marrow vascular niche is required for thrombopoiesis. *Nat Med*. Jan;10(1):64-71.

Awaya, N.; Baerlocher, G.M.; Manley, T.J.; Sanders, J.E.; Mielcarek ,M.; Torok-Storb, B. & Lansdorp, P.M. (2002). Telomere shortening in hematopoietic stem cell transplantation: a potential mechanism for late graft failure? *Biol Blood Marrow Transplant*. 8(11):597-600.

Baron, M.(2001). Induction of embryonic hematopoietic and endothelial stem/progenitor cells by hedgehog-mediated signals. *Differentiation*. Oct;68(4-5):175-85.

Bendall, S.C.; Stewart, M.H.; Menendez, P. George,D.; Vijayaragavan, K.; Werbowetski-Ogilvie, T.; Ramos-Mejia, V.; Rouleau, A.; Yang, J.; Bossé, M.; Lajoie, G.& Bhatia, M.(2007). IGF and FGF cooperatively establish the regulatory stem cell niche of pluripotent human cells in vitro. *Nature*. Aug 30; 448 (7157):1015-21.

Bhardwaj, G.; Murdoch, B.; Wu, D.; Baker, D.P.; Williams, K.P.; Chadwick, K.; Ling, L.E.; Karanu, F.N. & Bhatia, M.(2001). Sonic hedgehog induces the proliferation of primitive human hematopoietic cells via BMP regulation. *Nat Immunol*. Feb;2(2):172-80.

Bijl, J.; Thompson, A.; Ramirez-Solis, R.; Krosl, J.; Grier, D.G.; Lawrence, H.J. & Sauvageau,G.(2006). Analysis of HSC activity and compensatory Hox gene expression profile in Hoxb cluster mutant fetal liver cells. *Blood*. Jul 1;108(1):116-22.

Blank, U.; Karlsson, G. & Karlsson, S.(2008). Signaling pathways governing stem-cell fate. *Blood*. Jan 15;111(2):492-503.

Blackburn, E.H.(1991). Structure and function of telomeres. *Nature*. 350:569–573.

Blackburn, E.H. (2001). Switching and signaling at the telomere. *Cell* 106: 661–673.

Bowie, M.B.; McKnight, K.D.; Kent, D.G.; McCaffrey, L.; Hoodless, P.A. & Eaves, C.J.(2006).Hematopoietic stem cells proliferate until after birth and show a reversible phase-specific engraftment defect. *J Clin Invest*. Oct;116(10):2808-16.

Boyer, L.A.; Plath, K.; Zeitlinger, J.; Brambrink, T.; Medeiros, L.A.; Lee, T.I.; Levine, S.S.; Wernig, M.; Tajonar, A.; Ray, M.K.; Bell, G.W.; Otte, A.P.; Vidal, M.; Gifford, D.K.; Young, R.A.& Jaenisch, R.(2006). Polycomb complexes repress developmental regulators in murine embryonic stem cells. *Nature*. May 18;441(7091):349-53.

Bradford, G.B.; Williams, B.; Rossi, R. & Bertoncello, I.(1997). Quiescence, cycling, and turnover in the primitive hematopoietic stem cell compartment. *Exp Hematol*. May;25(5):445-53.

Brun, A.C.; Björnsson, J.M.; Magnusson, M.; Larsson, N.; Leveén, P.; Ehinger, M.; Nilsson, E. & Karlsson, S.(2004). Hoxb4-deficient mice undergo normal hematopoietic development but exhibit a mild proliferation defect in hematopoietic stem cells. *Blood*. Jun1;103(11):4126-33.

Burns, C.E.; Traver, D.; Mayhall, E.; Shepard, J.L. & Zon, L.I.(2005). Hematopoietic stem cell fate is established by the Notch-Runx pathway. *Genes Dev*. Oct 1;19(19):2331-42.

Buza-Vidas, N.; Antonchuk, J.; Qian, H.; Månsson, R.; Luc, S,; Zandi, S.; Anderson, K.; Takaki, S.; Nygren, J.M.; Jensen, C.T. & Jacobsen, S.E.(2006). Cytokines regulate postnatal hematopoietic stem cell expansion: opposing roles of thrombopoietin and LNK. *Genes Dev*.Aug 1;20(15):2018-23.

Calvi, L.M.; Adams, G.B.; Weibrecht, K.W.; Weber, J.M.; Olson, D.P.; Knight, M.C.; Martin, R.P.;Schipani, E.; Divieti, P.; Bringhurst, F.R.; Milner, L.A.; Kronenberg, H.M. & Scadden, D.T.(2003).Osteoblastic cells regulate the haematopoietic stem cell niche. *Nature*. Oct23;425(6960):841-6.

Cellot, S.; Krosl, J.; Chagraoui, J.; Meloche, S.; Humphries, R.K. & Sauvageau, G.(2007). Sustained in vitro trigger of self-renewal divisions in Hoxb4hiPbx1(10)hematopoietic stem cells. *Exp Hematol*. May;35(5):802-16.

Ceradini, D.J.; Kulkarni, A.R.; Callaghan, M.J.; Tepper, O.M.; Bastidas, N.; Kleinman, M.E.; Capla, J.M.; Galiano, R.D.; Levine, J.P.& Gurtner, G.C.(2004). Progenitor cell trafficking is regulated by hypoxic gradients through HIF-1 induction of SDF-1. *Nat Med*. Aug;10(8):858-64.

Cheng, T.; Rodrigues, N.; Shen, H.; Yang, Y.; Dombkowski, D.; Sykes, M.& Scadden, D.T.(2000). Hematopoietic stem cell quiescence maintained by p21cip1/waf1. *Science*. Mar 10;287(5459):1804-8.

Chia, W.; Somers, W.G. & Wang, H.(2008). Drosophila neuroblast asymmetric divisions: cell cycle regulators, asymmetric protein localization, and tumorigenesis. *J Cell Biol*. Jan 28;180(2):267-72.

Chiba, S.(2006). Notch signaling in stem cell systems. *Stem Cells*. Nov;24(11):2437-47.

Chien, W.M.; Rabin, S.; Macias, E.; Miliani de Marval, P.L.; Garrison, K.; Orthel, J.; Rodriguez-Puebla, M. & Fero, M.L.(2006). Genetic mosaics reveal both cell-autonomous and cell-nonautonomous function of murine p27Kip1. *Proc Natl Acad Sci U S A*. Mar 14;103(11):4122-7.

Choudhury, A.R.; Ju, Z.; Djojosubroto, M.W.; Schienke, A.; Lechel, A.; Schaetzlein, S.; Jiang, H.; Stepczynska, A.; Wang, C. ; Buer, J.; Lee, H.W.; von Zglinicki, T.; Ganser, A.; Schirmacher, P.; Nakauchi, H. & Rudolph, K.L.(2007). Cdkn1a deletion improves stem cell function and lifespan of mice with dysfunctional telomeres without accelerating cancer formation. *Nat Genet*. Jan;39(1):99-105.

Chung,Y.J.; Park, B.B.; Kang, Y.J.; Kim, T.M.; Eaves, C.J.& Oh, I.H.(2006). Unique effects of Stat3 on the early phase of hematopoietic stem cell regeneration. *Blood*. Aug 15;108(4):1208-15.

Clevers, H.(2006) Wnt/beta-catenin signaling in development and disease. *Cell*. Nov 3;127(3):469-80.

Coultas, L.; Chawengsaksophak, K. & Rossant, J.(2005). Endothelial cells and VEGF in vascular development. *Nature*. Dec 15;438(7070):937-45.

Crcareva, A.; Saito, T.; Kunisato, A.; Kumano, K.; Suzuki, T.; Sakata-Yanagimoto, M.;Kawazu, M.; Stojanovic, A.; Kurokawa, M.; Ogawa, S.; Hirai, H. & Chiba, S.(2005). Hematopoietic stem cells expanded by fibroblast growth factor-1 are excellent targets for retrovirus-mediated gene delivery. *Exp Hematol*.Dec;33(12):1459-69.

Czechowicz, A.; Kraft, D.; Weissman, I.L. & Bhattacharya, D.(2007). Efficient transplantation via antibody-based clearance of hematopoietic stem cell niches. *Science*. Nov 23;318(5854):1296-9.

Daria, D.; Filippi, M.D.; Knudsen, E.S.; Faccio, R.; Li, Z.; Kalfa, T. & Geiger, H.(2008).The retinoblastoma tumor suppressor is a critical intrinsic regulator for hematopoietic stem and progenitor cells under stress. *Blood*. Feb 15;111(4):1894-902.

Doe, C.Q.(2008). Neural stem cells: balancing self-renewal with differentiation. *Development*. May;135(9):1575-87.

Domen, J.; Gandy, K.L.& Weissman, I.L.(1998). Systemic overexpression of BCL-2 in the hematopoietic system protects transgenic mice from the consequences of lethal irradiation. *Blood*. Apr 1;91(7):2272-82.

Domen, J.; Cheshier, S.H.& Weissman, I.L.(2000). The role of apoptosis in the regulation of hematopoietic stem cells: Overexpression of Bcl-2 increases both their number and repopulation potential. *J Exp Med*. Jan 17;191(2):253-64.

Dufourcq, P.; Descamps, B.; Tojais, N.F.; Leroux, L.; Oses, P.; Daret, D.; Moreau, C.; Lamaziere, J.M.; Couffinhal, T. & Duplaa, D. (2008). Secreted frizzled-related protein-1 enhances mesenchymal stem cell function in angiogenesis and contributes to neovessel maturation. *Stem Cells* 26 (11) 2991–3001.

Dumble, M.; Moore, L.; Chambers, S.M.; Geiger, H.; Van Zant, G.; Goodell, M.A.& Donehower, L.A.(2007). The impact of altered p53 dosage on hematopoietic stem cell dynamics during aging. *Blood*. Feb 15;109(4):1736-42.

Duncan, A.W.; Rattis, F.M.; DiMascio, L.N.; Congdon, K.L.; Pazianos, G.; Zhao, C.; Yoon, K.; Cook, J.M.; Willert, K.; Gaiano, N. & Reya, T.(2005). Integration of Notch and Wnt signaling in hematopoietic stem cell maintenance. *Nat Immunol*. Mar;6(3):314-22.

Edling, C.E. & Hallberg, B.(2007). c-Kit--a hematopoietic cell essential receptor tyrosine kinase. *Int J Biochem Cell Biol*. 39(11):1995-8.

El-Hashash, A.H.; Turcatel, G.; Al Alam, D.; Buckley, S.; Tokumitsu, H.; Bellusci, S. & Warburton, D. (2011). Eya1 controls cell polarity, spindle orientation, cell fate and Notch signaling in distal embryonic lung epithelium. *Development*. Apr;138(7):1395-407.

Ficara, F.; Murphy, M.J.; Lin, M.& Cleary, M.L.(2008). Pbx1 regulates self-renewal of long-term hematopoietic stem cells by maintaining their quiescence. *Cell Stem Cell*. May 8;2(5):484-96.

Fleming, H.E.; Janzen, V.; Lo Celso, C.; Guo, J.; Leahy, K.M.; Kronenberg, H.M. & Scadden, D.T.(2008).Wnt signaling in the niche enforces hematopoietic stem cell quiescence and is necessary to preserve self-renewal in vivo. *Cell Stem Cell*. Mar 6;2(3):274-83.

Fuchs, E.(2008). Skin stem cells: rising to the surface. *J Cell Biol*. Jan 28;180(2):273-84.

Gekas, C.; Dieterlen-Lièvre, F.; Orkin, S.H. & Mikkola, H.K.(2005). The placenta is a niche for hematopoietic stem cells. *Dev Cell*. Mar;8(3):365-75.

Gering, M. & Patient R.(2005). Hedgehog signaling is required for adult blood stem cell formation in zebrafish embryos. *Dev Cell*. Mar;8(3):389-400.

Heissig, B.; Hattori, K.; Dias, S.; Friedrich, M.; Ferris, B; Hackett, N.R.; Crystal, R.G.; Besmer, P.; Lyden, D.; Moore, M.A.; Werb, Z. & Rafii, S.(2002). Recruitment of stem and progenitor cells from the bone marrow niche requires MMP-9 mediated release of kit-ligand.*Cell*. May 31;109(5):625-37.

Hock, H.; Meade, E.; Medeiros, S.; Schindler, J.W.; Valk, P.J.; Fujiwara, Y.& Orkin, S.H.(2004).Tel/Etv6 is an essential and selective regulator of adult hematopoietic stem cellsurvival. *Genes Dev.* Oct 1;18(19):2336-41.

Huang, X.; Cho, S. & Spangrude, G.J.(2007) Hematopoietic stem cells: generation and self-renewal. *Cell Death Differ.* Nov;14(11):1851-9.

Huntly, B.J. & Gilliland, D.G.(2005) Cancer biology: summing up cancer stem cells. *Nature.* Jun 30;435(7046):1169-70.

Ichikawa, M.; Asai, T.; Chiba, S.; Kurokawa, M. & Ogawa S.(2004) Runx1/AML-1 ranks as a master regulator of adult hematopoiesis. *Cell Cycle.* Jun;3(6):722-4.

Ikuta, K.& Weissman, I.L.(1992). Evidence that hematopoietic stem cells express mouse c-kit but do not depend on steel factor for their generation. *Proc Natl Acad Sci U S A.* Feb 15;89(4):1502-6.

Inman, K.E. & Downs, K.M.(2007). The murine allantois: emerging paradigms in development of the mammalian umbilical cord and its relation to the fetus. *Genesis.* May;45(5):237-58.

Ito, T.; Tajima, F.& Ogawa, M.(2000). Developmental changes of CD34 expression by murine hematopoietic stem cells. *Exp Hematol.* Nov;28(11):1269-73.

Ito, K.; Hirao, A.; Arai, F.; Matsuoka, S.; Takubo, K.; Hamaguchi, I.; Nomiyama, K.; Hosokawa, K.; Sakurada, K.; Nakagata, N.; Ikeda, Y.; Mak, T.W. & Suda, T.(2004). Regulation of oxidative stress by ATM is required for self-renewal of haematopoietic stem cells. *Nature.* Oct 21;431(7011):997-1002.

Ito, K.; Hirao, A.; Arai, F.; Takubo, K.; Matsuoka, S.; Miyamoto, K.; Ohmura, M.; Naka, K.;Hosokawa, K.; Ikeda, Y. & Suda T. (2006). Reactive oxygen species act through p38 MAPK to limit the lifespan of hematopoietic stem cells. *Nat Med.* Apr;12(4):446-51.

Iwama, A.; Oguro, H.; Negishi, M.; Kato, Y.; Morita, Y.; Tsukui, H.; Ema, H.; Kamijo, T.; Katoh-Fukui, Y.; Koseki, H.; van Lohuizen, M.& Nakauchi, H. (2004). Enhanced self-renewal of hematopoietic stem cells mediated by the polycomb gene product Bmi-1. *Immunity.* Dec;21(6):843-51.

Janzen, V. & Scadden, D.T.(2006). Stem cells: good, bad and reformable. *Nature.* May 25;441(7092):418-9.

Janzen, V.; Forkert, R.; Fleming, H.E.; Saito, Y.; Waring, M.T.; Dombkowski, D.M.; Cheng, T.; DePinho, R.A.; Sharpless, N.E. & Scadden, D.T.(2006). Stem-cell ageing modified by the cyclin-dependent kinase inhibitor p16INK4a. *Nature.* 2006 Sep 28;443(7110):421-6.

Ju, Z.; Zhang, J.; Gao, Y. & Cheng, T.(2011). Telomere dysfunction and cell cycle checkpoints in hematopoietic stem cell aging. *Int J Hematol.* Jul;94(1):33-43.

Kajiume, T.; Ninomiya, Y.; Ishihara, H.; Kanno, R.& Kanno, M.(2004). Polycomb group gene mel-18 modulates the self-renewal activity and cell cycle status of hematopoietic stem cells. *Exp Hematol.* Jun;32(6):571-8.

Karahuseyinoglu, S.; Cinar, O.; Kilic, E.; Kara, F.; Akay, G.G.; Demiralp, D.O.; Tukun, A.; Uckan, D.& Can, A.(2007).Biology of stem cells in human umbilical cord stroma: in situ and in vitro surveys. *Stem Cells.* Feb;25(2):319-31.

Kato, Y.; Iwama, A.; Tadokoro, Y.; Shimoda, K.; Minoguchi, M.; Akira, S.; Tanaka, M.; Miyajima, A.; Kitamura, T. & Nakauchi, H.(2005). Selective activation of STAT5 unveils its role in stem cell self-renewal in normal and leukemic hematopoiesis. *J Exp Med*. Jul 4;202(1):169-79.

Kawano, Y. & Kypta, R.(2003). Secreted antagonists of the Wnt signaling pathway. *J Cell Sci*. Jul 1;116(Pt 13):2627-34.

Kent, D.; Copley, M.; Benz, C.; Dykstra, B.; Bowie, M.& Eaves, C.(2008).Regulation of hematopoietic stem cells by the steel factor/KIT signaling pathway. *Clin Cancer Res*.Apr 1;14(7):1926-30.

Kiel, M.J.; Yilmaz, O.H.; Iwashita, T.; Yilmaz, O.H.; Terhorst, C. & Morrison, S.J.(2005). SLAM family receptors distinguish hematopoietic stem and progenitor cells and reveal endothelial niches for stem cells. *Cell*. Jul 1;121(7):1109-21.

Kiel, M.J.& Morrison, S.J.(2006). Maintaining hematopoietic stem cells in the vascular niche. *Immunity*. Dec;25(6):862-4.

Kiel, M.J.; He, S.; Ashkenazi, R.; Gentry, S.N.; Teta, M.; Kushner, J.A.; Jackson, T.L. & Morrison, S.J.(2007). Haematopoietic stem cells do not asymmetrically segregate chromosomes or retain BrdU. *Nature*. Sep 13;449(7159):238-42.

Kiel, M.J.; Radice, G.L. & Morrison, S.J.(2007). Lack of evidence that hematopoietic stem cells depend on N-cadherin-mediated adhesion to osteoblasts for their maintenance. *Cell Stem Cell*. Aug 16;1(2):204-17.

Kim, J.Y.; Sawada, A.; Tokimasa, S.; Endo, H.; Ozono, K.; Hara, J. & Takihara, Y.(2004). Defective long-term repopulating ability in hematopoietic stem cells lacking the Polycomb-group gene rae28. *Eur J Haematol*. Aug;73(2):75-84.

Kollet, O.; Dar, A.; Shivtiel, S.; Kalinkovich, A.; Lapid, K.; Sztainberg, Y.; Tesio, M.; Samstein, R.M.; Goichberg, P.; Spiegel, A.; Elson, A. & Lapidot T. (2006). Osteoclasts degrade endosteal components and promote mobilization of hematopoietic progenitor cells. *Nat Med*. Jun;12(6):657-64.

Kopp, H.G.; Avecilla, S.T.; Hooper, A.T. & Rafii, S.(2005). The bone marrow vascular niche: home of HSC differentiation and mobilization. *Physiology (Bethesda)*. Oct;20:349-56.

Kosodo, Y.; Röper, K.; Haubensak, W.; Marzesco, A.M.; Corbeil, D. & Huttner, W.B.(2004). Asymmetric distribution of the apical plasma membrane during neurogenic divisions of mammalian neuroepithelial cells. *EMBO J*. Jun 2;23(11):2314-24.

Konuma, T.; Oguro, H. & Iwama, A.(2010). Role of the polycomb group proteins in hematopoietic stem cells. *Dev Growth Differ*. Aug;52(6):505-16.

Krosl, J.; Austin, P.; Beslu, N.; Kroon, E.; Humphries, R.K. & Sauvageau, G.(2003). In vitro expansion of hematopoietic stem cells by recombinant TAT-HOXB4 protein. *Nat Med*.Nov;9(11):1428-32.

Kubota, Y.; Takubo, K. & Suda, T.(2008). Bone marrow long label-retaining cells reside in the sinusoidal hypoxic niche. *Biochem Biophys Res Commun*. 2008 Feb 8;366(2):335-9.

Kühn, R.; Schwenk, F.; Aguet, M. & Rajewsky, K.(1995). Inducible gene targeting in mice. *Science*. Sep 8;269(5229):1427-9.

Kumano, K.; Chiba, S.; Kunisato, A.; Sata, M.; Saito, T.; Nakagami-Yamaguchi, E.; Yamaguchi, T.; Masuda, S.; Shimizu, K.; Takahashi, T.; Ogawa, S.; Hamada, Y. & Hirai, H.(2003). Notch1 but not Notch2 is essential for generating hematopoietic stem cells from endothelial cells. *Immunity*. May;18(5):699-711.

Lacombe, J.; Herblot, S.; Rojas-Sutterlin, S.; Haman, A.; Barakat, S.; Iscove, N.N.; Sauvageau, G.& Hoang, T.(2010). Scl regulates the quiescence and the long-term competence of hematopoietic stem cells. *Blood*. Jan 28;115(4):792-803.

Laiosa, C.V.; Stadtfeld, M.; Xie, H.; de Andres-Aguayo, L. & Graf, T.(2006).Reprogramming of committed T cell progenitors to macrophages and dendritic cells by C/EBP alphaand PU.1 transcription factors. *Immunity*. 2006 Nov;25(5):731-44.

Lansdorp, P.M. (1995). Telomere length and proliferation potential of hematopoietic stem cells. *J. Cell Sci*. 108: 1-6.

Lansdorp, P.M. (1997). Self-renewal of stem cells. *Biol. Blood Marrow Transplant* 3: 171-178.

Lansdorp, P.M. (2005). Role of telomerase in Hematopoietic Stem Cells. *Ann. N.Y.Acad.Sci.* 220-227.

Li, J.(2011). Quiescence regulators for hematopoietic stem cell. *Exp Hematol*. May;39(5):511-20.

Lee, H.W.; Blasco, M.A.; Gottlieb, G.J.; Horner, J.W2nd.; Greider, C.W. & Depinho, R.A. (1998). Essential role of mouse telomerase in highly proliferative organs. *Nature*. 392:569-574.

Lee, T.I.; Jenner, R.G.; Boyer, L.A.; Guenther, M.G.; Levine, S.S.; Kumar, R.M.; Chevalier, B.; Johnstone, S.E.; Cole, M.F.; Isono, K.; Koseki, H.; Fuchikami, T.; Abe, K.; Murray, H.L.; Zucker, J.P.; Yuan, B.; Bell, G.W.; Herbolsheimer, E.; Hannett, N.M.; Sun, K.; Odom, D.T.; Otte, A.P.; Volkert, T.L.; Bartel, D.P.; Melton, D.A.; Gifford, D.K.; Jaenisch, R. & Young, R.A. (2006). Control of developmental regulators by Polycomb in human embryonic stem cells. *Cell*. Apr 21;125(2):301-13.

Lessard, J.& Sauvageau, G.(2003). Bmi-1 determines the proliferative capacity of normal and leukaemic stem cells. *Nature*. May 15;423(6937):255-60.

Lewis, J.(1998). Notch signaling and the control of cell fate choices in vertebrates. *Semin Cell Dev Biol*. Dec;9(6):583-9.

Li, J. (2011). Quiescence regulators for hematopoietic stem cell. *Exp Hematol*. May; 39(5):511-20.

Li, L. & Xie, T.(2005). Stem cell niche: structure and function. *Annu Rev Cell Dev Biol*. 21:605-31.

Li, Z. & Li, L.(2006). Understanding hematopoietic stem-cell microenvironments. *Trends Biochem Sci*. Oct;31(10):589-95.

Li, W.; Johnson, S.A.; Shelley, W.C. & Yoder, M.C.(2004). Hematopoietic stem cell repopulating ability can be maintained in vitro by some primary endothelial cells. *Exp Hematol*. Dec;32(12):1226-37.

Li, X.; Han, Y. & Xi, R. (2010). Polycomb group genes Psc and Su(z)2 restrict follicle stem cell self-renewal and extrusion by controlling canonical and noncanonical Wnt signaling. *Genes Dev*. May;24(9):933-46.

Liu, Y.; Elf, S.E.; Miyata, Y.; Sashida, G.; Liu, Y.; Huang, G.; Di Giandomenico, S.; Lee, J.M.; Deblasio, A.; Menendez, S.; Antipin, J.; Reva, B.; Koff, A. & Nimer, S.D.(2009). p53 regulates hematopoietic stem cell quiescence. *Cell Stem Cell*. Jan 9;4(1):37-48.

Lo Celso, C.; Fleming, H.E.; Wu, J.W.; Zhao, C.X.; Miake-Lye, S.; Fujisaki, J.; Côté, D.; Rowe,D.W.; Lin, C.P. & Scadden, D.T.(2009) Live-animal tracking of individual haematopoietic stem/progenitor cells in their niche. *Nature*. Jan 1;457(7225):92-6.

Luis, T.C.; Weerkamp, F.; Naber, B.A.; Baert, M.R.; de Haas, E.F.; Nikolic, T.; Heuvelmans, S.; De Krijger, R.R.; van Dongen, J.J.& Staal, F.J.(2009). Wnt3a deficiency irreversibly impairs hematopoietic stem cell self-renewal and leads to defects in progenitor cell differentiation. *Blood*. Jan 15;113(3):546-54.

Maillard, I.; He, Y. & Pear, W.S.(2003). From the yolk sac to the spleen: New roles for Notch in regulating hematopoiesis. *Immunity*. May;18(5):587-9.

Mancini, S.J.; Mantei, N.; Dumortier, A.; Suter, U.; MacDonald, H.R. & Radtke, F.(2005). Jagged1-dependent Notch signaling is dispensable for hematopoietic stem cell self-renewal and differentiation. *Blood*. Mar 15;105(6):2340-2.

Matsunaga, T.; Kato, T.; Miyazaki, H.& Ogawa, M.(1998). Thrombopoietin promotes the survival of murine hematopoietic long-term reconstituting cells: comparison with the effects of FLT3/FLK-2 ligand and interleukin-6. *Blood*. Jul 15;92(2):452-61.

Matsuyama, M.; Aizawa, S. & Shimono, A. (2009). Sfrp controls apicobasal polarity and oriented cell division in developing gut epithelium. *PLoS Genet*. 5 (3) e1000427.

Miyake, N.; Brun, A.C.; Magnusson, M.; Miyake, K.; Scadden, D.T.& Karlsson, S.(2006).HOXB4-induced self-renewal of hematopoietic stem cells is significantly enhanced by p21 deficiency. *Stem Cells*.Mar;24(3):653-61.

Miyamoto, K.; Araki, K.Y.; Naka, K.; Arai, F.; Takubo, K.; Yamazaki, S.; Matsuoka, S.; Miyamoto, T.; Ito, K.; Ohmura, M.; Chen, C.; Hosokawa, K.; Nakauchi, H.; Nakayama, K.; Nakayama, K.I.; Harada, M.; Motoyama, N.; Suda, T. & Hirao, A. (2007). Foxo3a is essential for maintenance of the hematopoietic stem cell pool. *Cell Stem Cell*. Jun 7;1(1):101-12.

Molofsky, A.V.; Pardal, R.; Iwashita, T.; Park, I.K.; Clarke, M.F. & Morrison, S.J.(2005). Bmi-1 dependence distinguishes neural stem cell self-renewal from progenitor proliferation. *Nature*. Oct 30;425(6961):962-7.

Moore, K.A. & Lemischka, I.R.(2006). Stem cells and their niches. *Science*. Mar 31;311(5769):1880-5.

Morisada, T.; Kubota, Y.; Urano, T.; Suda, T. & Oike Y.(2006). Angiopoietins and angiopoietin-like proteins in angiogenesis. *Endothelium*. Mar-Apr;13(2):71-9.

Morrison, S.J.& Spradling, A.C.(2008). Stem cells and niches: mechanisms that promote stem cell maintenance throughout life. *Cell*. Feb 22;132(4):598-611.

Müller, A.M.; Medvinsky, A.; Strouboulis, J.; Grosveld, F. & Dzierzak, E.(1994)Development of hematopoietic stem cell activity in the mouse embryo. *Immunity*.Jul;1(4):291-301.

Murdoch, B.; Chadwick, K.; Martin, M.; Shojaei, F.; Shah, K.V.; Gallacher, L.; Moon, R.T.& Bhatia, M.(2003). Wnt-5A augments repopulating capacity and primitive hematopoietic development of human blood stem cells in vivo. *Proc Natl Acad Sci U S A*. Mar 18;100(6):3422-7.

Nemeth, M.J.& Bodine, D.M.(2007). Regulation of hematopoiesis and the hematopoietic stem cell niche by Wnt signaling pathways. *Cell Res*. Sep;17(9):746-58.

Ohta, H.; Sawada, A.; Kim, J.Y.; Tokimasa, S.; Nishiguchi, S.; Humphries, R.K.; Hara, J. & Takihara, Y. (2002). Polycomb group gene rae28 is required for sustaining activity of hematopoietic stem cells. *J Exp Med*. Mar 18;195(6):759-70.

Opferman, J.T.; Iwasaki, H.; Ong, C.C.; Suh, H.; Mizuno, S.; Akashi, K.& Korsmeyer, S.J.(2005).Obligate role of anti-apoptotic MCL-1 in the survival of hematopoietic stem cells. *Science*. Feb 18;307(5712):1101-4.

Orkin, S.H. & Zon, L.I.(2008) Hematopoiesis: an evolving paradigm for stem cell biology.*Cell*. Feb 2;132(4):631-44.

Ottersbach, K. & Dzierzak, E. (2005). The murine placenta contains hematopoietic stem cells within the vascular labyrinth region. *Dev Cell*. Mar;8(3):377-87.

Papadimitriou, J.C.; Drachenberg, C.B.; Shin, M.L. & Trump, B.F.(1994). Ultrastructural studies of complement mediated cell death: a biological reaction model to plasma membrane injury. *Virchows Arch.* 424(6):677-85.

Pardanaud, L. & Dieterlen-Lièvre, F.(1999). Manipulation of the angiopoietic/hemangiopoietic commitment in the avian embryo. *Development.* Feb;126(4):617-27.

Park, I.K.; Morrison, S.J. & Clarke, M.F.(2004). Bmi1, stem cells, and senescence regulation. *J Clin Invest.* Jan;113(2):175-9.

Park, I.K.; Qian, D.; Kiel, M.; Becker, M.W.; Pihalja, M.; Weissman, I.L.; Morrison, S.J. & Clarke, M.F.(2003). Bmi-1 is required for maintenance of adult self-renewing haematopoietic stem cells. *Nature.* May 15;423(6937):302-5.

Parmar, K.; Mauch, P.; Vergílio, J.A.; Sackstein, R. & Down, J.D.(2007). Distribution of hematopoietic stem cells in the bone marrow according to regional hypoxia. *Proc Natl Acad Sci U S A.* Mar 27;104(13):5431-6.

Petit-Cocault, L.; Volle-Challier, C.; Fleury, M.; Péault, B.& Souyri M.(2007). Dual role of Mpl receptor during the establishment of definitive hematopoiesis. *Development.* Aug;134(16):3031-40.

Pimanda, J.E.; Donaldson, I.J.; de Bruijn, M.F.; Kinston, S.; Knezevic, K.; Huckle, L.; Piltz, S.; Landry, J.R.; Green, A.R.; Tannahill, D. & Göttgens, B.(2007). The SCL transcriptional network and BMP signaling pathway interact to regulate RUNX1 activity. *Proc Natl Acad Sci U S A.* Jan 16;104(3):840-5.

Pizzatti, L.; Binato, R.; Cofre, J.; Gomes, B.E.; Dobbin, J.; Haussmann, M.E.; D'Azambuja, D.; Bouzas, L.F. & Abdelhay, E.(2010). SUZ12 is a candidate target of the non-canonical WNT pathway in the progression of chronic myeloid leukemia. *Genes Chromosomes Cancer.* Feb;49(2):107-18.

Rekhtman, N.; Radparvar, .F; Evans, T. & Skoultchi, A.I.(1999). Direct interaction of hematopoietic transcription factors PU.1 and GATA-1: functional antagonism in erythroid cells. *Genes Dev.* Jun 1;13(11):1398-411.

Renstrom, J.; Kroger, M.; Peschel, C. & Robert, A.J.(2010). Oostendorp. How the niche regulates hematopoietic stem cells. *Chemico-Biological Interactions.* 184: 7-15.

Reya, T.& Clevers, H.(2005). Wnt signaling in stem cells and cancer. *Nature.* Apr 14;434(7035):843-50.

Reya, T.; Duncan, A.W.; Ailles, L.; Domen, J.; Scherer, D.C.; Willert, K.; Hintz, L.; Nusse, R. & Weissman, I.L.(2003). A role for Wnt signaling in self-renewal of haematopoietic stem cells. *Nature.* May 22;423(6938):409-14.

Rizzo, P.; Osipo, C.; Foreman, K.; Golde, T.; Osborne, B. & Miele, L.(2008). Rational targeting of Notch signaling in cancer. *Oncogene.* Sep 1;27(38):5124-31.

Robert-Moreno, A.; Espinosa, L.; de la Pompa, J.L. & Bigas, A.(2005). RBPjkappa-dependent Notch function regulates Gata2 and is essential for the formation of intra-embryonic hematopoietic cells. *Development.* Mar; 132(5):1117-26.

Rodriguez, J.; Esteve, P. ; Weinl, C. ; Ruiz, J.M.; Fermin, Y.; Trousse, F.; Dwivedy, A.; Holt, C. & Bovolenta, P. (2005). SFRP1 regulates the growth of retinal ganglion cell axons through the Fz2 receptor, *Nat. Neurosci.* 8 (10) 1301–1309.

Ross, J. & Li, L.(2006). Recent advances in understanding extrinsic control of hematopoietic stem cell fate. *Curr Opin Hematol.* ul;13(4):237-42.

Samper, E.; Fernández, P.; Eguía, R.; Martín-Rivera, L.; Bernad, A.; Blasco, M.A.& Aracil, M. (2002). Long-term repopulating ability of telomerase-deficient murine hematopoietic stem cells. *Blood*. Apr 15;99(8):2767-75.

Sato, T.; Laver,J.H. & Ogawa, M.(1999). Reversible expression of CD34 by murine hematopoietic stem cells. *Blood*. Oct 15;94(8):2548-54.

Sato, T.; Onai, N.; Yoshihara, H.; Arai, F.; Suda, T. & Ohteki, T. (2009). Interferon regulatory factor-2 protects quiescent hematopoietic stem cells from type I interferon-dependent exhaustion. *Nat Med*. Jun;15(6):696-700.

Sauvageau, G.; Thorsteinsdottir, U.; Eaves, C.J.; Lawrence, H.J.; Largman, C.; Lansdorp,P.M. & Humphries, R.K.(1995). Overexpression of HOXB4 in hematopoietic cells causes the selective expansion of more primitive populations in vitro and in vivo. *Genes Dev*. Jul 15;9(14):1753-65.

Scandura, J.M.; Boccuni, P.; Massagué, J. & Nimer, S.D.(2004). Transforming growth factor beta-induced cell cycle arrest of human hematopoietic cells requires p57KIP2 up-regulation. *Proc Natl Acad Sci U S A*. Oct 19;101(42):15231-6.

Schiedlmeier, B.; Santos, A.C.; Ribeiro, A.; Moncaut, N.; Lesinski, D.; Auer, H.; Kornacker,K.; Ostertag, W.; Baum, C.; Mallo, M. & Klump, H.(2007). HOXB4's road map to stem cell expansion. *Proc Natl Acad Sci U S A*. Oct 23;104(43):16952-7.

Scholl, C.; Gilliland, D.G. & Fröhling, S.(2008). Deregulation of signaling pathways in acute myeloid leukemia. *Semin Oncol*. Aug;35(4):336-45.

Seita, J.; Ema, H.; Ooehara, J.; Yamazaki, S.; Tadokoro, Y.; Yamasaki, A.; Eto, K.; Takaki,S.; Takatsu, K.& Nakauchi H.(2007). Lnk negatively regulates self-renewal of hematopoietic stem cells by modifying thrombopoietin-mediated signal transduction. *Proc Natl Acad Sci U S A*. Feb 13;104(7):2349-54.

Shao, Y.; Kim, S.Y.; Shin, D.; Kim, M.S.; Suh, H.W.; Piao, Z.H.; Jeong, M.; Lee, S.H.; Yoon, S.R.; Lim,B.H.; Kim, W.H.; Ahn, J.K. & Choi, I.(2010). TXNIP regulates germinal center generation by suppressing BCL-6 expression. *Immunol Lett*. Apr 8;129(2):78-84.

Shih, Ie.M. & Wang, T.L.(2007). Notch signaling, gamma-secretase inhibitors, and cancer therapy. *Cancer Res*. Mar 1;67(5):1879-82.

Silver, I.A.; Murrills, R.J.& Etherington, D.J.(1988). Microelectrode studies on the acid microenvironment beneath adherent macrophages and osteoclasts. *Exp Cell Res*.Apr;175(2):266-76.

Sirin, O.; Lukov, G.L.; Mao, R.; Conneely, O.M. & Goodell, M.A.(2010). The orphan nuclear receptor Nurr1 restricts the proliferation of haematopoietic stem cells. *Nat Cell Biol*. Dec;12(12):1213-9.

Snow, J.W.; Abraham, N.; Ma, M.C.; Abbey, N.W.; Herndier, B.& Goldsmith, M.A. (2002). STAT5 promotes multilineage hematolymphoid development in vivo through effects on early hematopoietic progenitor cells. *Blood*. Jan 1;99(1):95-101.

Solar, G.P.; Kerr, W.G.; Zeigler, F.C.; Hess, D.; Donahue, C.; de Sauvage, F.J. & Eaton, D.L.(1998).Role of c-mpl in early hematopoiesis. *Blood*. Jul 1;92(1):4-10.

Spike, B.T.; Dirlam, A.; Dibling, B.C.; Marvin, J.; Williams, B.O.; Jacks, T.& Macleod, K.F.(2004).The Rb tumor suppressor is required for stress erythropoiesis. *EMBO J*. Oct 27;23(21):4319-29.

Stein, M.I.; Zhu, J. & Emerson, S.G. (2004). Molecular pathways regulation the self-renewal of hematopoietic stem cells. *Exp Hematology*. 32- 1129-1136.

Stead, E.; White, J.; Faast, R.; Conn, S.; Goldstone, S.; Rathjen, J.; Dhingra, U.; Rathjen,P.; Walker, D. & Dalton, S.(2002). Pluripotent cell division cycles are driven by ectopic Cdk2, cyclin A/E and E2F activities. *Oncogene*. Nov 28;21(54):8320-33.

Stepanova, L.& Sorrentino, B.P.(2005). A limited role for p16Ink4a and p19Arf in the loss of hematopoietic stem cells during proliferative stress. *Blood*. Aug 1;106(3):827-32.

Stier, S.; Ko, Y.; Forkert, R.; Lutz, C.; Neuhaus, T.; Grünewald, E.; Cheng, T.; Dombkowski,D.; Calvi, L.M.; Rittling, S.R. & Scadden, D.T.(2005). Osteopontin is a hematopoietic stem cell niche component that negatively regulates stem cell pool size. *J Exp Med*. Jun 6;201(11):1781-91.

Suzuki, T.; Yokoyama, Y.; Kumano, K.; Takanashi, M.; Kozuma, S.; Takato, T.; Nakahata, T.;Nishikawa, M.; Sakano, S.; Kurokawa, M.; Ogawa, S.& Chiba S. (2006). Highly efficient ex vivo expansion of human hematopoietic stem cells using Delta1-Fc chimeric protein.*Stem Cells*. Nov;24(11):2456-65.

Tong, W.; Ibarra, Y.M. & Lodish, H.F.(2007). Signals emanating from the membrane proximal region of the thrombopoietin receptor (mpl) support hematopoietic stem cell self-renewal. *Exp Hematol*. Sep;35(9):1447-55.

Tothova, Z.; Kollipara, R.; Huntly, B.J.; Lee, B.H.; Castrillon, D.H.; Cullen, D.E.; McDowell, E.P.; Lazo-Kallanian, S.; Williams, I.R.; Sears, C.; Armstrong, S.A.; Passegué, E.; DePinho, R.A. & Gilliland, D.G.(2007). FoxOs are critical mediators of hematopoietic stem cell resistance to physiologic oxidative stress. *Cell*. Jan 26;128(2):325-39.

Utsugisawa, T.; Moody, J.L.; Aspling, M.; Nilsson, E.; Carlsson, L.& Karlsson, S.(2006). A road map toward defining the role of Smad signaling in hematopoietic stem cells. *Stem Cells*. Apr;24(4):1128-36.

Van der Lugt, N.M.; Alkema, M.; Berns, A. & Deschamps, J.(1996). The Polycomb-group homolog Bmi-1 is a regulator of murine Hox gene expression. *Mech Dev*. Aug;58(1-2):153-64.

Van Os, R.; Kamminga, L.M.; Ausema, A.; Bystrykh, L.V.; Draijer, D.P.; van Pelt, K.; Dontje, B. & de Haan. G. (2007). A Limited role for p21Cip1/Waf1 in maintaining normal hematopoietic stem cell functioning. *Stem Cells*. Apr;25(4):836-43.

Viatour, P.; Somervaille, T.C.; Venkatasubrahmanyam, S.; Kogan, S.; McLaughlin, M.E.; Weissman, I.L.; Butte, A.J.; Passegué, E.& Sage, J.(2008). Hematopoietic stem cell quiescence is maintained by compound contributions of the retinoblastoma gene family. *Cell Stem Cell*. Oct 9;3(4):416-28.

Vaziri, H.; Dragowska, W.; Allsopp, R.C.; Thomas, T.E.; Harley, C.B. & Lansdorp, P.M. (1994). Evidence for a mitotic clock in human hematopoietic stem cells: loss of telomeric DNA with age. *Proc Natl Acad Sci U S A*. Oct 11;91(21):9857-60.

Visnjic, D.; Kalajzic, Z.; Rowe, D.W.; Katavic, V.; Lorenzo, J. & Aguila, H.L.(2004). Hematopoiesis is severely altered in mice with an induced osteoblast deficiency. *Blood*. May 1;103(9):3258-64.

Walkley, C.R. & Orkin, S.H.(2006). Rb is dispensable for self-renewal and multilineage differentiation of adult hematopoietic stem cells. *Proc Natl Acad Sci U S A*. Jun 13;103(24):9057-62.

Walkley, C.R.; Fero, M.L.; Chien, W.M.; Purton, L.E.& McArthur, G.A.(2005). Negative cell-cycle regulators cooperatively control self-renewal and differentiation of haematopoietic stem cells. *Nat Cell Biol*. Feb;7(2):172-8.

Wang, Z.; Li, G.; Tse, W. & Bunting, K.D.(2009). Conditional deletion of STAT5 in adult mouse hematopoietic stem cells causes loss of quiescence and permits efficient nonablative stem cell replacement. *Blood*. May 14;113(20):4856-65.

Weissman, I.L. (2000).Stem cells: units of development, units of regeneration, and units in evolution. *Cell* Jan 7;100(1):157-68.

Willert, K.; Brown, J.D.; Danenberg, E.; Duncan, A.W.; Weissman, I.L.; Reya, T.; Yates, J.R3rd. & Nusse, R.(2003). Wnt proteins are lipid-modified and can act as stem cell growth factors. *Nature*. May 22;423(6938):448-52.

Wilson, A.& Trumpp, A.(2006). Bone-marrow haematopoietic-stem-cell niches. *Nat Rev Immunol*.Feb;6(2):93-106.

Wilson, A.; Murphy, M.J.; Oskarsson, T.; Kaloulis, K.; Bettess, M.D.; Oser, G.M.; Pasche, A.C.; Knabenhans, C.; Macdonald, H.R. & Trumpp, A.(2004). c-Myc controls the balance between hematopoietic stem cell self-renewal and differentiation. *Genes Dev*. Nov 15;18(22):2747-63.

Wu, M.; Kwon, H.Y.; Rattis, F.; Blum, J.; Zhao, C.; Ashkenazi, R.; Jackson, T.L.; Gaiano, N.; Oliver, T. & Reya, T.(2007). Imaging hematopoietic precursor division in real time. *Cell Stem Cell*.Nov;1(5):541-54.

Xie, Y.; Yin, T.; Wiegraebe, W.; He, X.C.; Miller, D.; Stark, D.; Perko, K.; Alexander, R.;Schwartz, J.; Grindley, J.C.; Park, J.; Haug, J.S.; Wunderlich, J.P.; Li, H.; Zhang, S.; Johnson,T.; Feldman, R.A.& Li, L.(2009). Detection of functional haematopoietic stem cell niche using real-time imaging. *Nature*. Jan 1;457(7225):97-101.

Yamashita, Y.M.& Fuller, M.T.(2008). Asymmetric centrosome behavior and the mechanisms of stem cell division. *J Cell Biol*. Jan 28;180(2):261-6.

Yeoh, J.S.; van Os, R.; Weersing, E.; Ausema, A.; Dontje, B.; Vellenga, E. & de Haan, G.(2006).Fibroblast growth factor-1 and -2 preserve long-term repopulating ability of hematopoietic stem cells in serum-free cultures. *Stem Cells*. Jun;24(6):1564-72.

Yoshihara, H.; Arai, F.; Hosokawa, K.; Hagiwara, T.; Takubo, K.; Nakamura, Y.; Gomei, Y.;Iwasaki, H.; Matsuoka, S.; Miyamoto, K.; Miyazaki, H.; Takahashi, T. & Suda, T.(2007).Thrombopoietin/MPL signaling regulates hematopoietic stem cell quiescence and interaction with the osteoblastic niche. *Cell Stem Cell*. Dec 13;1(6):685-97.

You, L.R.; Lin, F.J.; Lee, C.T.; DeMayo, F.J.; Tsai, M.J. & Tsai, S.Y.(2005). Suppression of Notch signaling by the COUP-TFII transcription factor regulates vein identity. *Nature*. May 5;435(7038):98-104.

Yu, H.; Yuan, Y.; Shen, H. & Cheng, T.(2006). Hematopoietic stem cell exhaustion impacted by p18 INK4C and p21 Cip1/Waf1 in opposite manners. *Blood*. Feb 1;107(3):1200-6.

Yuan, Y.; Shen, H.; Franklin, D.S.; Scadden, D.T. & Cheng, T.(2004). In vivo self-renewing divisions of haematopoietic stem cells are increased in the absence of the early G1-phase inhibitor, p18INK4C. *Nat Cell Biol*. May;6(5):436-42.

Zayas, J.; Spassov, D.S.; Nachtman, R.G. & Jurecic, R.(2008). Murine hematopoietic stem cells and multipotent progenitors express truncated intracellular form of c-kit receptor. *Stem Cells Dev*. Apr;17(2):343-53.

Zeng, H.; Yücel, R.; Kosan, C.; Klein-Hitpass, L. & Möröy T. (2004).Transcription factor Gfi1 regulates self-renewal and engraftment of hematopoietic stem cells. *EMBO J*.Oct 13;23(20):4116-25.

Zhang, C.C. & Lodish, H.F.(2004). Insulin-like growth factor 2 expressed in a novel fetal liver cell population is a growth factor for hematopoietic stem cells. *Blood*. Apr 1;103(7):2513-21.

Zhang, J.; Niu, C.; Ye, L.; Huang, H.; He, X.; Tong, W.G.; Ross, J.; Haug, J.; Johnson, T.; Feng,J.Q.; Harris, S.; Wiedemann, L.M.; Mishina, Y. & Li, L.(2003). Identification of the haematopoietic stem cell niche and control of the niche size. *Nature*. Oct 23;425(6960):836-41.

Zhang, P.; Behre, G.; Pan, J.; Iwama, A.; Wara-Aswapati, N.; Radomska, H.S.; Auron, P.E.; Tenen, D.G. & Sun, Z.(1999) Negative cross-talk between hematopoietic regulators: GATA proteins repress PU.1. *Proc Natl Acad Sci U S A*. Jul 20;96(15):8705-10.

Zhang, P.; Iwasaki-Arai, J.; Iwasaki, H.; Fenyus, M.L.; Dayaram, T.; Owens, B.M.; Shigematsu, H.; Levantini, E.; Huettner, C.S.; Lekstrom-Himes, J.A.; Akashi, K. & Tenen, D.G.(2004). Enhancement of hematopoietic stem cell repopulating capacity and self-renewal in the absence of the transcription factor C/EBP alpha. *Immunity*. Dec;21(6):853-63.

Zon, L.I.(2008). Self-renewal and differentiation at Cell Stem Cell. *Cell Stem Cell*. Jun 5;2(6):510.

4

Regulation of Hematopoietic Stem Cell Fate: Self-Renewal, Quiescence and Survival

Yasushi Kubota[1,2] and Shinya Kimura[1]
*[1]Division of Hematology, Respiratory Medicine and Oncology,
Department of Internal Medicine, Faculty of Medicine, Saga University
[2]Department of Transfusion Medicine, Saga University Hospital
Japan*

1. Introduction

Hematopoietic stem cells (HSCs) are probably the most extensively characterized somatic stem cells and are the only stem cells that have been clinically used to treat diseases such as leukemia, germ cell tumors, and congenital immunodeficiencies. Because of their capacity for self-renewal and their ability to differentiate into different lineages, HSCs are able to continually replenish the cells that make up the hematopoietic system (Kondo et al., 2003). Decades of intensive study using multicolor cell sorting techniques have allowed investigators to identify these cells within a small population in the mouse bone marrow (BM) (i.e., CD34[low/-], Kit[+] Sca-1[+] lineage marker-negative cells: CD34[low/-] KSL) and thereby allow the prospective isolation of nearly-homogenous HSC populations for further characterization (Osawa et al., 1996).

Under steady-state conditions, the majority of HSCs are maintained in a quiescent state in which they divide infrequently to produce proliferative progenitors that eventually give rise to the mature hematopoietic cells that sustain blood homeostasis (Cheshier et al., 1999). However, in response to external stresses such as bleeding, myeloablative chemotherapy and total body irradiation, HSCs proliferate extensively to produce very high numbers of primitive progenitor cells, thereby enabling rapid hematological regeneration (Randall et al., 1997). Once recovery from myelosuppression has been achieved, the activated HSCs return to a quiescent state via a number of negative feedback mechanisms (Venezia et al., 2004). The cell fate decisions (including life and death, self-renewal and differentiation) of HSCs are important processes that regulate the number and lifespan of the HSC pool within a host. Defects in these processes may contribute to hematopoietic failures and to the development of hematologic malignancies.

Understanding the molecular mechanisms underlying HSC regulation is of great importance to basic stem cell biology and for the development of HSCs for use in various clinical applications. Information regarding the regulation of HSC fate has been gained using conventional experimental approaches such as gene deletion, gene overexpression, and the direct stimulation of HSCs with cytokines. Although many studies have elucidated the factors controlling HSC fate using these methods, they can occasionally be misleading because they lack physiological relevance and do not identify phenomena such as genetic redundancy. For example, family genes or alternative pathways can compensate functionally for deleted genes in gene-ablated mouse models in a manner that masks the true physiology. One approach to identifying the individual components involved in the molecular pathways underlying HSC regulation is to define the molecular signature of the HSCs by comparative transcriptional profiling of distinct subsets of hematopoietic cells. Over the past decade, several attempts have been made by independent investigators, including ourselves, to define the molecular signature of HSCs (Park et al., 2002; Ramalho-Santos et al., 2002; Ivanova et al., 2002; Akashi et al., 2003; Venezia et al., 2004; Zhong et al., 2005; Forsberg et al., 2005; Ramos et al., 2006; Chambers et al., 2007; Kubota et al., 2009). A list of gene expression profiling studies using purified mouse HSCs performed to date is shown in Table 1. Although this information has, more or less, clarified the molecular makeup of HSCs and several critical factors have been identified based on the data reported in these studies, it is still extremely time-consuming to elucidate the physiological function of each individual gene involved in HSC regulation. The transcriptional regulation of stem cell fate, particularly by factors that have specific functions in HSCs, is only beginning to be understood.

In this chapter, we briefly review the recent advances in our knowledge of cell-intrinsic regulators of HSC self-renewal, differentiation, quiescence, cycling, and survival.

	Year	HSC phenotype	Compared population	References
Park et al.	2002	Rho^{low} KSL	Rho^{high} KSL	*Blood* 99(2):488-498.
Ramalho-Santos et al.	2002	CD34$^{-/low}$KSL-SP	MP	*Science* 298(5593):597-600.
Ivanova et al.	2002	Rho^{low} KSL	Rho^{high} KSL, LCP, MBC	*Science* 298(5593):601-604.
Akashi et al.	2003	Rho^{low}Thy-1.1^{low}KSL	MPP, CLP, CMP	*Blood* 101(2):383-389.
Venezia et al.	2004	Sca-1$^+$-SP	5-FU treated SP	*PLoS Biol* 2(10):e301.
Zhong et al.	2005	CD34$^-$CD38$^+$ KSL	CD38$^+$ or CD38$^-$CD34$^+$ KSL	*PNAS* 102(7):2448-2453.
Kiel et al.	2005	Thy1.1^{low}KSL	Thy-1.1^{lo}Sca-1$^+$Mac-1^{lo}CD4^{lo}B220$^-$	*Cell* 121(7):1109-1121.
Forsberg et al.	2005	Flk2$^-$Thy1.1^{low} KSL	Thy1.1^{low}, Thy1.1$^-$Flk2+ KSL	*PLoS Genet* 1(3):e28.
Ramos et al.	2006	Sca-1$^+$Gr1$^-$-SP	CD8$^+$ Tcell	*PLoS Genet* 2(9):e159.
Chambers et al.	2007	KSL-SP	Erythrocyte Granulocyte Native T Activated T B-cell Monocyte NK	*Cell Stem Cell* 1(5):578-591.
Kubota et al.	2009	CD34$^{-/low}$KSL	CD34$^+$KSL	*Blood* 114(20):4383-4392.

Rho, rhodamine; SP, side population; LCP, lineage-committed progenitor; MBC, mature blood cell;
MPP, multipotent progenitor; CLP, common lymphoid progenitor; CMP, common myeloid progenitor

Table 1. Gene expression profiling analyses of adult HSCs

2. Regulators of HSC fate

2.1 Regulation of HSC self-renewal and quiescence

The outstanding feature of adult stem cells is their relative quiescence (Orford et al., 2008; Wilson et al., 2008). Quiescence is critical for the maintenance and self-renewal of HSCs. Unscheduled HSC proliferation results in the loss of self-renewal or stem cell exhaustion (Orford et al., 2008; Wilson et al., 2009; Trumpp et al., 2010). Identification of the molecules that regulate adult HSCs has largely been achieved through the use of gene-targeted mouse models. Increasing or decreasing HSC cell-cycling results in the accelerated production of more committed progenitors at the expense of self renewal, or the insufficient production of progeny cells, which eventually results in BM failure.

2.1.1 Positive regulation

2.1.1.1 GATA-2

GATA-2 is highly expressed in immature progenitors within hematopoietic lineages (Tsai & Orkin, 1997; Akashi et al., 2000). The haploinsufficient $GATA-2^{+/-}$ mouse model shows mildly increased quiescence of both HSCs and progenitor cells (Rodrigues et al., 2005). However, Tipping et al. recently showed that enforced expression of GATA-2 in a murine cell line (Ba/F3), or human cord blood HSCs ($CD34^+CD38^-$) and progenitors ($CD34^+CD38^+$), increases quiescence and inhibits proliferation (Tipping, et al, 2009).

2.1.1.2 Bmi1

Bmi1 belongs to the polycomb group (PcG) of proteins, which play a role in the transcriptional repression of genes via histone modification (Rajasekhar et al., 2007). Bmi1 is highly expressed in HSCs. The expression of Bmi1 is maintained at high levels in lymphoid lineage cells but is downregulated during myeloid differentiation (Iwama et al., 2004). Although $Bmi1^{-/-}$ mice show normal fetal liver hematopoiesis, progressive pancytopenia emerges in postnatal $Bmi1^{-/-}$ mice. This hematopoietic defect can be attributed to impaired HSC self-renewal. Transplanted fetal liver and bone marrow cells from $Bmi1^{-/-}$ mice cannot contribute to long-term hematopoiesis, although they do maintain the ability to repopulate in the short-term (Park et al., 2003; Iwama et al., 2004). Conversely, enforced expression of Bmi1 promotes HSC self-renewal (Iwama et al., 2004). Thus, Bmi1 is essential for the maintenance of HSC self-renewal.

The activity of Bmi1 in HSCs largely depends on the silencing of its target, the $Ink4a$ locus (Jacobs et al., 1999). The expression of $p16^{INK4a}$ and $p19^{ARF}$ (both cell-cycle inhibitors encoded by the $Ink4a$ locus) is markedly upregulated in hematopoietic cells in $Bmi1$-deficient mice, and the overexpression of $p16^{INK4a}$ and $p19^{ARF}$ in HSCs induces cell-cycle arrest and p53-dependent apoptosis (Park et al., 2003). On the contrary, the deletion of both $p16^{INK4a}$ and $p19^{ARF}$ restores the self-renewal ability of $Bmi1^{-/-}$ HSCs (Oguro et al., 2006). Thus, Bmi1 prevents the premature loss of HSCs by repressing the $p16^{INK4a}$- and $p19^{ARF}$-dependent senescence pathways.

2.1.1.3 Gfi-1

Gfi1 is a SNAG-domain–containing zinc-finger transcriptional repressor, which plays a role in T cell proliferation and the development of lymphoid tumors (Gilks et al., 1993). It is suggested that Gfi-1 restricts proliferation and preserves functional integrity of hematopoietic stem cells. Gfi-1-null HSCs show excessive cell cycling and a decreased capacity for self-renewal in competitive repopulation assays (Hock et al., 2004; Zeng et al., 2004).

2.1.1.4 Pbx1

Pbx1 is a TALE class homeodomain transcription factor that critically regulates numerous embryonic processes, including hematopoiesis (DiMartino et al., 2001). Although a potential role was suggested by the observation that Pbx1 is preferentially expressed in long-term repopulating HSCs (LT-HSCs) compared with more mature progenitor cells (Forsberg et al., 2005), its functional analysis in adult HSCs has been hampered because Pbx1 mutant mice are embryonic lethal. Therefore, Pbx1-conditional knockout (KO) mice have been used to study the role of Pbx1 in the adult mouse hematopoietic system (Ficara et al., 2008). Conditional inactivation of Pbx1 in hematopoietic cells results in the loss of HSCs, which is associated with decreased quiescence. This leads to a defect in the maintenance of self-renewal in serial transplantation assays. Global gene expression profiling analyses show that a significant proportion (~8%) of the downregulated genes in Pbx1-deficient HSCs belong to the TGF-β signaling pathway, which has been implicated in maintaining HSC quiescence (Yamazaki et al., 2009). Also, in contrast to WT LT-HSCs, Pbx1-mutant LT-HSCs do not upregulate the expression of several downstream transcripts in response to TGF-β stimulation *in vitro*. These results suggest that Pbx1 regulates HSC self-renewal and quiescence, at least in part by affecting the response to TGF-β.

2.1.1.5 Evi-1

The ecotropic viral integration site-1 (Evi-1) was first identified in murine model systems as the integration site for the ecotropic retrovirus that causes myeloid leukemia (Morishita et al., 1988; Mucenski et al., 1988). Several studies using gene-targeting mice show that Evi-1 is required for HSC regulation. Yuasa et al. showed that Evi-1 is preferentially expressed in HSCs in embryos and adult BM. Evi-1–deficient embryonic HSCs are severely decreased in number, and show defective repopulating capacity. In addition, the expression of GATA-2 mRNA is markedly reduced in HSCs from Evi-1–null embryos. GATA-2 promoter analysis revealed that Evi-1 directly binds to the GATA-2 promoter and acts as an enhancer (Yuasa et al., 2005). Another study using conditional Evi-1 knockout mice showed that Evi-1 also regulates adult HSC proliferation in a dose-dependent manner. Evi-1–deficient BM HSCs did not maintain definitive hematopoiesis and lost their ability to reconstitute the cell population. Mutant mice heterozygous for Evi-1 exhibited an intermediate phenotype in terms of HSC activity (Goyama et al., 2008). Furthermore, gene expression profiling of Evi-1–deleted HSCs and leukemic cells identified Pbx1 as a downstream target for Evi-1 in HSCs (Shimabe et al., 2009).

2.1.1.6 JunB

The AP-1 transcription factor, JunB, is a transcriptional regulator of myelopoiesis and a potential tumor suppressor gene in mice (Passegue et al., 2001). Compared with normal HSCs, JunB-deficient LT-HSCs showed an average 2-fold increase in the percentage of cycling cells, suggesting that JunB functions to limit cell-cycle entry. Gene expression analyses revealed that JunB-deficient LT-HSCs show increased expression of cyclins and decreased expression of cyclin-dependent kinase inhibitors (Santaguida et al., 2009). These results suggest that the absence of JunB induces quiescent cells to enter the cell cycle.

2.1.1.7 p53

The p53 tumor suppressor protein functions as a transcription factor, regulating the transcription of genes that induce cell-cycle arrest, senescence, and apoptosis. LT-HSCs express high levels of p53 (Dumble et al., 2007). Although p53-deficient mice show almost normal hematopoiesis (Lotem & Suchs., 1993), a number of studies have identified a role for p53 in the proliferation, differentiation, apoptosis, and aging of HSCs (Kastan et al., 1991; Shounan et al., 1996; Park et al., 2003; Dumble et al., 2007). Recent detailed analyses of p53-null mice have unraveled other important functions of p53 in HSCs. Liu et al. found that p53 promotes HSC quiescence, and that p53-deficient HSCs enter the cell cycle more easily (Liu et al., 2009). Competitive BM repopulation assays revealed that p53-null cells out-compete wild-type cells (TeKippe et al., 2003; Chen et al., 2008; Liu et al., 2009), indicating that p53 is a negative regulator of HSC self-renewal. In addition, Liu et al. also identified Gfi-1 and necdin as p53 target genes by performing comparative transcriptional profiling of HSCs isolated from wild-type and p53-deficient mice. The results of *in vitro* overexpression and knockdown experiments identified a role for necdin in the maintenance of HSC quiescence and self-renewal. However, necdin appears to have a modest functional role in HSCs *in vivo* (Kubota et al., 2009), and necdin overexpression does not result in enhanced HSC quiescence (Sirin et al., 2010).

2.1.1.8 Nurr1

Gene expression profiling analyses identified Nurr1 (also known as Nr4a2), an orphan nuclear receptor, as a candidate molecule that may play a functional role in HSC quiescence (Venezia et al., 2004; Chambers et al., 2007). Overexpression of Nurr1 resulted in HSC quiescence. On the other hand, loss of one Nurr1 allele resulted in enhanced cycling and sensitivity to the chemotherapeutic agent 5-fluorouracil (5-FU). Molecular analysis showed that Nurr1 overexpression is positively correlated with the upregulation of the cell-cycle inhibitor $p18^{INK4C}$, suggesting a mechanism by which Nurr1 may regulate HSC quiescence (Sirin et al., 2010).

2.1.1.9 Reactive oxygen species, FoxOs

Reactive oxygen species (ROS) play an important role in the regulation of HSC quiescence. The forkhead O (FoxO) family of transcription factors (FoxO1, FoxO3, FoxO4, and FoxO6) participates in various cellular processes, including the induction of cell-cycle arrest, stress resistance, apoptosis, differentiation, and metabolism (Greer & Brunet., 2005). Two groups reported that FoxOs play a regulatory role in a number of physiologic processes that influence HSC numbers and function. Both aged germline FoxO3-deficient mice and conditional triple knockout (FoxO1, 3, 4) mice show a reduction in HSC numbers with a deficient repopulating capacity in competitive reconstitution assays and serial competitive transplantation assays (Tothova et al., 2007; Miyamoto et al., 2007). These phenotypes correlate with increased cell-cycling and apoptosis of HSCs, caused by increased levels of ROS. Furthermore, treatment with the antioxidant, N-acetyl-L-cysteine (NAC), rescues the FoxO-deficient HSC phenotype.

2.1.1.10 Fbxw7

Fbxw7 is the F-box protein subunit of an SCF-type ubiquitin ligase complex that targets positive regulators of the cell-cycle, including Notch, c-Myc, cyclin E, and c-Jun. Two independent groups investigated the functions of Fbxw7 in HSCs using conditional Fbxw7 knockout mice (Matsuoka et al., 2008; Thompson et al., 2008). Conditional ablation of Fbxw7 rapidly and severely affects hematopoietic progenitor maintenance within the BM. *Fbxw7-/-* HSCs show increased cycling and defective long-term repopulation capacity in competitive transplantation assays. As Fbxw7 is able to ubiquitinate several target proteins, studies were conducted to examine the protein expression of Notch1, c-Myc, and cyclin E. The results showed that c-Myc protein was substantially overexpressed in *Fbxw7-/-* HSCs, suggesting that the activation of the cell-cycle in Fbxw7-null HSCs induced by excess c-Myc causes the premature exhaustion of HSCs.

2.1.1.11 HIF-1α

Leukemic stem cells (LSCs) reside in the niches near epiphysis of the bone (Ishikawa et al., 2007) and oxygen concentration of this area is quite low. Thus, it may be very important for leukemic cells, especially for LSCs to survive and adapt to hypoxia (Takeuchi et al., 2010). Cellular responses to hypoxia are mediated by hypoxia-inducible factors (HIFs), which regulate gene expression to facilitate adaptation to hypoxic conditions (Kaelin & Ratcliffe., 2008). Hypoxia inducible factor-1α (HIF-1α) is stabilized under low-oxygen conditions, such as those present in the BM. Recently, two groups investigated the importance of hypoxia and its related signaling pathways in HSC function using different approaches (Simsek et al., 2010; Takubo et al., 2010). HIF-1α levels are elevated in adult HSCs and its transcription is regulated by the homeodomain protein Meis1, which is essential for hematopoiesis (Hisa et al., 2004; Simsek et al., 2010). HIF-1α conditional knockout mice show that HIF-1α–deficient HSCs have an increased cell cycling rate and show progressive loss of long-term repopulation ability in serial transplantation assays (Takubo et al., 2010). Taken together, these data indicate that the precise regulation of HIF-1α levels is required to maintain HSC quiescence.

2.1.1.12 Lkb1

The control of energy metabolism within HSCs is poorly understood, although they are highly sensitive to oxidative stress. Recently, several groups examined the role of the protein, Lkb1, in the metabolic regulation of HSCs (Nakada et al., 2010; Gurumurthy et al., 2010; Gan et al., 2010). Lkb1 is a kinase enzyme that regulates the activity of AMP-activated protein kinase (AMPK). Conditional inactivation of Lkb1 (*Mx1-Cre; LKB1$^{fl/fl}$* or *RosaCreERT2; LKB1$^{L/L}$*) in adult mice causes the loss of HSC quiescence, rapid HSC depletion, and pancytopenia. Interestingly, Lkb1 seems to regulate HSC homeostasis primarily through pathways that are independent of its downstream effectors, AMPK and mTORC1.

2.1.1.13 Cyclin-dependent kinase inhibitors

p21$^{cip1/waf1}$ (hereafter referred to as p21) is a mammalian member of the CIP/KIP family and was the first cyclin-dependent kinase inhibitor to be identified (Serrano et al., 1993; Harper et al., 1993; Stier et al., 2003). Serial transplantation assays using p21-deficient cells showed premature HSC exhaustion; also, p21-null mice were more sensitive to 5-FU (Cheng et al., 2000). These results suggest that p21 restricts HSC entry into the cell cycle and regulates the size of the HSC pool under conditions of stress. However, a later study demonstrated that p21 plays a minor role in regulating HSC quiescence under conditions of steady-state hematopoiesis (van Os et al., 2007).

Although p57^{kip2} (hereafter referred to as p57) is highly expressed in HSCs (Table 2) (Kubota et al., 2009; Umemoto et al., 2005), little is known about its functional role. Microarray analysis studies of human CD34+ HSC/progenitor cells identified p57 as the only cyclin-dependent kinase inhibitor induced by TGFβ (Scandura et al., 2004). Knockdown of p57 in hematopoietic cell lines using small interfering RNA (siRNA) results in more rapid proliferation of hematopoietic cells in the absence of TGF-β. These results suggest that p57 is required for the TGF-β–mediated cell cycle entry of hematopoietic cells and for repressing the proliferation of these cells.

Gene Name	Gene Symbol
Apoptosis	
serine (or cysteine) peptidase inhibitor, clade A, member 3G	Serpina3g
Cell surface	
adhesion molecule with Ig like domain 2	Amigo2
claudin 5	Cldn5
junction adhesion molecule 2	Jam2
vascular cell adhesion molecule 1	Vcam1
Cell Cycle Regulation	
cyclin-dependent kinase inhibitor 1C (P57)	Cdkn1c
Cell Signaling	
frizzled homolog 4 (Drosophila)	Fzd4
insulin-like growth factor 1	Igf1
interferon inducible GTPase 1	Iigp
multiple PDZ domain protein	Mpdz
nik related kinase	Nrk
regulator of G-protein signaling 4	Rgs4
ras homolog gene family, member J	Rhoj
suppressor of cytokine signaling 2	Socs2
Cellular Metabolism	
cytochrome P450, family 4, subfamily b, polypeptide 1	Cyp4b1
fatty acid binding protein 4, adipocyte	Fabp4
RIKEN cDNA 4432416J03 gene	4432416J03Rik
Endocytosis	
intersectin 1 (SH3 domain protein 1A)	Itsn
Extracellular	
bone morphogenetic protein 2	Bmp2
connective tissue growth factor	Ctgf
nidogen 1	Nid1
tissue factor pathway inhibitor	Tfpi
tissue inhibitor of metalloproteinase 3	Timp3
Transcription Factor	
forkhead box A3	Foxa3
kruppel-like factor 9	Klf9
myeloid/lymphoid or mixed lineage-leukemia translocation to 3 homolog (Drosophila)	Mllt3
necdin	Ndn
nuclear protein 1 (p8)	Nupr1
retinoid X receptor gamma	Rxrg
Unknown	
tripartite motif-containing 47	Trim47
RIKEN cDNA 2310051E17 gene	2310051E17Rik
RIKEN cDNA 2810432L12 gene	2810432L12Rik

Table 2. Genes expressed at higher levels in HSCs than in other subsets.

Genes showing at least 2-fold higher expression in CD34-/low KSL cells than in CD34+ KSL cells were selected by microarray analysis. The selected genes were then evaluated by Q-PCR, and genes whose transcripts were expressed at ≥ 2-foltd higher levels in CD34-/low KSL cells than all other samples are listed.

2.1.2 Negative regulation

2.1.2.1 E3 ubiquitin ligase

The E3 ubiquitin ligase, c-Cbl, is a member of the RING finger-type ubiquitin ligase Cbl (casitas B-cell lymphoma) family. The c-Cbl protein is thought to implement the degradation of various cellular proteins, receptors, and signaling molecules including Notch1, STAT5, and c-Kit (Jehn et al., 2002; Goh et al., 2002; Zeng et al., 2005). c-Cbl–deficient mice were used to study the role of c-Cbl in HSCs (Rathinam et al., 2008). The number of HSCs and progenitors was significantly higher in the BM of c-Cbl-null mice due to increased proliferation. Interestingly, detailed analyses revealed augmented STAT5 phosphorylation in c-Cbl-/- HSCs in response to TPO/c-MPL signaling which is crucial for the proliferation and self-renewal of HSCs (Kimura et al., 1998), and this led to enhanced c-Myc expression. C-Cbl–deficient HSCs also showed an increased repopulating ability in competitive reconstitution assays, including serial transplantation. These results suggest that c-Cbl acts as a negative regulator of both the size of the HSC pool and self-renewal (Rathinam et al., 2008).

Recently, Itch, another E3 ligase belonging to the HECT family (Bernassola et al., 2008), was also identified as a negative regulator of HSC homeostasis and function. The phenotype of $Itch$-/- HSCs was similar to that of c-Cbl-/- HSCs. However, unlike c-Cbl, Itch-deficient HSCs showed augmented Notch1 signaling. Furthermore, knockdown of Notch1 in Itch-null HSCs resulted in the reversion of the phenotype (Rathinam et al., 2011). Taken together, these studies underscore the pivotal roles of E3 ubiquitin ligases and the importance of post-translational modification of HSCs in the molecular control of HSC self-renewal.

2.1.2.2 Egr1

Egr1 is a member of the immediate early response gene family (Gashler et al., 1995). Egr1 is highly expressed in LT-HSCs under steady-state conditions and is downregulated upon proliferative stimulation and migration in response to pharmacological mobilization (Min et al., 2008). Egr1-deficient mice show a significant increase in the frequency of cycling HSCs. This phenomenon results in a slightly higher frequency of HSCs in the BM of $Egr1$-/- mice. Interestingly, loss of Egr1 results in a striking increase (up to 10-fold) in the number of circulating HSCs. Importantly, HSCs isolated from both the BM and peripheral blood of $Egr1$-/- mice show a greater degree of long-term multi-lineage repopulation after transplantation, although their life span is slightly reduced. Quantitative RT-PCR analysis shows that Bmi1 is upregulated in $Egr1$-/- HSCs. In addition, $Egr1$-/- HSCs also show the downregulation of p21[CIP1/WAF1] and increased expression of cyclin-dependent kinase 4 (cdk4), which is consistent with their increased cell-cycling status (Min et al., 2008). Taken together, the deletion of Egr1 causes an increase in the number of cycling HSCs but does not lead to stem cell exhaustion. This may be due to Bmi1 upregulation.

2.1.2.3 Lnk

Lnk is a member of an adaptor protein family that possesses a number of protein-protein interaction domains: a proline-rich amino-terminus, a pleckstrin homology (PH) domain, a Src homology 2 (SH2) domain, and many potential tyrosine phosphorylation motifs (Rudd., 2001). Studies using Lnk-deficient mice show that Lnk-null HSCs are expanded during post-natal development (Ema et al., 2005; Buza-Vidas et al., 2006). The Lnk-/- HSC population contains an increased proportion of quiescent cells and shows decelerated cell cycle kinetics and enhanced resistance to repeat treatment with 5-FU *in vivo* compared with wild-type HSCs. Genetic evidence demonstrates that Lnk controls HSC self-renewal and quiescence, predominantly through c-Mpl. Furthermore, Lnk-deficient HSCs show higher levels of symmetric proliferation in response to thrombopoietin (TPO) in *ex vivo* culture than wild-type HSCs (Seita et al., 2007). Biochemical analyses revealed that Lnk directly binds to phosphorylated tyrosine residues in JAK2 after TPO stimulation (Bersenev et al., 2008). Therefore, Lnk is a physiologic negative regulator of JAK2 in HSCs, and TPO/c-Mpl/JAK2/Lnk constitute a major regulatory pathway controlling HSC quiescence and self-renewal.

2.1.2.4 Myc

Human c-MYC was the second proto-oncogene to be identified and encodes a basic helix-loop-helix leucine zipper transcription factor (c-Myc) (Sheiness et al., 1978). Overexpression of one of the three family members has been detected in numerous human cancers including Burkitt's lymphoma (c-MYC), neuroblastoma (N-MYC), and small cell lung cancer (L-MYC) (Nesbit et al., 1999). Conditional deletion of c-Myc in the BM results in cytopenia and the accumulation of functionally defective HSCs. In the absence of c-Myc, HSC differentiation into more committed progenitors is inhibited because they upregulate a number of adhesion molecules, such as N-cadherin, that anchor them in the niche. Conversely, enforced c-Myc expression in HSCs causes marked repression of N-cadherin and integrin expression leading to the loss of self-renewal ability at the expense of differentiation (Wilson et al., 2004). These results suggest that c-Myc activity controls the first differentiation step of LT-HSCs *in vivo*. Unexpectedly, conditional ablation of both c-myc and N-myc results in pancytopenia and rapid lethality due to HSC apoptosis via the accumulation of the cytotoxic molecule, Granzyme B (Laurenti et al., 2008). Thus, Myc activity controls important aspects of HSC function such as proliferation, survival and differentiation.

2.1.2.5 MEF/ELF4

MEF (also known as ELF4), an Ets transcription factor, was identified as a novel component of the transcriptional circuit that dynamically regulates HSC quiescence (Lacorazza et al., 2006). Mef-deficient HSCs grow more slowly than wild-type HSCs in response to cytokine stimulation Pyronin Y staining and BrdU incorporation show increased quiescence. Enhanced HSC quiescence in Mef-null mice also increases HSC resistance to cytotoxic agents that target dividing cells and allows more rapid hematological recovery after chemotherapy or irradiation. These findings suggest that Mef normally functions to induce or facilitate the entry of quiescent HSCs into the cell cycle and imply that Mef expression and/or activity may be dynamically regulated in HSCs. To explain this, Lacorazza et al. proposed a model in which Mef acts at an earlier stage than p18 and antagonizes p21.

2.2 Survival of HSCs

HSC self-renewal and apoptosis represent major factors that determine the size of the HSC mass. The number of HSCs is also controlled by their capacity to survive during homeostasis or under conditions of stress.

2.2.1 Bcl-2 family

Accumulating evidence suggests that the suppression of apoptosis is required for HSC survival. Forced expression of Bcl-2 increases the number of HSCs and provides them with enhanced competitive repopulation ability (Domen et al., 1998, 2000), suggesting that cell death plays a role in regulating HSC homeostasis.

Mcl-1, another anti-apoptotic Bcl-2 family member, is also an essential regulator of HSC survival. Mcl-1 is highly expressed in LT-HSCs, and conditional deletion of MCl-1 results in the loss of the early BM progenitor population, including HSCs, leading to fatal hematopoietic failure (Opferman et al., 2005). Recently, it was reported that Mcl-1 is an indispensable regulator of self-renewal in human stem cells and that functional dependence on Mcl-1 defines the human stem cell hierarchy (Campbell et al., 2010).

2.2.2 Scl, Lyl1

Scl/Tal1 is a basic helix-loop-helix (bHLH) transcription factor that is essential for the development of HSCs in the embryo (Robb et al., 1995; Shivdasani et al., 1995). During adult hematopoiesis, Scl/Tal1 is highly expressed in LT-HSCs compared with short-term HSCs and progenitor cells (Lacombe et al., 2010). However, a study using conditional Scl/Tal1 knockout mice revealed that Scl/Tal1 is required for the generation of, but not the maintenance of, adult HSCs (Mikkola et al., 2003). Another group showed that conditional deletion of Scl/Tal1 in adult HSCs has a relatively mild effect: Scl-null HSCs show impaired short-term repopulating ability, but no defect in long-term repopulating capacity (Curtis et al., 2004). Redundant activity caused by the expression of Lyl1, a related bHLH transcription factor, in adult HSCs may provide an explanation for these "mild" phenotypes. While adult HSCs in single-knockout mice show no or only a mild phenotype, Lyl1;Scl-conditional double-knockout mice show a gene dosage defect on HSC survival, as HSCs and progenitor cells are immediately lost due to apoptosis (Souroullas et al., 2009).

Recently, Lacombe et al. demonstrated that Scl/Tal1 is required for the maintenance of the quiescent stem cell pool (Lacombe et al., 2010). Cell-cycle analyses revealed that Scl/Tal1 negatively regulates the G0-G1 transit of LT-HSCs; however, these phenomena were specific to adult HSCs and were not observed in perinatal HSCs. The reconstituting ability of $Scl^{+/-}$ HSCs or HSCs with decreased Scl protein expression induced by RNA interference was impaired in various transplantation assays. Furthermore, gene expression analysis and chromatin immunoprecipitation experiments revealed that the Cdkn1a and Id1 genes are direct SCL targets.

2.2.3 Tel/Etv6

The transcription factor Tel (also known as Etv6), an Ets-related transcriptional repressor, is a frequent target of the diverse chromosomal translocations observed in leukemias (Golub et al., 1994). Tel/ETV6 is also required for HSC survival in adult hematopoiesis. Following conditional inactivation of Tel/Etv6, HSCs are rapidly lost from the adult BM. However, Tel/Etv6 is not required for the maintenance of lineage-committed progenitors. Conditional deletion of Tel/Etv6 after lineage commitment does not affect the differentiation or survival of these progenitors, although it does impair the maturation of megakaryocytes (Hock et al., 2004).

2.2.4 Zfx

Zfx is a zinc finger protein belonging to the Zfx/ZFy family. Mammalian Zfx is encoded on the X chromosome and contains an acidic transcriptional activation domain, a nuclear localization sequence, and a DNA binding protein domain consisting of 13 C2H2-type zinc fingers (Schneider-Gadicke et al., 1989). Zfx is highly expressed in both HSCs and undifferentiated embryonic stem cells (ESCs). Using conditional gene targeting, Zfx was identified as an essential transcriptional regulator of HSC function (Galan-Caridad et al., 2007). Constitutive or inducible deletion of Zfx in HSCs (using *Tie2-Cre* and *Mx1-Cre* deletion strains, respectively) impairs self-renewal, resulting in increased apoptosis and the upregulation of stress-inducible genes.

2.2.5 ADAR1

ADAR (adenosine deaminase acting on RNA) catalyzes the deamination of adenosine to inosine in double-stranded RNA. Conventional *Adar-/-* mice die around embryonic day 11.5–12 because of widespread apoptosis and defective hematopoiesis (Hartner et al., 2004; Wang et al., 2004). Conditional deletion of Adar in HSCs shows that ADAR1 is essential for the maintenance of both fetal and adult HSCs, and leads to global upregulation of type I and II interferon-inducible transcripts and rapid apoptosis (Hartner et al., 2009). Interferon regulatory factor-2 (Irf2), a transcriptional suppressor of type I interferon signaling, is a positive regulator of HSC quiescence (Sato et al., 2009). Irf2-deficient HSCs are unable to restore hematopoiesis in irradiated mice, but the reconstituting capacity of *Irf2-/-* HSCs can be restored in these cells by disabling type I IFN signaling.

2.3 Response to hematopoietic emergency

Various external stresses, such as myelosuppressive chemotherapy, bleeding, infection, and total body irradiation, put HSCs under stress, as they must proliferate to produce large numbers of primitive progenitor cells, thereby enabling rapid hematologic regeneration. Although this property has long been recognized, the molecular basis underlying the reaction of HSCs to hematologic emergency remains enigmatic. However, some key players have been identified.

2.3.1 Heme oxygenase-1

Heme promotes the proliferation and differentiation of hematopoietic progenitor cells (HPCs) (Chertkov et al., 1991) and stimulates hematopoiesis (Porter et al., 1979; Abraham, 1991). The degradation of heme is catalyzed by heme oxygenase (HO). HO-1, encoded by the *Hmox1* gene, is the stress-inducible isozyme of HO and is highly expressed in the spleen and BM (Abraham, 1991). Heterozygous HO-1–deficient mice (*HO-1+/-*) show accelerated hematologic recovery from myelotoxic injury induced by 5-FU treatment, and mice transplanted with *HO-1+/-* BM cells show more rapid hematopoietic repopulation than those transplanted with *Ho-1+/+* BM cells. However, *HO-1+/-* HSCs show a reduced capacity to rescue lethally irradiated mice and to serially repopulate irradiated recipients (Cao et al., 2008). These results suggest that HO-1 limits the proliferation and differentiation of HPCs under stressful conditions, and that the failure of this mechanism can lead to the premature exhaustion of the HSC pool.

2.3.2 Necdin

Necdin is a member of the melanoma antigen family of molecules, whose physiological roles have not been well characterized (Xiao et al., 2004). Necdin acts as a cell cycle regulator in post-mitotic neurons (Yoshikawa, 2000). Intriguingly, recent genetic analyses show that aberrant genomic imprinting of *NDN* on the human 15q11-q13 chromosomal region is, at least in part, responsible for the pathogenesis of Prader-Willi syndrome (MacDonald & Wevrick, 1997; Nakada et al., 1998; Barker et al., 2002), a disorder associated with a mildly increased risk of myeloid leukemia (Davies et al., 2003). Necdin interacts with multiple cell-cycle related proteins, such as SV-40 large T antigen, adenovirus E1A, E2F1, and p53 (Taniura et al., 1998, 1999, 2005; Hu et al., 2003). As shown in Table 2, necdin is one of 32 genes that show higher expression in HSCs than in differentiated hematopoietic cells (Kubota et al., 2009). Other groups also found that necdin is highly expressed in HSCs (Forsberg et al., 2005; Liu et al., 2009). Necdin-deficient mice show accelerated recovery of hematopoietic systems after myelosuppressive stress, such as 5-FU treatment and BM transplantation, whereas no overt abnormality is seen under conditions of steady-state hematopoiesis. Considering necdin as a potential negative cell-cycle regulator, it was reasoned that the enhanced hematologic recovery in necdin-null mice could be the result of an increased number of proliferating HSCs and progenitor cells. As expected, after 5-FU treatment, necdin-deficient mice had an increased number of HSCs, but this was only transiently observed during the recovery phase (Kubota et al., 2009). These data suggest that the repression of necdin function in HSCs may present a novel strategy for accelerating hematopoietic recovery, thus providing therapeutic benefits after clinical myelosuppressive treatments (e.g., cytoablative chemotherapy or HSC transplantation).

2.3.3 Slug

Slug belongs to the highly conserved Slug/Snail family of zinc-finger transcriptional repressors found in diverse species ranging from *C. elegans* to humans. SLUG is a target gene for the E2A-HLF chimeric oncoprotein in pro-B cell acute leukemia (Inukai et al., 1999). Slug-deficient mice show normal peripheral blood counts, but they are very sensitive to γ-irradiation (Inoue et al., 2002). Slug is induced by p53 and protects primitive hematopoietic cells from apoptosis triggered by DNA damage. Slug exerts this function by repressing Puma, a proapoptotic target of p53 (Wu et al., 2005). Sun et al. recently showed that Slug negatively regulates the repopulating ability of HSCs under conditions of stress. Slug deficiency increases HSC proliferation and reconstitution potential *in vivo* after myelosuppressive treatment, and accelerates HSC expansion during *in vitro* culture (Sun et al., 2010).

3. Cancer stem cells

Accumulating evidence strongly suggests that tumors are organized into cellular hierarchies initiated and maintained by a small pool of self-renewing cancer stem cells (CSCs) (Dick, 2008; Reya et al., 2001). CSCs are thought to be resistant to various cancer treatments because of their relative quiescence (Komarova & Wodarz., 2007). Cancer relapses may occur because the dormancy of CSCs protects them from elimination by various cancer therapies (Dick, 2008). In an acute myelogenous leukemia (AML) xenograft model, AML leukemic stem cells (LSCs) localized in the endosteal region of the BM show cellular quiescence and resistance to chemotherapy (Ishikawa et al., 2007; Saito et al., 2010). In patients with chronic myelogenous leukemia (CML), CD34+ progenitor cells contain dormant cells that are resistant to BCR/ABL tyrosine kinase inhibitors (Bhatia et al., 2003).

It is well documented that regulators of HSC maintenance are also involved in the development of leukemias (Rizo et al., 2006). A number of cancer-related proteins, such as Bmi1, c-Myc, p53, Gfi-1, and PTEN, are key participants in HSC regulation, demonstrating the close relationship between normal HSCs and CSCs. Therefore, further understanding the mechanisms regulating HSC fate is needed if we are to develop new strategies for targeting CSCs and successfully treat cancer.

4. Conclusions

In this review, we have briefly summarized a number of critical regulators involved in the control of HSC self-renewal, quiescence, survival, and responses to external insults. Recent evidence strongly suggests that the BM niche also plays an integral role by providing critical signals that maintain HSCs in a stat of hibernation, thus preventing them from exhausting themselves. However, HSCs are critical for the maintenance and regeneration of an organism after injury/illness. This process must be tightly regulated and coordinated. Intensive studies have uncovered the molecular signatures and key molecules regulating HSC behavior. Moreover, new systems approaches, such as microRNA expression profiling and protein expression profiling, are expected to provide further useful information about HSC biology in the future. However, the overall picture of the molecular mechanisms that govern HSC fate is still unclear. Further understanding of the systems that regulate HSCs will enable the manipulation of stem cells for use in tissue engineering and cell-based therapies.

5. Acknowledgments

This work was supported by a Grant-in-Aid for Young Scientists to Y.K. (no. 23791083) from the Ministry of Education, Culture, Sports, Science and Technology (MEXT), Japan.

6. References

Abraham, N.G. (1991) Molecular regulation--biological role of heme in hematopoiesis. *Blood Rev* 5(1):19-28.
Akashi, K., Traver, D., Miyamoto, T., & Weissman, I.L. (2000) A clonogenic common myeloid progenitor that gives rise to all myeloid lineages. *Nature* 404(6774):193-197.
Akashi, K., He, X., Chen, J., Iwasaki, H., Niu, C., Steenhard, B., Zhang, J., Haug, J., & Li, L. (2003) Transcriptional accessibility for genes of multiple tissues and hematopoietic lineages is hierarchically controlled during early hematopoiesis. *Blood* 101(2):383-389.
Barker, P.A., & Salehi, A. (2002) The MAGE proteins: emerging roles in cell cycle progression, apoptosis, and neurogenetic disease. *J Neurosci Res* 67(6):705-712.

Bernassola, F., Karin, M., Ciechanover, A., & Melino, G. (2008) The HECT family of E3 ubiquitin ligases: multiple players in cancer development. *Cancer Cell* 14(1):10-21.

Bersenev, A., Wu, C., Balcerek, J., & Tong, W. (2008) Lnk controls mouse hematopoietic stem cell self-renewal and quiescence through direct interactions with JAK2. *J Clin Invest* 118(8):2832-2844.

Bhatia, R., Holtz, M., Niu, N., Gray, R., Snyder, D.S., Sawyers, C.L., Arber, D.A., Slovak, M.L., & Forman, S.J. (2003) Persistence of malignant hematopoietic progenitors in chronic myelogenous leukemia patients in complete cytogenetic remission following imatinib mesylate treatment. *Blood* 101(12):4701-4707.

Buza-Vidas, N., Antonchuk, J., Qian, H., Månsson, R.,Luc, S., Zandi, S., Anderson, K., Takaki, S., Nygren, J.M., Jensen, C.T., & Jacobsen S.E. (2006) Cytokines regulate postnatal hematopoietic stem cell expansion: opposing roles of thrombopoietin and LNK. *Genes Dev* 20(15):2018-2023.

Campbell, C.J.V., Lee, J.B., Levadoux-Martin, M., Wynder, T., Xenocostas, A., Leber, B., & Bhatia, M. (2010) The human stem cell hierarchy is defined by a functional dependence on Mcl-1 for self-renewal capacity. *Blood* 116(9):1433-1442.

Cao, Y.A., Wagers, A.J., Karsunky, H., Zhao, H., Reeves, R., Wong, R.J., Stevenson, D.K., Weissman, I.L., & Contag, C.H. (2008) Heme oxygenase-1 deficiency leads to disrupted response to acute stress in stem cells and progenitors. *Blood* 112(12):4494-4502.

Chambers, S.M., Boles, N.C., Lin, K.Y., Tierney, M.P., Bowman, T.V., Bradfute, S.B., Chen, A.J., Merchant, A.A., Sirin, O., Weksberg, D.C., Merchant, M.G., Fisk, C.J., Shaw, C.A., & Goodell, M.A. (2007) Hematopoietic fingerprints: an expression database of stem cells and their progeny. *Cell Stem Cell* 1(5): 578-591.

Chen, J., Ellison, F.M., Keyvanfar, K., Omokaro, S.O., Desierto, M.J., Eckhaus, M.A., & Young, N.S. (2008) Enrichment of hematopoietic stem cells with SLAM and LSK markers for the detection of hematopoietic stem cell function in normal and Trp53 null mice. *Exp Hematol* 36(10):1236-1243.

Cheng, T., Rodrigues, N., Shen, H., Yang, Y., Dombkowski, D., Sykes, M., & Scadden D.T. (2000) Hematopoietic stem cell quiescence maintained by p21$^{cip1/waf1}$. *Science* 287(5459):1804-1808.

Chertkov, J.L., Jiang, S., Lutton, J.D., Levere, R.D., & Abraham, N.G. (1991) Hemin stimulation of hemopoiesis in murine long-term bone marrow culture. *Exp Hematol* 19(9):905-909.

Cheshier, S.H., Morrison, S.J., Liao, X., & Weissman, I.L. In vivo proliferation and cell cycle kinetics of long-term self-renewing hematopoietic stem cells. (1999) *Proc Natl Acad Sci U S A* 96(6):3120-3125.

Curtis, D.J., Hall, M.A., Van Stekelenberg, L.J., Robb, L., Jane, S.M., & Begley, C.G. (2004) SCL is required for normal function of short-term repopulating hematopoietic stem cells. *Blood* 103(9):3342-3348.

Davies, H.D., Leusink, G.L., McConnell, A., Deyell, M., Cassidy, S.B., Fick, G.H., & Coppes, M.J. (2003) Myeloid leukemia in Prader-Willi syndrome. *J Pediatr* 142(2):174-178.

Dick, J.E. (2008) Stem cell concepts renew cancer research. *Blood* 112(13):4793-4807.

DiMartino, J.F., Selleri, L., Traver, D., Firpo, M.T., Rhee, J., Warnke, R., O'Gorman, S., Weissman, I.L., & Cleary, M.L. (2001) The Hox cofactor and protooncogene Pbx1 is required for maintenance of definitive hematopoiesis in the fetal liver. *Blood* 98:618-626.

Domen, J., Gandy, K.L., & Weissman, I.L. (1998) Systemic overexpression of BCL-2 in the hematopoietic system protects transgenic mice from the consequences of lethal irradiation. *Blood* 91(7):2272-2282.

Domen, J., Cheshier, S.H., & Weissman, I.L. (2000) The role of apoptosis in the regulation of hematopoietic stem cells: Overexpression of Bcl-2 increases both their number and repopulation potential. *J Exp Med* 191(2):253-264.

Dumble, M., Moore, L., Chambers, S.M., Geiger, H., Zant, G.V., Goodell, M.A. & Donehower, L.A. (2007) The impact of altered p53 dosage on hematopoieitic stem cell dynamics during aging. *Blood* 109(4):1736-1742.

Ema, H., Sudo, K., Seita, J., Matsubara, A., Morita, Y., Osawa, M., Takatsu, K., Takaki, S., & Nakauchi, H. (2005) Quantification of self-renewal capacity in single hematopoietic stem cells from normal and Lnk-deficient mice. *Dev Cell* 8(6):907-914.

Ficara, F., Murphy, M.J., Lin, M., & Cleary, M.L. (2008) Pbx1 regulates self-renewal of long-term hematopoietic stem cells by maintaining their quiescence. *Cell Stem Cell* 2(5):484-496.

Forsberg, E.C., Prohaska, S.S., Katzman, S., Heffner, G.C., Stuart, J.M., & Weissman, I.L. (2005) Differential expression of novel potential regulators in hematopoietic stem cells. *PLoS Genet* 1(3):e28.

Galan-Caridad, J.M., Harel, S., Arenzana, T.L., Hou, Z.E., Doetsch, F.K., Mirny, L.A., & Reizis, B. (2007) Zfx controls the self-renewal of embryonic and hematopoietic stem cells. *Cell* 129(2):345-357.

Gan, B., Hu, J., Jiang, S., Liu, Y., Sahin, E., Zhuang, L., Fletcher-Sananikone, E., Colla, S., Wang, Y.A., Chin, L., & Depinho, R.A. (2010) Lkb1 regulates quiescence and metabolic homeostasis of haematopoietic stem cells. *Nature* 468(7324):701-704.

Gashler, A., & Sukhatme, V.P. (1995) Early growth response protein 1 (Egr-1): prototype of a zinc-finger family of transcription factors. *Prog Nucleic Acid Res Mol Biol* 50:191-224.

Gilks, C.B., Bear, S.E., Grimes, H.L., & Tsichlis, P.N. (1993) Progression of interleukin-2 (IL-2)-dependent rat T cell lymphoma lines to IL-2-independent growth following activation of a gene (Gfi-1) encoding a novel zinc finger protein. *Mol Cell Biol* 13(3): 1759-1768.

Golub,T.R., Barker, G.F., Lovett, M., & Gilliland, D.G. (1994) Fusion of PDGF receptor β to a novel ets-like gene, tel, in chronic myelomonocytic leukemia with t(5;12) chromosomal translocation. *Cell* 77(2): 307-316.

Goh, E.L., Zhu, T., Leong, W.Y., & Lobie, P.E. (2002) c-Cbl is a negative regulator of GH-stimulated STAT5-mediated transcription. *Endocrinology* 143(9):3590-3603.

Goyama, S., Yamamoto, G., Shimabe, M., Sato, T., Ichikawa, M., Ogawa, S., Chiba, S., & Kurokawa, M. (2008) Evi-1 is a critical regulator for hematopoietic stem cells and transformed leukemic cells. *Cell Stem Cell* 3(2):207-220.

Greer, E.L., & Brunet, A. (2005) FOXO transcription factors at the interface between longevity and tumor suppression. *Oncogene* 24(50):7410-7425.

Gurumurthy, S., Xie, S.Z., Alagesan, B., Kim, J., Yusuf, R.Z., Saez, B., Tzatsos, A., Ozsolak, F., Milos, P., Ferrari, F., Park, P.J., Shirihai, O.S., Scadden, D.T., & Bardeesy, N. (2010) The Lkb1 metabolic sensor maintains haematopoietic stem cell survival. *Nature* 468(7324):659-663.

Harper, J.W., Adami, G.R., Wei, N., Keyomarsi, K., & Elledge, S.J. (1993) The p21 Cdk-interacting protein Cip1 is a potent inhibitor of G1 cyclin-dependent kinases. *Cell* 75(4):805-816.

Hartner, J.C., Schmittwolf, C., Kispert, A., Müller, A.M., Higuchi, M., & Seeburg, P.H. (2004) Liver disintegration in the mouse embryo caused by deficiency in the RNA-editing enzyme ADAR1. *J Biol Chem* 279(6):4894-4902.

Hartner,J.C., Walkley, C.R., Lu, J., & Orkin, S.H. (2009) ADAR1 is essential for the maintenance of hematopoiesis and suppression of interferon signaling. *Nat Immunol* 10(1):109-115.

Hisa, T., Spence, S.E., Rachel, R.A., Fujita, M., Nakamura, T., Ward, J.M., Devor-Henneman, D.E., Saiki, Y., Kutsuna, H., Tessarollo, L., Jenkins, N.A., & Copeland, N.G. (2004) Hematopoietic, angiogenic and eye defects in Meis1 mutant animals. *EMBO J* 23(2):450-459.

Hock, H., Meade, E., Medeiros, S., Schindler, J.W., Valk, P.J.M., Fujiwara, Y., & Orkin, S.H. (2004) Tel/Etv6 is an essential and selective regulator of adult hematopoietic stem cell survival. *Genes Dev* 18(19):2336-2341.

Hock, H., Hamblen, M.J., Rooke, H.M., Schindler, J.W., Saleque, S., Fujiwara, Y., & Orkin, S.H. (2004) Gfi-1 restricts proliferation and preserves functional integrity of haematopoietic stem cells. *Nature* 431(7011):1002-1007.

Hu, B., Wang, S., Zhang, Y., Feghali, C.A., Dingman, J.R., & Wright, T.M. (2003) A nuclear target for interleukin-1alpha: interaction with the growth suppressor necdin modulates proliferation and collagen expression. *Proc Natl Acad Sci U S A* 100(17):10008-10013.

Inoue, A., Seidel, M.G., Wu, W., Kamizono, S., Ferrando, A.A., Bronson, R.T., Iwasaki, H., Akashi, K., Morimoto, A., Hitzler, J.K., Pestina, T.I., Jackson, C.W., Tanaka, R., Chong, M.J., McKinnon, P.J., Inukai, T., Grosveld, G.C., & Look, A.T. (2002) Slug, a highly conserved zinc finger transcriptional repressor, protects hematopoietic progenitor cells from radiation-induced apoptosis in vivo. *Cancer Cell* 2(4):279-288.

Inukai, T., Inoue, A., Kurosawa, H., Goi, K., Shinjyo,T., Ozawa, K., Mao, M., Inaba, T., & Look, A.T. (1999) SLUG, a ces-1-related zinc finger transcription factor gene with antiapoptotic activity, is a downstream target of the E2A-HLF oncoprotein. *Mol Cell* 4(3):343-352.

Ishikawa, F., Yoshida, S., Saito, Y., Hijikata, A., Kitamura, H., Tanaka, S., Nakamura, R., Tanaka, T., Tomiyama, H., Saito, N., Fukata, M., Miyamoto, T., Lyons, B., Ohshima, K., Uchida, N., Taniguchi, S., Ohara, O., Akashi, K., Harada, M., & Shultz, L.D. (2007) Chemotherapy-resistant human AML stem cells home to and engraft within the bone-marrow endosteal region. *Nat Biotechnol* 25(11):1315-1321.

Ivanova, N.B., Dimos, J.T., Schaniel, C., Hackney, J.A., Moore, K.A., & Lemischka, I.R. (2002) A stem cell molecular signature. *Science* 298(5593):601-604.

Iwama, A., Oguro, H., Negishi, M., Kato, Y., Morita, Y., Tsukui, H., Ema, H., Kamijo, T., Katoh-Fukui, Y., Koseki, H., van Lohuizen, M., & Nakauchi, H. (2004) Enhanced self-renewal of hematopoietic stem cells mediated by the polycomb gene product Bmi-1. *Immunity* 21(6):843-851.

Jacobs, J.J.L., Kieboom, K., Marino, S., DePinho, R.A., & van Lohuizen, M. (1999) The oncogene and Polycomb-group gene bmi1 regulates proliferation and senescence through the ink4a locus. *Nature* 397(6715):164-168.

Jehn, B.M., Dittert, I., Beyer, S., von der Mark, K., & Bielke, W. (2002) c-Cbl binding and ubiquitin-dependent lysosomal degradation of membrane-associated Notch1. *J Biol Chem* 277(10):8033-8040.

Kaelin, W.G., Jr., & Ratcliffe, P.J. (2008) Oxygen sensing by metazoans: the central role of the HIF hydroxylase pathway. *Mol Cell* 30(4):393-402.

Kastan, M.B., Radin, A.I., Kuerbitz, S.J., Onyekwere, O., Wolkow, C.A., Civin, C.I., Stone, K.D., Woo, T., Ravindranath, Y., & Craig, R.W. (1991) Levels of p53 protein increase with maturation in human hematopoietic cells. *Cancer Res* 51(16):4279-4286.

Kiel, M.J., Yilmaz, O.H., Iwashita, T., Yilmaz, O.H., Terhorst, C., & Morrison, S.J. (2005) SLAM family receptors distinguish hematopoietic stem and progenitor cells and reveal endothelial niches for stem cells. *Cell* 121(7):1109-1121.

Kimura, S., Roberts, A.W., Metcalf, D., & Alexander, W.S. (1998) Hematopoietic stem cell deficiencies in mice lacking c-Mpl, the receptor for thrombopoietin. *Proc Natl Acad Sci USA* 95(3):1195-1200.

Komarova, N.L., & Wodarz, D. (2007) Effect of cellular quiescence on the success of targeted CML therapy. *PLoS One* 2(10):e990.

Kondo, M., Wagers, A.J., Manz, M.G., Prohaska, S.S., Scherer, D.C., Beilhack, G.F., Shizuru, J.A., & Weissman, I.L. (2003) Biology of hematopoietic stem cells and progenitors: implications for clinical application. *Annu Rev Immunol* 21:759-806.

Kubota, Y., Osawa, M., Jakt, L.M., Yoshikawa, K., & Nishikawa, S-I. (2009) Necdin restricts proliferation of hematopoietic stem cells during hematopoietic regeneration. *Blood* 114(20):4383-4392.

Lacombe, J., Herblot, S., Rojas-Sutterlin, S., Haman, A., Barakat, S., Iscove, N.N., Sauvageau, G., & Hoang, T. (2010) Scl regulates the quiescence and the long-term competence of hematopoietic stem cells. *Blood* 115(4):792-803.

Lacorazza, H.D., Yamada, T., Liu, Y., Miyata, Y., Sivina, M., Nunes, J., & Nimer, S.D. (2006) The transcription factor MEF/ELF4 regulates the quiescence of primitive hematopoietic cells. *Cancer Cell* 9(3):175-187.

Laurenti, E., Varnum-Finney, B., Wilson, A., Ferrero, I., Blanco-Bose, W.E., Ehninger, A., Knoepfler, P.S., Cheng, P.F., MacDonald, H.R., Eisenman, R.N., Bernstein, I.D., & Trumpp, A. (2008) Hematopoietic stem cell function and survival depend on c-Myc and N-Myc activity. *Cell Stem Cell* 3(6):611-624.

Liu, Y., Elf, S.E., Miyata, Y., Sashida, G., Liu, Y., Huang, G., Di Giandomenico, S., Lee, J.M., Deblasio, A., Menendez, S., Antipin, J., Reva, B., Koff, A., & Nimer, S.D. (2009) p53 regulates hematopoietic stem cell quiescence. *Cell Stem Cell* 4(1):37-48.

Lotem, J., & Sachs, L. (1993) Hematopoietic cells from mice deficient in wild-type p53 are more resistant to induction of apoptosis by some agents. *Blood* 82(4):1092-1096.

MacDonald, H.R. & Wevrick, R. (1997) The necdin gene is deleted in Prader-Willi syndrome and is imprinted in human and mouse. *Hum Mol Genet* 6(11):1873-1878.

Matsuoka, S., Oike, Y., Onoyama, I., Iwama, A., Arai, F., Takubo, K., Mashimo, Y., Oguro, H., Nitta, E., Ito, K., Miyamoto, K., Yoshiwara, H., Hosokawa, K., Nakamura, Y., Gomei, Y., Iwasaki, H., Hayashi, Y., Matsuzaki, Y., Nakayama, K., Ikeda, Y., Hata, A., Chiba, S., Nakayama, K.I., & Suda, T. (2008) Fbxw7 acts as a critical fail-safe against premature loss of hematopoietic stem cells and development of T-ALL. *Genes Dev* 22(8):986-991.

Mikkola, H.K., Klintman, J., Yang, H., Hock, H., Schlaeger, T.M., Fujiwara, Y., & Orkin, S.H. (2003) Haematopoietic stem cells retain long-term repopulating activity and multipotency in the absence of stem-cell leukaemia SCL/tal-1 gene. *Nature* 421(6922):547-551.

Min, I.M., Pietramaggiori, G., Kim, F.S., Passegué, E., Stevenson, K.E., & Wagers, A.J. (2008) The transcription factor EGR1 controls both the proliferation and localization of hematopoietic stem cells. *Cell Stem Cell* 2(4):380-391.

Miyamoto, K., Araki, K.Y., Naka, K., Arai, F., Takubo, K., Yamazaki, S., Matsuoka, S., Miyamoto, T., Ito, K., Ohmura, M., Chen, C., Hosokawa, K., Nakauchi, H., Nakayama, K., Nakayama, K.I., Harada, M., Motoyama, N., Suda, T., & Hirao, A. (2007) Foxo3a is essential for maintenance of the hematopoietic stem cell pool. *Cell Stem Cell* 1(1):101-112.

Morishita, K., Parker, D.S., Mucenski, M.L., Jenkins, N.A., Copeland, N.G., & Ihle, J.N. (1988) Retroviral activation of a novel gene encoding a zinc finger protein in IL-3-dependent myeloid leukemia cell lines. *Cell* 54(6):831-840.

Mucenski, M.L., Taylor, B.A., Ihle, J.N., Hartley, J.W., Morse, H.C., Jenkins, N.A., Copeland, N.G. (1988) Identification of a common ecotropic viral integration site, Evi-1, in the DNA of AKXD murine myeloid tumors. *Mol Cell Biol* 8(1):310-308.

Nakada, D., Saunders, T.L., & Morrison, S.J. (2010) Lkb1 regulates cell cycle and energy metabolism in haematopoietic stem cells. *Nature* 468(7324):653-658.

Nakada, Y., Taniura, H., Uetsuki, T., Inazawa, J., & Yoshikawa, K. (1998) The human chromosomal gene for necdin, a neuronal growth suppressor, in the Prader-Willi syndrome deletion region. *Gene* 213(1-2):65-72.

Nesbit, C.E., Tersak, J.M., & Prochownik, E.V. (1999) MYC oncogenes and human neoplastic disease. *Oncogene* 18(19):3004-3016.

Oguro, H., Iwama, A., Morita, Y., Kamijo, T., van Lohuizen, M., & Nakauchi, H. (2006) Differential impact of *Ink4a* and *Arf* on hematopoietic stem cells and their bone marrow microenvironment in *Bmi1*-deficient mice. *J Exp Med* 203(10):2247-2253.

Opferman, J.T., Iwasaki, H., Ong, C.C., Suh, H., Mizuno, S., Akashi, K., & Korsmeyer, S.J. (2005) Obligate role of anti-apoptotic MCL-1 in the survival of hematopoietic stem cells. *Science* 307(5712):1101-1104.

Orford, K.W., & Scadden, D.T. (2008) Deconstructing stem cell self-renewal: genetic insights into cell-cycle regulation. *Nat Rev Genet* 9(2):115-128.

Osawa, M., Hanada, K., Hamada, H., & Nakauchi, H. (1996) Long-term lymphohematopoietic reconstitution by a single CD34-low/negative hematopoietic stem cell. *Science* 273(5272):242-245.

Park, I.K., He, Y., Lin, F., Laerum, O.D., Tian, Q., Bumgarner, R., Klug, C.A., Li, K., Kuhr, C., Doyle, M.J., Xie, T., Schummer, M., Sun, Y., Goldsmith, A., Clarke, M.F., Weissman, I.L., Hood, L., & Li, L. (2002) Differential gene expression profiling of adult murine hematopoietic stem cells. *Blood* 99(2):488-498.

Park, I.K., Qian, D., Kiel, M., Becker, M.W., Pihalja, M., Weissman, I.L., Morrison, S.J., & Clarke, M.F. (2003) Bmi-1 is required for maintenance of adult self-renewing haematopoietic stem cells. *Nature* 423(6937):302-305.

Passegué E., Jochum W., Schorpp-Kistner M., Möhle-Steinlein U., & Wagner E.F. (2001) Chronic Myeloid Leukemia with Increased Granulocyte Progenitors in Mice Lacking JunB Expression in the Myeloid Lineage. *Cell* 104(1):21-32.

Porter, P.N., Meints, R.H., & Mesner,K. (1979) Enhancement of erythroid colony growth in culture by hemin. *Exp Hematol* 7(1):11-16.

Rajasekhar, V.K., Begemann, M. (2007) Concise review: roles of polycomb group proteins in development and disease: a stem cell perspective. *Stem Cells* 25(10):2498-2510.

Ramalho-Santos, M., Yoon, S., Matsuzaki, Y., Mulligan, R.C., & Melton, D.A. (2002) "Stemness": transcriptional profiling of embryonic and adult stem cells. *Science* 298(5593):597-600.

Ramos, C.A., Bowman, T.A., Boles, N.C., Merchant, A.A., Zheng, Y., Parra, I., Fuqua, S.A., Shaw, C.A., & Goodell, M.A. (2006) Evidence for diversity in transcriptional profiles of single hematopoietic stem cells. *PLoS Genet* 2(9):e159.

Randall, T.D., & Weissman, I.L. (1997) Phenotypic and functional changes induced at the clonal level in hematopoietic stem cells after 5-fluorouracil treatment. *Blood* 89(10):3596-3606.

Rathinam, C., Thien, C.B., Langdon, W.Y., Gu,H., & Flavell, R.A. (2008) The E3 ubiquitin ligase c-Cbl restricts development and functions of hematopoietic stem cells. *Genes Dev* 22(8):992-997.

Rathinam, C., Matesic, L.E., & Flavell, R.A. (2011) The E3 ligase Itch is a negative regulator of the homeostasis and function of hematopoietic stem cells. *Nat Immunol* 12(5):399-407.

Reya, T., Morrison, S.J., Clarke, M.F., & Weissman, I.L. (2001) Stem cells, cancer, and cancer stem cells. *Nature* 414(6859):105-111.

Rizo, A., Vellenga, E., de Haan, G., & Schuringa, J.J. (2006) Signaling pathways in self-renewing hematopoietic and leukemic stem cells: do all stem cells need a niche? *Hum Mol Genet* 15 Spec No 2:R210-9.

Robb, L., Lyons, I., Li, R., Hartley, L., Köntgen, F., Harvey, R.P., Metcalf, D., & Begley, C.G. (1995) Absence of yolk sac hematopoiesis from mice with a targeted disruption of the scl gene. *Proc Natl Acad Sci U S A* 92(15):7075-7079.

Rodrigues, N.P., Janzen, V., Forkert, R., Dombkowski, D.M., Boyd, A.S., Orkin, S.H., Enver, T., Vyas, P., & Scadden, D.T. (2005) Haploinsufficiency of GATA-2 perturbs adult hematopoietic stem cell homeostasis. *Blood* 106(2):477-484.

Rudd, C.E. (2001) Lnk adaptor: novel negative regulator of B cell lymphopoiesis. *Sci STKE* 2001(85):pe1

Saito, Y., Uchida, N., Tanaka, S., Suzuki, N., Tomizawa-Murasawa, M., Sone, A., Najima, Y., Takagi, S., Aoki, Y., Wake, A., Taniguchi, S., Shultz, L.D., & Ishikawa, F. (2010) Induction of cell cycle entry eliminates human leukemia stem cells in a mouse model of AML. *Nat Biotechnol* 28(3):275-280.

Santaguida, M., Schepers, K., King, B., Sabnis, A.J., Forsberg, E.C., Attema, J.L., Braun, B.S., & Passegué, E. (2009) JunB protects against myeloid malignancies by limiting hematopoietic stem cell proliferation and differentiation without affecting self-renewal. *Cancer Cell* 15(4):341-352.

Sato, T., Onai, N., Yoshihara, H., Arai, F., Suda, T., & Ohteki, T. (2009) Interferon regulatory factor-2 protects quiescent hematopoietic stem cells from type I interferon-dependent exhaustion. *Nat Med* 15(6):696-700.

Scandura, J.M., Boccuni, P., Massagué, J., Nimer, S.D. (2004) Transforming growth factor beta-induced cell cycle arrest of human hematopoietic cells requires p57KIP2 up-regulation. *Proc Natl Acad Sci U S A* 101(42):15231-15236.

Schneider-Gadicke, A., Beer-Romero, P., Brown, L.G., Mardon, G., Luoh, S.W., & Page, D.C. (1989) Putative transcription activator with alternative isoforms encoded by human ZFX gene. *Nature* 342(6250):708-711.

Seita, J., Ema, H., Ooehara, J., Yamazaki, S., Tadokoro, Y., Yamasaki, A., Eto, K., Takaki, S., Takatsu, K., & Nakauchi, H. (2007) Lnk negatively regulates self-renewal of hematopoietic stem cells by modifying thrombopoietin-mediated signal transduction. *Proc Natl Acad Sci U S A* 104(7):2349-2354.

Serrano, M., Hannon, G.j., & Beach, D. (1993) A new regulatory motif in cell-cycle control causing specific inhibition of cyclin D/CDK4. *Nature* 366(6456):740-707.

Sheiness, D., Fanshier, L., & Bishop, J.M. (1978) Identification of nucleotide sequences which may encode the oncogenic capacity of avian retrovirus MC29. *J Virol* 28(2):600-610.

Shimabe, M., Goyama, S., Watanabe-Okochi, N., Yoshimi, A., Ichikawa, M., Imai, Y., & Kurokawa, M. (2009) Pbx1 is a downstream target of Evi-1 in hematopoietic stem/progenitors and leukemic cells. *Oncogene* 28(49):4364-4374.

Shivdasani, R.A., Mayer, E.L., & Orkin, S.H. (1995) Absence of blood formation in mice lacking the T-cell leukaemia oncoprotein tal-1/SCL. *Nature* 373(6513):432-434.

Shounan, Y., Dolnikov, A., MacKenzie, K.L., Miller, M., Chan, Y.Y., & Symonds, G. Retroviral transduction of hematopoietic progenitor cells with mutant p53 promotes survival and proliferation, modifies differentiation potential and inhibits apoptosis. *Leukemia* 10(10):1619-1628.

Simsek, T., Kocabas, F., Zheng, J., Deberardinis, R.J., Mahmoud, A.I., Olson, E.N., Schneider, J.W., Zheng, C.C., & Sadek, H.A. (2010) The distinct metabolic profile of hematopoietic stem cells reflects their location in a hypoxic niche. *Cell Stem Cell* 7(9):380-390.

Sirin, O., Lukov, G.L., Mao, R., Conneely, O.M., & Goodell, M.A. (2010) The orphan nuclear receptor Nurr1 restricts the proliferation of haematopoietic stem cells. *Nat Cell Biol* 12(12):1213-1219.

Souroullas. G.P., Salmon, J.M., Sablitzky, F., Curtis, D.J., & Goodell, M.A. (2009) Adult hematopoietic stem and progenitor cells require either *Lyl1* or *Scl* for survival. *Cell Stem Cell* 4(2):180-186.

Stier S, Cheng T, Forkert R, Lutz C, Dombkowski DM, Zhang JL, Scadden DT. (2003) Ex vivo targeting of p21Cip1/Waf1 permits relative expansion of human hematopoietic stem cells. *Blood* 102(4):1260-1266.

Sun, Y., Shao, L., Bai, H., Wang, Z.Z., & Wu, W.S. (2010) Slug deficiency enhances self-renewal of hematopoietic stem cells during hematopoietic regeneration. *Blood* 115(9):1709-1717.

Takeuchi, M., Kimura, S., Kuroda, J., Ashihara, E., Kawatani, M., Osada, H., Umezawa, K., Yasui, E., Imoto, M., Tsuruo, T., Yokota, A., Tanaka, R., Nagao, R., Nakahara, T., Fujiyama, Y., & Maekawa, T. (2010) Glyoxalase-I is a novel target against Bcr-Abl⁺ leukemic cells acquiring stem-like characteristics in hypoxic environment. *Cell Death Diff* 17(7):1211-1220.

Takubo, K., Goda, N., Yamada, W., Iriuchishima, H., Ikeda, E., Kubota, Y., Shima, H., Johnson, R.S., Hirao, A., Suematsu, M., & Suda, T. (2010) Regulation of the HIF-1α level is essential for hematopoietic stem cells. *Cell Stem Cell* 7(9):391-402.

Taniura, H., Taniguchi, N., Hara, M., & Yoshikawa, K. (1998) Necdin, a postmitotic neuron-specific growth suppressor, interacts with viral transforming proteins and cellular transcription factor E2F1. *J Biol Chem* 273(2):720-728.

Taniura, H., Matsumoto, K., & Yoshikawa, K. (1999) Physical and functional interactions of neuronal growth suppressor necdin with p53. *J Biol Chem* 274(23):16242-16248.

Taniura, H., Kobayashi, M., & Yoshikawa, K. (2005) Functional domains of necdin for protein-protein interaction, nuclear matrix targeting, and cell growth suppression. *J Cell Biochem* 94(4):804-815.

TeKippe, M., Harrison, D.E., & Chen, J. (2003) Expansion of hematopoietic stem cell phenotype and activity in Trp53-null mice. *Exp Hematol* 31(6):521-527.

Thompson, B.J., Jankovic, V., Gao, J., Buonamici, S., Vest, A., Lee, J.M., Zavadil, J., Nimer, S.D., & Aifantis, I. (2008) Control of hematopoietic stem cell quiescence by the E3 ubiquitin ligase Fbw7. *J Exp Med* 205(6):1395-1408.

Tipping, A. J., Pina, C., Caster, A., Hong, D., Rodrigues, N.P., Lazzari, L., May, G.E., Jacobsen, S.E., & Enver, T. (2009) High GATA-2 expression inhibits human hematopoietic stem and progenitor cell function by effects on cell cycle. *Blood* 113(12): 2661-2672.

Tothova, Z., Kollipara, R., Huntly, B.J., Lee, B.H., Castrillon, D.H., Cullen, D.E., McDowell, E.P., Lazo-Kallanian, S., Williams, I.R., Sears, C., Armstrong, S.A., Passegué, E., DePinho, R.A., & Gilliland, D.G. (2007) FoxOs are critical mediators of hematopoietic stem cell resistance to physiologic oxidative stress. *Cell* 128(2):325-339.

Trumpp, A., Essers, M., & Wilson, A. (2010) Awakening dormant haematopoietic stem cells. *Nat Rev Immunol* 10(3):201-209.

Tsai, F. Y. & Orkin, S. H. (1997) Transcription factor GATA-2 is required for proliferation/survival of early hematopoietic cells and mast cell formation, but not for erythroid and myeloid terminal differentiation. *Blood* 89(10): 3636-3643.

Umemoto, T., Yamato, M., Nishida, K., Yang, J., Tano, Y., & Okano, T. (2005) p57Kip2 is expressed in quiescent mouse bone marrow side population cells. *Biochem Biophys Res Commun* 337(1):14-21.

van Os, R., Kamminga, L.M., Ausema, A., Bystrykh, L.V., Draijer, D.P., van Pelt, K., Dontje, B., & de Haan, G. (2007) A Limited role for p21Cip1/Waf1 in maintaining normal hematopoietic stem cell functioning. *Stem Cells* 25(4):836-843.

Venezia, T.A., Merchant,A.A., Ramos, C.A., Whitehouse, N.L., Young, A.S., Shaw, C.A., & Goodell, M.A. (2004) Molecular signatures of proliferation and quiescence in hematopoietic stem cells. *PLoS Biol* 2(10): e301.

Wang, Q., Miyakoda, M., Yang, W., Khillan, J., Stachura, D.L., Weiss, M.J., & Nishikura, K. (2004) Stress-induced apoptosis associated with null mutation of ADAR1 RNA editing deaminase gene. *J Biol Chem* 279(6):4952-4961.

Wilson, A., Murphy, M.J., Oskarsson, T., Kaloulis, K., Bettess, M.D., Oser, G.M., Pasche, A-C., Knabenhans, C., MacDonald, H.R., & Trumpp, A. (2004) c-Myc controls the balance between hematopoietic stem cell self-renewal and differentiation. *Genes Dev* 18(22):2747-2763.

Wilson, A., Laurenti, E., Oser, G., van der Wath, R.C., Blanco-Bose, W., Jaworski, M., Offner, S., Dunant, C.F., Eshkind, L., Bockamp, E., Lió, P., Macdonald, H.R., & Trumpp, A.

(2008) Hematopoietic stem cells reversibly switch from dormancy to self-renewal during homeostasis and repair. *Cell* 135(6):1118-1129.

Wilson, A., Laurenti, E., & Trumpp, A. (2009) Balancing dormant and self-renewing hematopoietic stem cells. *Curr Opin Genet Dev* 19(5):461-468.

Wu, W.S., Heinrichs, S., Xu, D., Garrison, S.P., Zambetti, G.P., Adams, J.M., & Look, A.T. (2005) Slug antagonizes p53-mediated apoptosis of hematopoietic progenitors by repressing puma. *Cell* 23(4):641-653.

Xiao, J., & Chen, H.S. (2004) Biological functions of melanoma-associated antigens. *World J Gastroenterol* 10(13):1849-1853.

Yamazaki, S., Iwama, A., Takayanagi, S., Eto, K., Ema, H., & Nakauchi, H. (2009) TGF-beta as a candidate bone marrow niche signal to induce hematopoietic stem cell hibernation. *Blood* 113(6):1250-1256.

Yoshikawa, K. (2000) Cell cycle regulators in neural stem cells and postmitotic neurons. *Neurosci Res* 37:1–14.

Yuasa, H., Oike, Y., Iwama, A., Nishikata, I., Sugiyama, D., Perkins, A., Mucenski, M.L., Suda, T., & Morishita, K. (2005) Oncogenic transcription factor Evi1 regulates hematopoietic stem cell proliferation through GATA-2 expression. *EMBO J* 24(11):1976-1987.

Zeng, H., Yücel, R., Kosan, C., Klein-Hitpass, L., & Möröy, T. (2004) Transcription factor Gfi1 regulates self-renewal and engraftment of hematopoietic stem cells. *EMBO J* 23(20): 4116-4125.

Zeng, S., Xu, Z., Lipkowitz, S., & Longley, J.B. (2005) Regulation of stem cell factor receptor signaling by Cbl family proteins (Cbl-b/c-Cbl). *Blood* 105(1):226-232.

Zhong, J.F., Zhao, Y., Sutton, S., Su, A., Zhan, Y., Zhu, L., Yan, C., Gallaher, T., Johnston, P.B, Anderson, W.F., & Cooke, M.P. (2005) Gene expression profile of murine long-term reconstituting vs. short-term reconstituting hematopoietic stem cells. *Proc Natl Acad Sci U S A* 102(7):2448-2453.

Part 2

Regulation of Hematopoietic Stem Cells

5

Interferon Regulatory Factor-2 Regulates Hematopoietic Stem Cells in Mouse Bone Marrow

Atsuko Masumi[1], Shoichiro Miyatake[2],
Tomoko Kohno[3] and Toshifumi Matsuyama[3]
[1]*Department of Safety Research on Blood and Biological Products,
National Institute of Infectious Diseases, Tokyo,*
[2]*Laboratory of Self Defense Gene Regulation, Tokyo Metropolitan
Institute of Medical Science, Tokyo,*
[3]*Department of Molecular Microbiology and Immunology, Nagasaki
University Graduate School of Biomedical Sciences, Nagasaki,
Japan*

1. Introduction

Hematopoiesis is regulated by intrinsic gene-regulatory networks, ensuring the rapid production of differentiated blood cells for the immediate needs of embryos and generation of definitive hematopoietic stem cells (HSCs) that are required for life-long hematopoiesis. Homeostasis in bone marrow is dependent on the ability of HSCs to faithfully self-renew and to generate progenitor cells that undergo limited proliferation and give rise to terminally differentiated cells in the peripheral blood. HSCs are specialized to give rise to all elements of the blood system throughout life (Orkin & Zon, 2002, 2008a, 2008b) and are capable of self-renewal and differentiation into various lineages of the hematopoietic system to form all types of blood cells. Self-renewal is a tightly controlled process through which stem cells divide and generate daughter stem cells with properties identical to those of the mother cells. However, under certain conditions, HSCs differentiate into progenitor cells with less ability to self-renew. Since the discovery of stem cells, intense research aimed at understanding the genetic and molecular bases of self-renewal has identified candidate regulatory factors involved in the process of HSC self-renewal. These include cell-intrinsic regulators, such as transcription factors, signal transducers, cell-cycle inhibitors and surface receptors and cell-extrinsic regulators, such as the bone marrow niche and cytokines (He et al., 2009).

Interferon (IFN) is produced by cells of the immune system in response to challenges by agents, such as viruses, bacteria and tumor cells. IFNs suppress viral replication, have immunomodulatory activities and are used clinically to treat viral diseases and malignancies, such as chronic myeloid leukemia (CML)(Stark, 1998). Type I IFNs are induced by the genomes of many RNA viruses, and this induction can be mimicked by the double-stranded RNA mimetic polyinosinic-polycytidylic acid (poly [I:C]) (Darnell et al.

1994, Pichlmair et al. 2007). However, under steady-state conditions in the absence of infection, small amount of IFN are produced constitutively (Taniguchi & Takaoka, 2001). Recently, Essers et al demonstrated that chronic activation of IFN-α pathway impairs function of HSCs and acute IFN-α treatment promotes the proliferation of dormant HSCs in vivo, and the possibility for new application of type I IFN to target cancer stem cells is expected (Essers et al. 2009) .

Interferon regulatory factors (IRFs) constitute a family of transcription factors involved in regulating the development and functions of the immune system (Honda et al., 2006; Taniguchi et al., 2001). Interferon regulatory factor-2 (IRF-2) is a transcriptional repressor in the interferon system and is thought to function by competing with IRF-1. While IRF-2 acts as a repressor for interferon production, IRF-2 exists ubiquitously and is a positive regulator for H4, vascular adhesion molecule-1 (VCAM-1), CIITA, gp91 phox, Fas ligand, TPO receptor (Vaughan et al.1995, Jesse et al. 1998 , Xi et al. 1999, Luo & Skalnik 1996, Chow et al. 2000, Stellacci et al. 2004, Masumi et al, 2001). Previously, we demonstrated that IRF-2 expression into mouse bone marrow hematopoietic stem/progenitor cells induced megakaryopoiesis through CD41 promoter activation in an inflammatory states (Masumi et al. 2009). IRF-2 regulates cell growth and differentiation through the target gene promoters.

There are several studies of hematopoietic approaches using IRF-2-/- mice. The physiological role in lymphoid and hematopoietic development has been investigated in IRF-2-/-mice, in which a general bone marrow suppression of hematopoiesis and B lymphopoiesis has been reported (Matsuyama et al. 1993). Recently, a marked reduction of hematopoietic stem cells in IRF-2-/- mice involving a type I interferon-dependent mechanism was reported (Sato et al. 2009). The population of bone marrow Lin-c-Kit+Sca-1+ (KSL) cells is increased in IRF-2-/- mice because of the general enhancement of Sca-1-positive cells.

Herein, we show that an enhanced population of Sca-1-positive cells and reduced HSC activity in the Lin-Sca-1+c-kit+ fraction were detected in IRF-2-/-mouse bone marrow cells. HSC abnormalities in IRF-2-/- mice have been demonstrated to be due to elevated type I IFN signaling (Sato et al. 2009). IFN signaling enhances the Sca-1 expression and cell cycle progression of HSCs. It was shown that chronic IFN signaling enhances cell cycle progression of HSCs in IRF-2-/-mice, resulting in the loss of quiescent HSCs. However, our results reveal unknown HSC markers in bone marrow from IRF-2-/- mice. Our present findings demonstrate that IRF-2 acts on long-term (LT)-HSCs, not only through protective type I IFN responses, but also by directly regulating HSC cell-surface molecules.

2. Hematopoietic stem cells in bone marrow derived from interferon regulatory factor-2-deficient mice

To analyze the expression of IRFs in mouse bone marrow cells, Gr1/Mac1-positive, B220-positive, Ter119-positive/lineage (Lin)-negative and KSL (c-kit+Sca-1+Lin-) cells were isolated from mouse bone marrow cells by flow cytometry. Real-time polymerase chain reaction (PCR) analysis and in situ hybridization showed that IRF-2 was present in especially high levels in the CD34-KSL fraction compared with fractions from other lineages (Masumi et al., 2009). The CD34-KSL cells from mouse bone marrow were stained with anti-IRF-2 antibody and DAPI (Fig. 1).

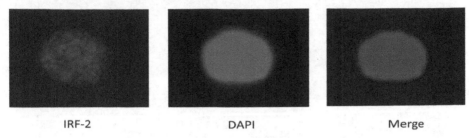

| IRF-2 | DAPI | Merge |

Fig. 1. CD34-KSL cells were stained with anti-IRF-2 as the primary antibody and then with anti-rabbit Alexa594 as the secondary antibody. Concurrently, cells were stained with DAPI.

2.1 Isolation and characterization of KSL cells

We showed that IRF-2 was highly localized in the mouse HSCs (CD34-Lin-c-kit+Sca-1+) in Fig. 1. To examine the role of IRF-2 in mouse hematopoietic stem cells, we isolated Lin-c-kit+sca-1+ (KSL) cells from the bone marrow of IRF-2-/-mice (Fig. 2A). The IRF-2-/- mice had a larger population of KSL cells than did wild-type mice because of enhanced expression Sca-1, which is downstream of interferon-α-receptor (IFNAR)-STAT1 signaling. Enhanced type I IFN signaling in IRF-2-/- mice induces Sca-1. Sca-1 cell-surface glycoprotein is used routinely as a marker of adult HSCs, allowing a >100-fold enrichment of these rare cells from the bone marrow of adult mice. The Sca-1 protein is encoded by the Ly-6A/E gene. This protein is highly inducible by IFNs -α, -β, and -γ, tumor necrosis factor (TNF) and interleukin-1 (IL-1) (Khan et al., 1990, 1993). The presence of a consensus sequence for IFN-γ-responsive elements has been reported to be localized to the Ly-6A/E genes promoter (Ma et al., 2001). Ito et al investigated that competitive repopulation assay using HSC from Sca-1-deficient mice and colony formation assay for Sca-1-deficient bone marrow. They demonstrated that Sca-1 is required for regulating HSC self-renewal and development of committed progenitor cells, megakaryocytes, and platelets (Ito et al. 2003). Bradfute et al investigated the effect of Sca-1 on HSC function and demonstrated that Sca-1 affects c-kit expression, the lineage fate of peripheral blood cells after transplantation, and may be dispensable for HSC self-renewal (Bradfute et al., 2005).We also observed higher populations of KSL cells in the spleens of IRF-2-/- mice (data not shown).

HSCs are contained within the CD150+CD48- population of KSL cells. There were far fewer CD150+CD48- cells in the KSL fraction in IRF-2-/- mice than in wild-type mice (0.97% versus 0.001%). In contrast, within the CD150+ CD48-Lin- subset, the fraction of KSL cells in wild-type mice and IRF-2-/- mice was 31.58% and 0.001%, respectively. Thus, the population of CD150+CD48-KSL cells was very low in IRF-2-/- mice (Fig. 2B). IRF-2 is known to be a transcription factor that attenuates type I IFN (IFN-α/IFN-β) signaling as indicated by the up-regulation of IFN-inducible genes in IRF-2-/-mice. IFN-α/IFN-β produced by plasmacytoid dendritic cells (DCs) in IRF-2-/- mice may have stimulated HSC proliferation, which resulted in loss of stem cells (Fig. 2C).

The number of KSL side-population (SP) cells was much lower in bone marrow cells from IRF-2-/- mice compared to those from wild-type mice (Fig. 3). We observed an increased cell number in the KSL fraction and a great reduction in the number of HSCs in the KSL fraction among the bone marrow cells of IRF-2-/- mice.

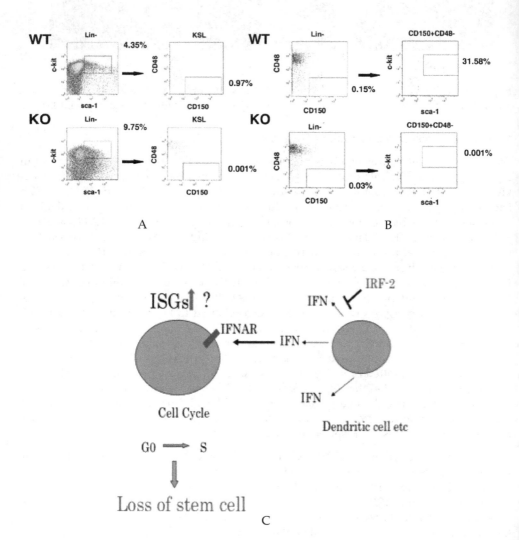

Fig. 2. (A) Lin-c-kit+sca-1+ cells were isolated from wild-type (WT) and IRF-2-/- bone marrow cells (KO), and then Lin-CD48-CD150+ cells were isolated from the KSL fraction. (B) Lin-c-kit+sca-1+ cells were isolated from Lin-CD48-CD150+ cells derived from the bone marrow cells of IRF-2-/- mice. (C) Chronic IFN stress model in KSL cells of IRF-2-/- mice. ISGs : Interferon-stimulated genes

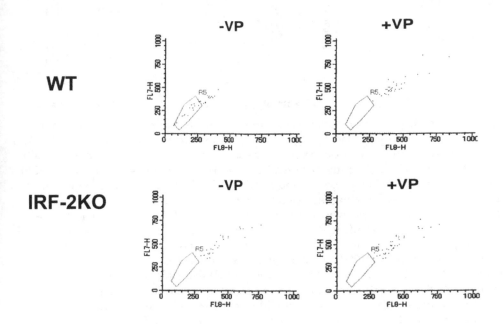

Fig. 3. Reduction in side population of KSL cells in the bone marrow cells from wild-type (WT) and IRF-2-/- mice (IRF-2KO). VP (verapamil) treatment eliminated the side population.

2.1.1 In vitro differentiation of KSL

To analyze the population of the KSL fraction in bone marrow from IRF-2-/- mice, an in vitro colony-forming assay was performed. The assay showed enhanced granulocyte/macrophage progenitor activity and reduced numbers of megakaryocyte progenitors in KSL derived from bone marrow of IRF-2-/- mice (Fig. 4). We did not see any difference for erythrocyte progenitors in the bone marrow derived-KSL cells in either wild-type or IRF-2-/-mice.

To compare ex vivo expansion of HSC between wild type and IRF-2-/-mice, KSL cells were plated at a density of 1 cell/well in Terasaki plates in 20 µL serum-free medium. The Terasaki single colony assay showed the significant colony formation activity in KSL cells from IRF-2-/- mice although its activity is less than that of wild-type mice (Fig. 5). In vitro culture assay, KSL cells from IRF-2-/- mice make colonies in the presence of cytokines, despite of near complete reduction of HSC population (Fig.2).

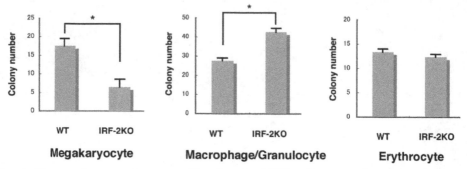

Megakaryocyte   **Macrophage/Granulocyte**   **Erythrocyte**

Fig. 4. Clonogenic progenitor assay. Two hundred KSL cells were subjected to a colony-forming unit-granulocyte/macrophage CFU-GM assay in methylcellulose medium M3231 (Stem Cell Technologies, Vancouver, BC, Canada) consisting of 1% methylcellulose, 30% fetal calf serum (FCS), 1% bovine serum albumin (BSA), 10 ng/mL stem cell factor (SCF), 25 ng/mL Flt ligand, 25 ng/mL thrombopoietin (TPO), 5 ng/mL IL-3 and 25 ng/mL granulocyte colony-stimulating factor (G-CSF). For the burst-forming units-erythroid (BFU-E) assay, 200 KSL cells were cultured in M3231 consisting of 1% methylcellulose, 30% FCS, 1% BSA, 50 ng/mL SCF, 50 ng/mL TPO and 5U/mL erythropoietin (EPO) for 7 days. To perform the mouse CFU-megakaryocytic (Mk) assays, 4×10^3 KSL cells were mixed with Megacult-C 04900 together with 1.1 mg/mL collagen, 50 ng/mL TPO and 10 ng/mL IL-3 in 0.75 mL and added to the wells of chamber slides (177429, LAB-TEK Brand Products). Cells were cultured at 37°C in an incubator with an atmosphere of 5% CO_2 and >95% humidity for 7 days. The chamber slides were placed in acetone solution to fix the cells and dried, and the dried slides were then stained with acetylthiocholiniodide solution (Sigma, St Louis, MO). After they were stained with hematoxylin, megakaryocyte colonies were counted. *$P<0.05$ (Student t test). Data are representative of two independent experiments (mean ±SD).

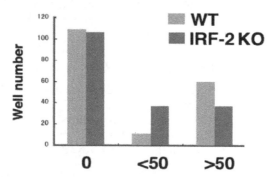

Fig. 5. Terasaki single colony assay. The KSL fraction from wild-type and IRF-2-/- bone marrow cells was fractionated to single cells in Terasaki plates by cell sorter (JSAN). Single cells were cultured with cytokines (hTPO, mSCF, mIL-3 and mFlt-3 ligand) containing 10% BSA and 2-mercaptethanol (0.01 M) in X-VIVO medium for 10 days. Colonies in each well were analyzed. <50 indicates wells that contain under 50 colonies in one well. >50 indicates wells that contain over 50 colonies. 0 indicates the wells containing no colony.

HSCs in wild-type mice were predominantly in a quiescent, intracellular Ki67-negative (icKi67 Hoechst low) G_0 phase. Quiescent cells were observed more frequently in KSL cells derived from IRF-2-/- mice, although the population of HSCs was much smaller than that of wild-type mice (Fig. 6).

2.1.2 Gene expression of KSL cells

Next, we investigated the KSL-specific gene expression in KSL cells derived from bone marrow cells of IRF-2-/-mice. Expression levels of GATA-2 and Tie2 in IRF-2-/- mice were similar to those of wild-type, but p57 expression was much lower than that of wild-type (Fig. 7A). Reduced p57 gene expression is associated with decreased numbers of HSCs in the KSL population, and the increased number of cells in G_0 phase may be associated with an increased frequency of quiescent KSL cells in bone marrow cells from IRF-2-/- mice (Fig. 6). When types I and II IFN were analyzed, expression of IFN-γ, but not of IFN-α and -β was decreased in the KSL fraction of IRF-2-/- mice under no stimulation (Fig. 7BC). Expression of Sca-1 was enhanced in the KSL fraction and in whole bone marrow in the IRF-2-/- mice. We examined PKR, TNF-a, adenosine deaminase 1 (ADAR1) expression which is known to be a suppressor of interferon signaling (Hartner et al. 2009) and Bmi1, which is down regulated in IRF-2 deficient HSC (Sato et al 2009). Expressions of ADAR1, PKR, Bmi1 and TNF-α were comparable between wild-type and IRF-2-deficient mice (Fig. 7C).

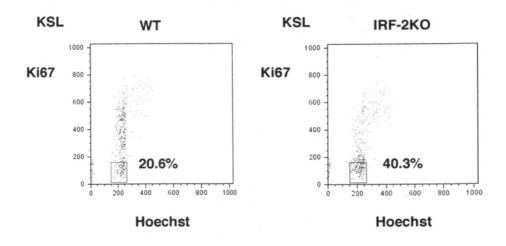

Fig. 6. Cell cycle analysis. Populations of KSL cells were isolated from bone marrow cells of IRF-2-/-mice and stained with Ki67 and Hoechst. Numbers indicate the percentage of cells in G_0 phase. Data are representative of two independent experiments.

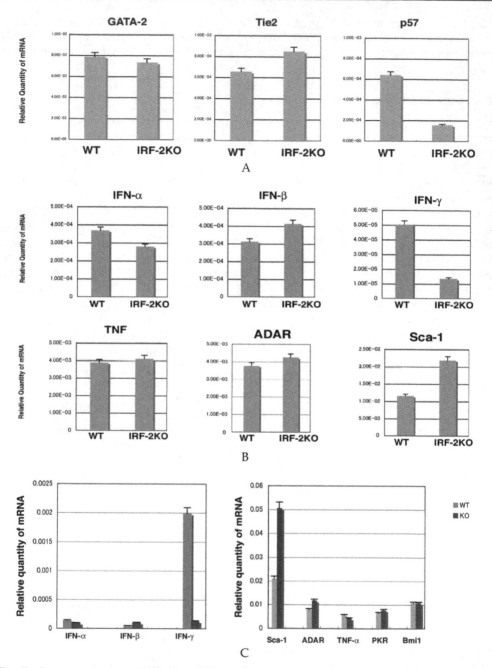

Fig. 7. Gene expression in KSL (A and B) and bone marrow cells (C) from wild-type and IRF-2-/- mice. Data represent the mean ± SD of triplicate reactions and are representative of two independent experiments.

2.1.3 Transplantation

To examine the functional properties of IRF-2-/- KSL cells, transplantation analysis was performed. In competitive repopulation assays, a constant number (1×10^5) of wild-type competitor cells was mixed with 1,500 KSL cells from IRF-2-/- mice and injected into lethally irradiated Ly5.1 mice. Engraftment analysis by peripheral blood chimerism (CD45.2 versus CD45.1 x CD45.2) at 4, 8 and 12 weeks after transplantation showed a profound deficit in wild-type recipient marrow, as peripheral blood elements derived from IRF-2-/- HSCs were progressively lost in favor of wild-type cells (Fig. 8A). Many more KSL cells could be engrafted into recipient mice if HSCs existed in the KSL fraction. However, a 24-fold larger number of cells also failed to rescue the recipients (Fig. 8B). When cells from the lineage-CD48 fraction were injected into recipients, no engraftment was shown in the recipients injected with cells from IRF-2-/- mice (Fig. 8C). The proportions of cells in the lineage-CD48 fraction isolated from both wild-type and IRF-2-/- mice were very similar (3.4% versus 2.9%). However, the number of CD150-positive cells was much lower in the IRF-2-/- mice compared to the wild-type mice (Fig.1).

To examine whether HSCs existed in fractions other than the KSL fraction of bone marrow cells in IRF-2-/- mice, whole bone marrow cells were injected into recipient mice and noncompetitive transplant assays were also performed. Transplantation of 1×10^5 wild-type bone marrow cells is normally sufficient to rescue and fully repopulate the hematopoietic systems of all lethally irradiated recipients. This dose of cells from KO donors failed to rescue any recipients from lethal irradiation, indicating impaired self-renewal of HSCs in whole bone marrow cells derived from IRF-2-/- cells. A dose of 2×10^6 cells from IRF-2-/- mice could rescue recipients from lethal irradiation, although the engraftment efficiency was poorer than that of wild-type at 1 month after transplantation (Fig. 8D).

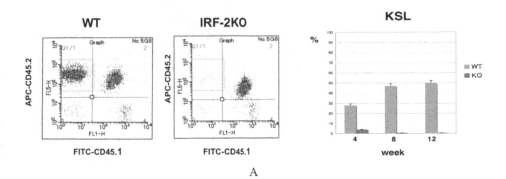

A

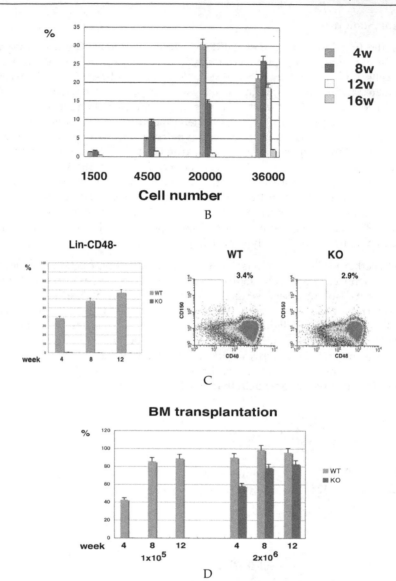

Fig. 8. Transplantation analysis. Cells in the KSL population were isolated from IRF-2-/-
mice (Ly5.2) and injected into X-irradiated mice. Peripheral blood cells were analyzed 4, 8
and 12 weeks after transplantation. (A) Percentage of donor-derived KSL cells (1500-cell
injection) in the blood. (B) Percentage of KSL derived from IRF-2-/- mice (injection of
indicated cell numbers) in the blood. (C) Percentage of Lin-CD48- cells from bone marrow of
wild-type and IRF-2-/- mice in the blood. (D) Percentage of donor-derived whole bone
marrow cells in the blood. Cells were grown in one of three mice injected with 2x10⁶ whole
bone marrow cells derived from IRF-2-/- mice. Representative data are shown from three
independent experiments.

An IRF-2-expressing retrovirus (Masumi et al. 2009) was transduced into the KSL fraction of IRF-2-deficient mouse bone marrow cells. When these IRF-2-expressing KSL cells were injected into lethally irradiated recipients, no sufficient rescue of engraftment was observed (data not shown). KSL cells from IRF-2-deficient mice may be distinct from those of wild-type mice. IRF-2 expression does not contribute to rescue the HSC function in KSL cells from IRF-2-/- mice in vivo.

IRF-2-/- mice were previously reported to be more sensitive to 5-fluorouracil (5-FU) than IRF-2+/- mice because of a progressive decrease in functional HSCs in IRF-2-/- mice (Sato et al., 2009). We treated both IRF-2-/- and wild-type mice weekly with 5-FU. Four of the IRF-2-/- mice died after the initial injection, but one mouse lived after three injections. We conclude that quiescent HSCs are present in whole bone marrow from IRF-2-/- mice, although the IRF-2-/- mice are more sensitive than wild-type (Fig. 9). As seen in Fig. 8D and Fig. 9, HSC-like cells, which may be isolated using cell surface markers distinct from KSL cells, are thought to be present in IRF-2-/-mice bone marrow cells (Fig. 10).

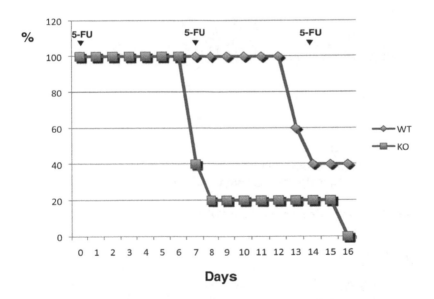

Fig. 9. Rate of survival (%) of wild-type and IRF-2-/- mice that were injected weekly with 150 mg/kg body weight of 5-FU (Sigma Chemical Co.); n= 5 for each group.

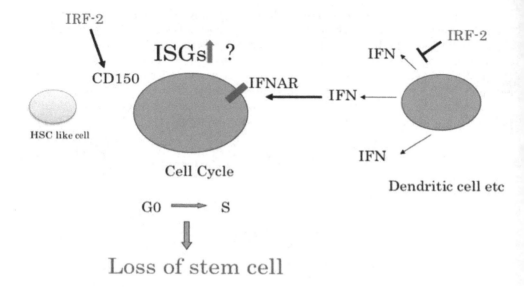

Fig. 10. HSC-like cells will be appeared in IRF-2-/- mice bone marrow cells (Refer to Fig.2C). IRF-2 may inhibit the down-regulation of CD150 gene expression by type I IFN.

2.2 Progenitors in bone marrow cells from IRF-2-/- mice

Next we analyzed the progenitor population in bone marrow cells from IRF-2-/- mice. Akashi et al proposed the model of major hematopoietic maturation pathways from HSCs (Akashi et al. 2000). According to his proposal, granulocyte/macrophage lineage progenitor (GMP), megakaryocyte/erythrocyte lineage progenitor (MEP), and common myeloid progenitor (CMP) and common lymphoid progenitor (CLP) were isolated from wild-type and IRF-2-deficient mice bone marrow. The frequencies of MEPs (Lin-ckit^{lo}sca-1-FcRg^{lo}CD34-) and CMPs (Lin-ckit^{lo}sca-1-FcRg^{lo}CD34+) were slightly decreased in IRF-2-deficient mice compared to wild-type mice. By contrast, GMPs (Lin-ckit^{lo}sca-1-FcRg^{high}CD34+) were slightly increased in IRF-2-deficient mice (Fig. 11A). The frequency of the CLP compartment in IRF-2-/- mouse bone marrow cells was lower than that from wild-type bone marrow (Fig. 11B).

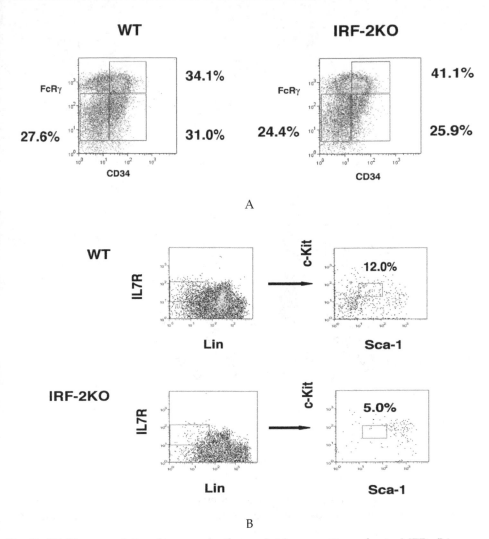

Fig. 11. (A) Lineage relationships among the myeloid progenitor subsets. MEPs (Lin-ckit\[lo\]sca-1-FcRg\[lo\]CD34-), CMPs (Lin-ckit\[lo\]sca-1-FcRg\[lo\]CD34+), and GMPs (Lin-ckit\[lo\]sca-1-FcRg\[high\]CD34+) are indicated. (B) Common lymphoid progenitors in bone marrow from IRF-2-/- mice.

2.2.1 Mouse colony-forming cell (CFC) assays with bone marrow derived from IRF-2-/- mice

The size of the GMP population from IRF-2-/- mice was higher than that from wild-type. We analyzed bone marrow and spleen cells from IRF-2-/- mice with CFU-GM assay. Colony numbers were higher in the bone marrow and spleen cells from IRF-2-/- mice, likely to the KSL population (Fig. 12 and Fig. 4).

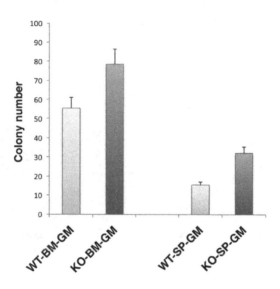

Fig. 12. Clonogenic progenitor assay with bone marrow and spleen cells from wild-type and IRF-2-/- mice. Assays performed as described in methods for Fig. 4. BM: bone marrow; SP: spleen

2.3 IRF-2 is required for bone marrow lymphopoiesis

To confirm the direct effect of IRF-2 deficiency in KSL cells, complementary DNA microarray analysis was performed on sorted Lin-c-Kit+Sca-1+ cells from bone marrow of wild-type and IRF-2-/- mice. This analysis showed that the up-regulated genes included IFN-inducible genes, such as Ly6s and Ifits, and the pre-B lymphocyte gene family (data not shown). As shown in Fig.13, when bone marrow B cell progenitors are analyzed, severe reduction in the frequency of mature IgM+ B cells was detected in the IRF-2-/- mice; and an enhanced frequency of pre-pro-B cells was detected in young IRF-2-deficient mice. These defects were correlated with the KSL array data (not shown). These data indicate a requirement for IRF-2 in maintaining bone marrow B homeostasis and B cell differentiation.

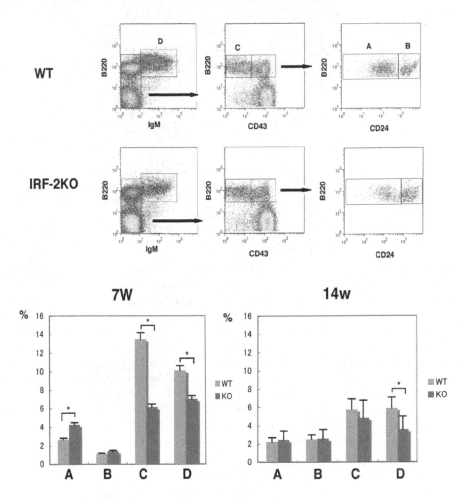

A: pre pro-B, B: pro-B, C: pre-B, D: Mature B

Fig. 13. Loss of IRF-2 in hematopoietic cells results in impaired B cell homeostasis. Top panel: FACS analysis of frequencies of B-cell subsets in bone marrow of IRF-2-/- and age-matched littermate control mice, for expression of B220, IgM, CD43 and CD24. Bottom panel: Four to five (each) young (7W) and old (14W) mice were analyzed. The frequency of mature B220+IgM+B cells (D) was significantly reduced in both young and old IRF-2-/-mice. Young, but not old, IRF-2-/- mice exhibited significant reductions in pre-B fractions (C) and increases in pre pro-B fractions (A).

Fluorescence-activated cell sorting (FACS) analysis of peripheral blood indicated that any significant differences in lineage between wild-type and IRF-2-/- mice were not observed (data not shown). However, an increase in Gr1+Mac1+ neutrophils and a decrease in B220+ cells were detected in the bone marrow and spleens IRF-2-/- mice (Fig.14). These lineage populations almost reflect to that of progenitors in IRF-2-/-mice (Fig.11).

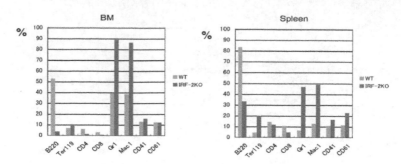

Fig. 14. Lineage populations in IRF-2-/- mouse bone marrow and spleens. Mononuclear cells from mouse bone marrow (BM) or spleen cells were stained with each antibody conjugated to PE and analyzed by FACS. Percentage indicates relative counts per whole mononuclear cells in each surface marker analysis.

2.4 Effect of type I IFN in IRF-2-/- mice

To assess the role of IRF-2 in the regulation of type I IFN signaling, we analyzed gene expression in IRF-2-/- mice compared to IRF-2-/- IFNAR-/- dKO mice, which do not respond to type I IFN. Sca-1 gene expression was enhanced in the bone marrow of IRF-2-/- mice, but not in IRF-2-/-/IFNAR-/- dKO mice. However, reduced expression of IFN-γ in IRF-2-/- mice was not rescued in IRF-2-/-IFNAR-/- dKO mice. Sca-1 expression is regulated by IRF-2 and the type I IFN response. However, IFN-γ may be regulated by IRF-2, independent of the type I IFN response. Arakura et al. reported the up-regulation of IFN-γ resulting from aberrant IFN-α/IFN-β responses in abdominal skin from IRF-2-/- mice (Arakura et al., 2007). In the bone marrow and KSL cells of our IRF-2-/- mice, IFN-γ expression was extremely low and the defect in IFN-α/IFN-β signaling did not rescue the expression. IFN-α/IFN-β expression was not enhanced in bone marrow and KSL cells in IRF-2-/- mice in the absence of stimulation (Fig. 8).

IFN-γ expression decreased in the bone marrow of both IRF-2-/- mice and IRF-2-/- IFNAR-/-dKO mice (Fig. 8B and Fig. 15). IFN-γ reduction is independent of type I IFN signaling in bone marrow cells from IRF-2-/- mice. IRF-2 may regulate IFN-γ gene expression through its promoter or other factors.

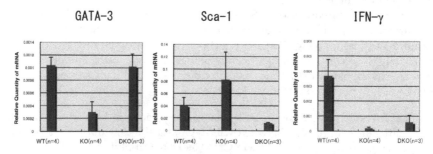

Fig. 15. Real-time PCR analysis for Sca-1, IFN-γ and GATA-3 gene expression in bone marrow cells from wild-type (WT), IRF-2-/- (KO)and IRF-2-/- IFNAR-/- dKO (DKO)mice.

A FACS analysis revealed the reduction of the CD150 surface marker in IRF-2-/- mice. Using real-time RT-PCR for expression of the CD150 gene in IRF-2-deficent mouse bone marrow, we demonstrated a profound decrease of CD150 gene expression (Fig. 16). However, the CD150 expression level in IRF-2-/- IFNAR-/- dKO bone marrow was comparable to wild-type mice. These results indicate that CD150 expression is regulated by the type I IFN response and is transcriptionally regulated in IRF-2-/-mice (Fig. 16). Sato et al. reported that the HSC population, including CD150-positive cells, was reduced through the induction of HSC proliferation by type I IFN signaling. However, we revealed another mechanism in which IRF-2 or type I IFN signaling directly mediated CD150 gene expression. In contrast, more depressed expression of Sca-1 was detected in IRF-2-/- IFNAR-dKO mice compared to that in wild type, supporting that Sca-1 expression was regulated by the type I IFN system (Fig. 16).

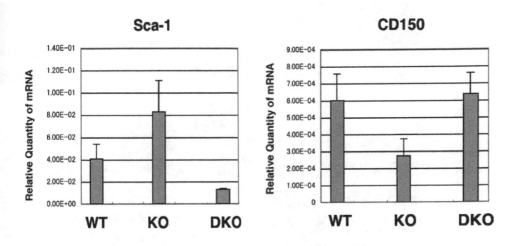

Fig. 16. Real-time PCR analysis for CD150 in bone marrow cells from wild-type (WT), IRF-2-/- (KO) and IRF-2-/- IFNAR-/- dKO (DKO) mice.

2.5 IRF-2 interaction with transcription factors in KSL

We investigated IRF-2-interacting transcription factors that are associated with hematopoiesis. TF(Transcriptional factor)-TF analysis indicates that IRF-2 associates GATA-1/2. However, we did not observe any difference of GATA-1 (data not shown) and GATA-2 (Fig.7A) expressions between wild-type and IRF-2-/- mice mice by KSL array data and real-time PCR analysis. We performed in vitro protein interaction analysis using 293T culture cells. IRF-2 interacted with GATA-2, but not GATA-1, when Flag-tagged IRF-2 and HA-tagged GATAs were transfected into 293T cells. To examine which region of IRF-2 interacts with GATA-2, IRF-2 DNA binding domain (DBD) and IRF-2 without DBD were incubated with several deletion constructs of GATA-2. The IRF-2 DNA-binding domain associated with GATA-2, specifically the N-terminal transcription activation domain in 293T cells (Fig. 17).

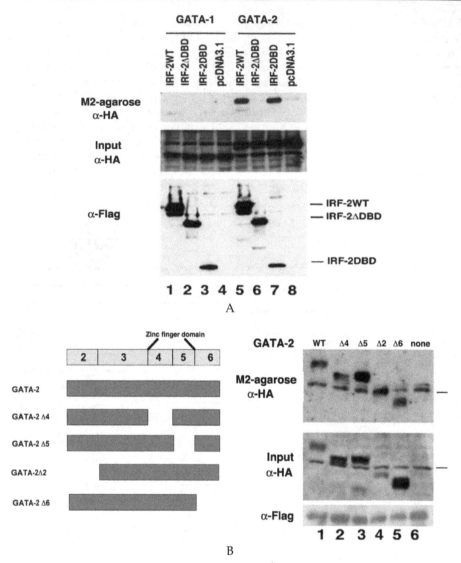

Fig. 17. IRF-2 interacts with GATA-2, but not GATA-1. (A) Flag-tagged IRF-2, Flag-tagged-IRF-2 DNA binding domain (IRF-2DBD) or Flag-tagged IRF-2 without DBD (IRF-2ΔDBD) and HA-tagged GATA-1 or HA-tagged GATA-2 were transfected to 293T cells. Cell lysate were incubated with M2-agarose, and agarose were washed and eluted with Flag peptide solution. Eluted fraction were electrophoresed and Western blot analysis was performed. (B) Protein structure of mouse GATA-2 and its mutants (GATA-2Δ4, GATA-2Δ5, GATA-2Δ2 and GATA-2Δ6) were shown (left) and numbers indicate exons of GATA-2. Each exon deletion mutants tagged with HA was incubated with Flag-tagged IRF-2. Exon2 (transcriptional activation domain) in GATA-2 has high affinity for binding with IRF-2 (right). - indicates non-specific bands.

We found that GATA-3 gene expression was decreased in IRF-2-deficient bone marrow and KSL cells by KSL array data and real-time PCR analysis (Fig. 15). GATA-3 gene expression was comparable to that in IRF-2-/- IFNAR-/- dKO mice, suggesting that the type I IFN response affects GATA-3 expression in IRF-2-/- mice. To examine GATA-3 interacts with IRF-2, Flag-tagged IRF-2 and myc-GATA-3 expression vectors were transfected to 293T cells. We show that GATA-3 interacted with IRF-2 in 293T cells (Fig. 18).

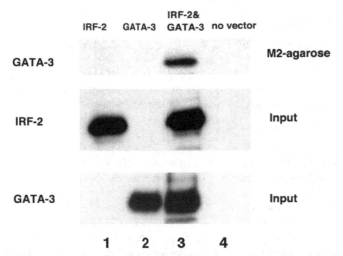

Fig. 18. IRF-2 interacts with GATA-3. Flag-tagged IRF-2 and Myc-tagged GATA-3 were transfected to 293T cells. Western blot analysis was performed as described in Fig.17.

In our investigation, GATA-2 and GATA-3 associated with IRF-2 in the in vitro cell culture system. GATA-2 is expressed abundantly in the mouse HSC population and is necessary for hematopoietic differentiation (Kitajima et al. 2006). GATA-1 is expressed in megakaryocyte/erythrocyte precursors (MEP) and their progenitors, and GATA-3 is expressed in common lymphoid precursors (CLPs) and T cells. There are very few reports regarding GATA-3 expression in HSCs, although we found that the GATA-3 expression level changed in IRF-2-deficient bone marrow and KSL in microarray and real time PCR analysis. Previous reports have shown that forced GATA-3 expression into mouse HSCs induces differentiation toward erythrocytes and megakaryocytes (Chen and Zhang 2001). As indicated by our investigation, GATA-3 may be important for the maintenance of HSC cooperation with IRF-2 or IFN signaling. These findings indicate that the interactions between IRF-2 and the GATAs are required to maintain HSC function in mouse bone marrow cells. Interactions between GATA-2 and GATA-3 with IRF-2 in HSCs should be clarified in future experiments.

3. Conclusion

IRF-2 exists high in the mouse bone marrow HSC population and helps maintain the protective immune response, which responds to viral or bacterial infection and inflammation, resulting in IFN producing system. HSCs are essential for the production of immune cells, such as myeloid or lymphoid cells. Recently, interferon treatment has been reported to be a target for cancer stem cells. Under chronic interferon stimulation, such as in an IRF-2-deficient condition, not only HSCs, but also cancer stem cells can be activated. Blocking the IRF-2 function may induce to eliminate of cancer stem cell through IFN signaling. However, the possibility of the presence of HSC-like cells in IRF-2 deficient mice cell population necessitates further investigation because IRF-2 in part regulates HSC populations independent of the type I IFN system in an another possible mechanism.

4. Acknowledgments

We thank Dr. I. Hamaguchi, Dr. T. Mizukami, Dr. H. Momose, Dr. M. Kuramitsu, Dr. K. Takizawa, and Dr. K. Yamaguchi for their experimental support and useful discussions. Ms. K. Furuhata for cell sorting and Ms. M. Tsuruhara for molecular technical assistance. This work was supported in part the Japan Society for the Promotion of Science and the Ministry of Education, Science, Sports and culture of Japan.

5. References

Akashi, K., Traver, D., Miyamoto, T. & Weissman I (2000). A clonogenic common myeloid progenitor that gives rise to all myeloid lineages. *Nature* Vol.404, 6774, (Mar 2000), pp. 193-197.

Arakura, F., Hida, S., Ichikawa, E., Yajima, C., Nakajima, S., Saida T. & Taki, S. (2007). Genetic control directed toward spontaneous IFN-alpha/IFN-beta responses and downstream IFN-gamma expression influences the pathogenesis of a murine psoriasis-like skin disease. *J Immunol* Vol.179, No.5, (Sep 2007), pp. 3249-3257.

Bradfute, S.B., Graubert, T.A. & Goodell, M.A. (2005). Roles of Sca-1 in hematopoietic stem/progenitor cell function. *Exp Hematol* Vol.33, No.7, (Jul 2005), pp. 836-843.

Chen, D. & Zhang, G. (2001). Enforced expression of the GATA-3 transcription factor affects cell fate decisions in hematopoiesis. *Exp Hematol* Vol.29, No.29, (Aug 2001), pp. 971-980.

Chow, W., Fang, J. & Yee, J. (2000). The IFN regulatory factor family participates in regulation of Fas ligand gene expression in T cells. *J Immunol* Vol. 164, No.7, (Apr 2000), pp. 3512-3518.

Darnell, JE Jr., Kerr, IM. & Stark, G.R. (1994). Jak-STAT pathways and transcriptional activation in response to IFNs and other extracellular signaling proteins. *Science* Vol. 264, 5164, (Jun 1994), pp. 1415-1421.

Essers, M., Offner, S., Blanco-Bose, W., Waibler, Z., Kalinke, U., Duchosal, M. & Trumpp, A. (2009). IFNa activates dormant hematopoietic stem cells in vivo. *Nature* Vol. 458, 7240, (Apr 2009), pp. 904-908.

Hartner, J., Walkley, C., Lu, J.& Orkin, S. (2009). ADAR1 is essential for the maintenance of hematopoiesis and suppression of interferon signaling. *Nat Immunol* Vol.10, No.1, (Jan 2009), pp. 109-115.

He, S., Nakada, D. & Morrison, S.J. (2009). Mechanisms of stem cell self-renewal. *Annu Rev Cell Dev Biol* Vol.25, (2009), pp. 377-406.

Honda, K., Takaoka, A. & Taniguchi, T. (2006). Type I interferon gene induction by the interferon regulatory factor family of transcription factors. *Immunity* Vol.25, No.3, (Sep 2006), pp. 349-360.

Ito, C.Y., Li, C.Y., Bernstein, A., Dick, J.E. & Stanford, W.L. (2003). Hematopoietic stem cell and progenitor defects in Sca-1/Ly-6A-null mice. *Blood* Vol.101, No.2, (Jan 2003), pp. 517-523.

Jesse, T.L, LaChance, R., Iademarco, M.F. & Dean, D.C. (1998). Interferon regulatory factor-2 is a transcriptional activator in muscle where it regulates expression of vascular cell adhesion molecule-1. *J Cell Biol* Vol.140, No.5, (Mar 1998), pp. 1265-1276.

Khan, K.D., Lindwall, G., Maher, S.E. & Bothwell, A.L. (1990). Characterization of promoter elements of an interferon-inducible Ly-6E/A differentiation antigen, which is expressed on activated T cells and hematopoietic stem cells. *Mol Cell Biol* Vol.10, No.10, (Oct 1990), pp. 5150-5159.

Khan, K.D., Shuai, K., Lindwall, G., Maher, S.E., Darnell, J.E., Jr., & Bothwell, A.L. (1993). Induction of the Ly-6A/E gene by interferon alpha/beta and gamma requires a DNA element to which a tyrosine-phosphorylated 91-kDa protein binds. *Proc Natl Acad Sci U S A* Vol.90, No.14, (July 1993), pp. 6806-6810.

Kitajima, K., Tanaka, M., Zheng, J., Yen, H., Sato, A., Sugiyama D., Umehara, H., Sakai, E. & Nakano, T. (2006). Redirecting differentiation of hematopoietic progenitors by a transcription factor, GATA-2. *Blood* Vol.107, No.5, (Mar 2006), pp. 1857-1863.

Luo, W. & Skalnik D (1996). Interferon regulatory factor-2 directs transcription from the gp91phox promoter. *J Biol Chem* Vol.271, No.38, (September 1996), pp. 23445-23451.

Ma, X., Ling, K.W. & Dzierzak, E. (2001). Cloning of the Ly-6A (Sca-1) gene locus and identification of a 3' distal fragment responsible for high-level gamma-interferon-induced expression in vitro. *Br J Haematol* Vol.114, No.3, (Sep 2001), pp. 724-730.

Masumi, A. & Ozato, K. (2001). Coactivator p300 acetylates the interferon regulatory factor-2 in U937 cells following phorbol ester treatment. *J Biol Chem* Vol.276, No.24, (Jun 2001), pp. 20973-20980.

Masumi, A., Hamaguchi, I., Kuramitsu, M., Mizukami, T., Takizawa, K., Momose, H., Naito, S. & Yamaguchi, K. (2009). Interferon regulatory factor-2 induces megakaryopoiesis in mouse bone marrow hematopoietic cells. *FEBS Lett* Vol.583, No.21, (Nov 2009), pp. 3493-3500.

Matsuyama, T., Kimura, T., Kitagawa, M., Pfeffer, K., Kawakami, T., Watanabe, N., Kundig, T. M., Amakawa, R., Kishihara, K., Wakeham, A., Potter, J., Fulonger, C.L., Narendan, A., Suzuki, H., Ohashi, P.S., Paige, C.J., Taniguchi, T. & Mak, T.W. (1993). Targeted disruption of IRF-1 or IRF-2 results in abnormal type I IFN gene induction and aberrant lymphocyte development. *Cell* Vol.75, No.1, (Oct 1993), pp. 83-97.

Orkin, S.H., & Zon, L.I. (2002). Hematopoiesis and stem cells: plasticity versus developmental heterogeneity. *Nat Immunol* Vol.3, No.4, (Apr 2002), pp. 323-328.

Orkin, S.H., & Zon, L.I. (2008a). SnapShot: hematopoiesis. *Cell* Vol. 132, No. 4, (Feb 2008), pp. 712.

Orkin, S.H. & Zon, L.I. (2008b). Hematopoiesis: an evolving paradigm for stem cell biology. *Cell* Vol.132, No.4, (Feb 2008), pp. 631-644.

Pichlmair A & Reis e Sousa C (2007). Innate recognition of viruses. *Immunity* Vol. 27, No.3, (Sep 2007), pp. 370-383.

Sato, T., Onai, N., Yoshihara, H., Arai, F., Suda, T. & Ohteki, T. (2009). Inteferon regulatory factor-2 protects quiescent hematopoietic stem cells from type 1 interferon-dependent exhaustion. *Nat Med* Vol.15, No.6, (Jun 2009), pp. 696-700.

Stark, G.R., Kerr, I.M., Williams B.R, Silverman, RH. & Schreiber, R.D. (1998). How cells respond to interferons. *Annu Rev Biochem* Vol. 67, pp. 227-264.

Stellacci, E., Testa, U., Petrucci, E., Benedetti, E., Orsatti, R., Feccia, T., Stafsnes, M., Marziali, G. & Battistini, A. (2004). Interferon regulatory factor-2 drives megakaryocytic differentiation. *Biochem J* Vol. 377, Pt2, (Jan 2004), pp. 367-378.

Taniguchi, T., Ogasawara, K., Takaoka, A. & Tanaka N. (2001). IRF family of transcription factors as regulators of host defense. *Annu Rev Immunol* Vol.19, pp. 623-655.

Taniguchi, T. & Takaoka, A. (2001). A weak signal for strong responses: interferon-α/β revisited. *Nat. Rev. Mol. Cell Biol* Vol. 2, No.5, (May 2001), pp. 378-386.

Vaughan, P., Aziz, F., van Wijnen, A., Wu, S., Harada, H., Taniguchi ,T., Soprano, K.J., Stein, J.L. & Stein, G.S. (1995). Activation of a cell-cycle-regulated histone gene by the oncogenic transcription factor IRF-2. *Nature* Vol.377, 6547, (Sep 1995), pp. 362-365.

Xi, H., Eason, D., Ghosh, D., Dovhey, S., Wright, K. & Blanck, G. (1999). Co-occupancy of the interferon regulatory element of the class II transactivator (CIITA) type IV promoter by interferon regulatory factors 1 and 2. *Oncogene* Vol.18, No.43, (Oct 1999), pp. 5889-5903.

6

The Hypoxia Regulatory System in Hematopoietic Stem Cells

Keiyo Takubo

Department of Cell Differentiation, The Sakaguchi Laboratory of Developmental Biology,
Keio University School of Medicine, Tokyo,
Japan

1. Introduction

Stem cells localize to specific sites called 'niches' in various tissues, where they are preferentially maintained by growth factors from the environment. Mammalian bone marrow (BM) has been shown to be relatively hypoxic compared to other tissues, and primitive hematopoietic cells, including hematopoietic stem cells (HSCs), are thought to localize to the most hypoxic microenvironments in the BM. The hypoxic *ex vivo* culture of BM cells or primitive hematopoietic progenitors results in the maintenance of the primitive phenotype and cell cycle quiescence (Mohyeldin et al., 2010; Suda et al., 2011). *Ex vivo* culture of human HSCs under hypoxia also stabilizes hypoxia-inducible factor-1α (HIF-1α), a master transcriptional regulator of the cellular and systemic hypoxic response, and induces various downstream effectors of HIF-1α (Danet et al., 2003). However, the regulatory mechanisms and functional effects of BM hypoxia on HSCs *in vivo* have not been fully elucidated.

In the stem cell niche, HSCs are quiescent and show slow cell cycling. Various extracellular ligands, including CXCL12 (Sugiyama et al., 2006), angiopoietin-1 (Arai et al., 2004), and/or thrombopoietin (TPO) (Qian et al., 2007; Yoshihara et al., 2007), contribute to the quiescence of HSCs. Quiescent HSCs are maintained at a lower oxidative stress state to avoid their differentiation and exhaustion (Jang & Sharkis 2007). HIF-1α is a bHLH-PAS–type transcription factor (Semenza, 2007, 2009, 2010). Under normoxic conditions, prolyl residues in the HIF-1α oxygen-dependent degradation domain (ODD) are hydroxylated by HIF prolyl hydroxylases (PHDs). The hydroxylated ODD domain of HIF-1α protein is recognized by an E3 ubiquitin ligase, the von Hippel-Lindau protein (VHL). In the autosomal dominant hereditary disorder von Hippel Lindau disease, VHL is mutated, resulting in overstabilized HIF-1α protein by the impaired ubiquitin-proteasome pathway. Under hypoxic conditions, PHDs are inactivated and HIF-1α protein escapes degradation. Several niche factors, such as thrombopoietin (TPO) (Kirito et al., 2005) and stem cell factor (SCF) (Pedersen et al., 2008), also stabilize HIF-1α protein in hematopoietic cells even under normoxic conditions.

Stabilized HIF-1α protein forms a heterodimeric transcriptional complex with the oxygen-independent subunit HIF-1β, translocates to the nucleus, and directly binds hypoxia-responsive elements found in the promoter regions of numerous downstream regulators, thereby activating their transcription. HIF-1β is reportedly required for hematopoietic cell generation during ontogeny. However, a detailed analysis of the contribution of HIF-1α to the maintenance of adult HSCs has not yet been reported.

We analyzed HSCs in HIF-1α– and VHL-deficient mice and found that the cellular pool and cell cycle status of HSCs were regulated by the HIF-1α level (Takubo et al., 2010). Our analysis revealed that the regulation of the HIF-1α dose is critical for HSC maintenance in the hypoxic niche microenvironment of the BM. The critical role for HIF-1α in HSC cell cycle regulation broadens the involvement of oxygen status in the stem cell niche. It also implies a novel strategy for maintaining and expanding HSC resources based on cellular oxygen metabolism reprogramming, including the modulation of HSC quiescence through the oxygenation status of HIF-1α.

2. Quiescence of hematopoietic stem cells

Somatic stem cells contribute to tissue homeostasis throughout life (Suda et al., 2011). Because proliferation will induce senescence, the proper maintenance of stem cells without senescence is mandatory. There are two states for tissue stem cells in terms of the cell cycle. One is the quiescent state. Stem cells in the quiescent state are out of the active cell cycle (S/G2/M phase) and in the G0 phase. The other is the cycling state. Cycling stem cells actively reproduce themselves (self-renewal) to generate progeny. Cycling cells are in the non-G0 phase of the cell cycle. Quiescence is thought to be an effective strategy for stem cells to avoid various forms of cytotoxic damage. If stem cells lost quiescence, they would become susceptible to intrinsic and extrinsic stresses.

Mammalian HSCs are included in the heterogeneous population of lineage marker-, Sca-1+, and c-Kit+ (LSK) cells. LSK cells are a mixture of progenitors and HSCs. Within the LSK population, CD34-CD150hiCD48-CD41-Flt3- cells, as well as side population (SP) cells (Osawa et al, 1996; Kiel et al, 2005; Goodell et al, 1996), are quiescent.

Measurement of the cell cycle in HSCs by the staining of DNA with Hoechst 33342, DAPI, and/or anti-Ki67 indicates that more than 70% of highly purified HSC (CD34-CD48-CD150hi LSK) are in the G0 phase, whereas less than 10% of CD34+ LSK cells (differentiated progenitors) are in the quiescent phase (Wilson et al, 2008).

Slow-cycling HSCs have long-term (LT) reconstitution activity when they are transplanted into lethally irradiated recipient mice. In contrast, actively cycling HSCs and progenitors exhibit only short-term (ST) reconstitution activity and only maintain hematopoiesis for 3–4 months. Thus, the former are termed "LT-HSC(s)" and the latter are "ST-HSC(s)". LT-HSCs produce ST-HSCs, multipotent progenitors (MPPs), lineage-restricted progenitors, and terminally differentiated hematopoietic cells including erythrocytes, platelets, lymphocytes, granulocytes, and macrophages (Figure 1).

Because slow-cycling stem cells are not in the S or M phase of the cell cycle, they are more resistant to cytotoxic agents such as ultraviolet (UV) light, ionizing radiation and chemicals, compared with actively cycling cells. Recent reports indicate that quiescent stem cell fractions are present in several tissues. For example, in the hair follicle, cell cycle progression of stem cells in bulge regions is suppressed by Wnt inhibitors (Fuchs and Horsley, 2011). In contrast, stem cells in the murine intestinal and gastric epithelia divide every 24 hours

(Snippert and Clevers, 2011). Therefore, quiescence itself is not the only strategy for the long-term maintenance of stem cells.

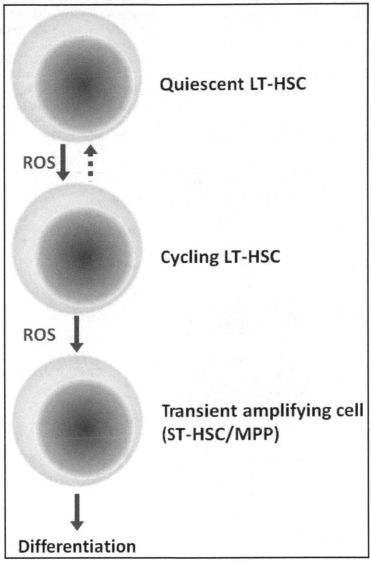

Life-long hematopoiesis is maintained by long-term (LT)-HSCs and their progeny. LT-HSCs have a two cell cycle states: a quiescent state (G0 phase) and a cycling state (non-G0; i.e., G1/S/G2/M phase). LT-HSCs in the former state are resistant to various cytotoxic stresses. Reactive oxygen species (ROS) change the cell cycle state of LT-HSCs from quiescent to cycling. Cycling LT-HSCs are also promoted to differentiate into short-term (ST)-HSCs and multipotent progenitors (MPPs). These differentiated progenitors actively produce various terminally differentiated hematopoietic cells.

Fig. 1. Quiescent and cycling hematopoietic stem cells (HSCs)

One important regulator for the quiescence of HSCs is reactive oxygen species (ROS). ROS are an intrinsic and extrinsic stress for HSCs (Figure 2). Intrinsically, ROS are mainly produced by mitochondria, the energy factory of the cell, as a by-product of the electron transport chain. Because anaerobic energy metabolism in mitochondria utilizes oxygen to generate ATP, oxygen-rich conditions produce intracellular ROS in HSCs. In addition, various immune cells utilize oxygen to generate ROS as an anti-microbial agent. ROS have favourable and unfavourable effects on HSCs. ROS are a signal transducer for essential cytokine signalling in HSCs (Sattler et al., 1999). However, excessive or prolonged ROS exposure is detrimental to HSCs (Naka et al., 2008). Aberrant exposure to ROS induces senescence, apoptosis, or the accumulation of DNA damage in HSCs. These damaged cells are dysfunctional and a potential source for leukemic transformation. Therefore, it is reasonable to hypothesize that HSCs reside in a hypoxic microenvironment.

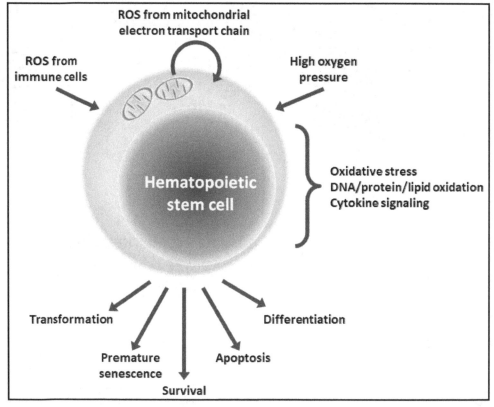

HSCs are exposed to ROS from various sources, including endogenous mitochondria and adjacent immune cells. High O2 pressure in the microenvironment also promotes ROS generation. This ROS burden results in the oxidation of DNA, protein, and lipid in HSCs. Also, the appropriate dose of ROS mediates cytokine signalling in HSCs. These balances determine the fate of HSCs: survival, premature senescence, apoptosis, differentiation, or malignant transformation.

Fig. 2. Intrinsic and extrinsic oxidative stresses and HSCs

3. Hypoxic nature of bone marrow

Although molecular oxygen is critically important for living organisms, HSCs are susceptible to reactive oxygen species or oxidative stresses that are derived from molecular oxygen. To maintain life-long hematopoiesis, it is reasonable for HSCs to avoid high-oxygen conditions. Although classical observations and theoretical studies supported these views, experimental evidence has only been recently provided.

Classically, bone marrow has been thought to be hypoxic. Recently, its exact nature and dynamic regulation were studied. This section will summarize the classical and recent studies related to the functional anatomy of bone marrow oxygenation.

Genetic studies have postulated that LT-HSCs reside primarily in the endosteal zone of the bone marrow (BM) (Calvi et al, 2003; Zhang J, 2003; Arai et al, 2004). Vascular organization around the endosteal zone is unique (Draenert and Draenert, 1980). Nutrient arteries penetrate the cortical bone, enter the medullary canal, and then proceed in a spiral pattern into the metaphyseal region of the bone marrow. The blood in arterial capillaries drains into sinusoids, which are fenestrated and loosely organized.

As a result, hematopoietic cells can easily move across the sinusoidal endothelium. Accordingly, the perfusion of the BM is limited and the partial oxygen pressure (PO2) in the endosteal region is very low.

In addition to hypoperfusion, the BM is tightly packed with blood cells. Oxygen consumption by hematopoietic cells is relatively high, and a simulation of O2 diffusion in the bone marrow suggested that the PO2 is decreased 10-fold at a distance of several cells from the nearest capillary (Chow et al, 2001). The average PO2 in the BM is approximately 55 mmHg and the mean O2 saturation is 87.5% (Harrison et al, 2002). Thus, based on this simulation study, HSCs may well reside in a severely hypoxic environment.

In support of this idea, it has also been reported that murine HSCs live in a hypoxic BM niche. By administering a perfusion tracer into mice, one group found that HSCs accumulated in a hypoperfusion cellular fraction in the BM (Parmar et al, 2007). These hypoperfused cells retained pimonidazole, a probe that selectively binds and forms adducts with protein thiol groups in a hypoxic environment. Administration of a toxin selective for hypoxic cells (tirapazamine) resulted in the depletion of HSCs *in vivo*. It was also shown that LT-HSCs are positive for pimonidazole in mice (Takubo et al, 2010). Moreover, human cord blood stem cells transplanted into super-immunodeficient NOD/scid/IL-2Rγ (NOG) mice homed to the BM niche and became both hypoxic and quiescent after BM transplantation (Shima et al, 2010).

Collectively, these findings suggest the hypoxic nature of HSCs. The hypoxic character of LT-HSCs is potentially determined by their position within the BM. However, in contrast to the simple O2 gradient model for the BM hypoxic niche, immunohistochemical observation of a two-dimensional segment of the murine BM suggests that 60% of LT-HSCs localize closely to BM endothelial cells (Kiel et al, 2005; Sugiyama et al, 2006). These findings do not fit the simple O2 gradient model for the hypoxic status of HSCs in the niche. However, as noted above, the vasculature in the niche near the endosteal zone of the BM may perfuse the bone marrow very poorly. Four-dimensional tracking (time-lapse and three-dimensional observation with a multi-photon microscope) of single LT-HSCs in the BM has shed light on this paradox. Real-time tracking of murine BM revealed that HSCs gradually move away from bone marrow blood vessels and then detach from them and translocate to the osteoblastic zone of the BM after transplantation (Lo Celso et al, 2009; Xie et al, 2009). Based on these observations, it is possible that subpopulations of HSCs residing in different specific locations have different oxygenation statuses.

In parallel with the hypoxic microenvironment for HSCs *in vivo*, hypoxic culture phenotypically and functionally sustained HSCs more effectively than normoxic culture (20% oxygen). Also, hypoxic culture enhances the colony-forming ability (progenitor ability) and transplantation capacity (HSC capacity) of cultured BM cells or isolated HSCs (Cipolleschi et al, 1993; Danet et al, 2003; Ivanovic et al, 2004). Hypoxic treatment also induces cell cycle quiescence in cultured HSC (Hermitte et al, 2006; Shima et al, 2010). Quiescent HSCs are defined by a high amount of efflux of the DNA-binding dye Hoechst 33342 from the cytosol (Goodell et al, 1996). These cells are called "side population (SP)" cells due to their specific staining pattern by flow cytometric analysis. Hypoxic treatment also sustains the SP phenotype in HSC *in vitro* (Krishnamurthy et al, 2004). Exclusion of Hoechst dye from the HSC cytosol is supported by Bcrp1/ABCG2, an ATP-dependent transporter, at the plasma membrane. When HSCs were cultured under hypoxic conditions, mRNA expression of Bcrp1/ABCG2 was significantly increased and the number of SP cells was also increased as compared to HSCs cultured at normoxia. Interestingly, because Bcrp1-/- mice show no significant defect in hematopoiesis (Zhou et al, 2001), the functional role of Bcrp1 in HSCs is still uncharacterized.

4. Hypoxia response system in HSCs

Cells sense, respond, and adapt to hypoxia using hypoxia-responsive regulatory pathways. HSCs utilize the same hypoxia response pathways as a number of other cell types. A central component of these pathways is hypoxia-inducible factor-1 (HIF-1), a transcription factor that is essential for cellular and systemic responses to a low oxygen microenvironment (Semenza, 2010) (Figure 3). HIF-1 is a heterodimeric transcription factor consisting of the oxygen-dependent HIF-1α subunit and an oxygen-independent HIF-1β subunit (Wang and Semenza, 1995). HIF-1α is hydroxylated at proline (Pro) 402 and/or 564 in the oxygen-dependent degradation (ODD) domain under normoxic conditions (Kaelin and Ratcliffe, 2008). HIF-1α is hydroxylated by three prolyl hydroxylases (PHD1-3) which require molecular oxygen, Fe^{2+}, 2-oxoglutarate, and ascorbic acid for their full enzymatic activity (Epstein et al, 2001). Prolyl-hydroxylated HIF-1α protein is recognized by the von Hippel-Lindau (VHL) tumor suppressor protein, which recruits the Elongin C/Elongin B/Cullin2/E3 ubiquitin ligase complex. As a result, prolyl-hydroxylated HIF-1α protein is ubiquitinated and degraded by the proteasome. Under a hypoxic environment, prolyl hydroxylases lose their enzymatic activity. Thus, prolyl hydroxylation of HIF-1α is suppressed, and HIF-1α protein is stabilized without degradation (Kaelin and Ratcliffe, 2008). HIF-1 heterodimers (HIF-1α:HIF-1β) are recruited and bind to hypoxia response elements (HREs) in various target genes and activate transcription programs (Semenza, 2010).

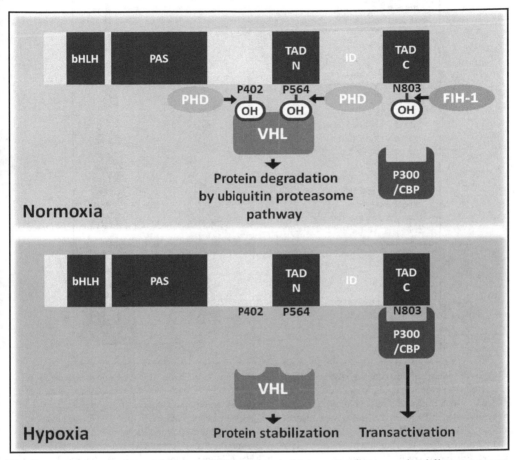

The diagrams represent the regulation of HIF-1α protein and interacting factors under different oxygen conditions. HIF-1α is a substrate for both prolyl and asparaginyl hydroxylases. Under normoxia, proline and asparagine residues are hydroxylated. These modifications regulate the stability and transcriptional activity of HIF-1α. bHLH, basic-helix-loop-helix domain; PAS, Per-ARNT-Sim domain; TAD-N, transactivation domain N-terminal; ID, inhibitory domain; TAD-C, C-terminal transactivation domain; PHD, prolyl hydroxylase domain-containing protein; and FIH-1, factor-inhibiting HIF-1.

Fig. 3. Regulation of hypoxia-inducible factor-1α (HIF-1α)

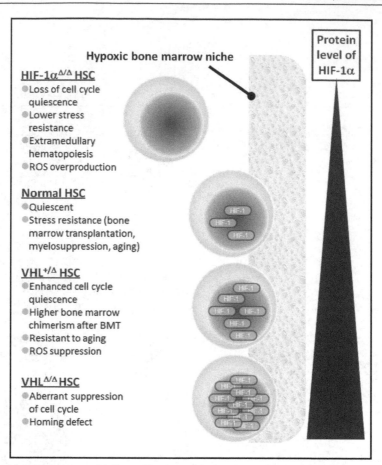

Scheme of biological outcomes of different HIF-1α protein levels in HSCs. This is achieved by HIF-1α or VHL deletion in HSCs using knockout mouse models. Normal HSCs (the second from the top) stabilize HIF-1α, which maintains cell cycle quiescence at the hypoxic bone marrow niche in the endosteum. Preferential stabilization of HIF-1α was observed in HSCs under hypoxia. HIF-1α$^{\Delta/\Delta}$ HSCs (top) lose cell cycle quiescence and stress resistance against transplantation, chemotherapeutic agents, and aging. In addition, HIF-1α$^{\Delta/\Delta}$ HSCs leave the bone marrow niche and drive extramedullary hematopoiesis in the spleen. Production of ROS is accelerated in HIF-1α$^{\Delta/\Delta}$ HSCs. Heterozygous deletion of VHL results in a slight increase in HIF-1α protein. Under these conditions, cell cycle quiescence in HSCs is enhanced. The VHL$^{+/\Delta}$ HSC (the second from the bottom) is resistant to transplantation and aging. ROS production is also suppressed in VHL$^{+/\Delta}$ HSCs. The homozygous VHL mutant (VHL$^{\Delta/\Delta}$) HSC has a maximal dose of HIF-1α protein. In contrast to heterozygous VHL mutant HSCs, VHL$^{\Delta/\Delta}$ HSCs completely lost stem cell capacity potentially due to aberrant suppression of the cell cycle and/or homing capacity to the niche. This defect is HIF-1α–dependent because the co-deletion of HIF-1α in homozygous VHL-deficient hematopoietic cell rescued the defect. Thus, the precise regulation of HIF-1α levels coordinates stem cell proliferation and differentiation. Recently, it has been reported that vascular endothelial growth factor, heat shock proteins, and GRP78 and its ligand Cripto regulate HSC quiescence and maintain HSCs in hypoxia as downstream factors of HIF-1α (Rehn et al, 2011; Miharada et al, 2011).

Fig. 4. Features of HIF-1α or VHL knockout HSCs

HIF-1α mRNA and protein are highly expressed in LT-HSCs (Takubo et al, 2010; Simsek et al, 2010) (Figure 4). HSCs derived from conditional HIF-1α knockout (HIF-1α$^{Δ/Δ}$) mice have a defective capacity for marrow reconstitution during serial BM transplantation (Takubo et al., 2010). HIF-1α$^{Δ/Δ}$ LT-HSCs lost cell cycle quiescence, entered the cell cycle from G0 phase, proliferated, and showed reduced tolerance to stresses such as 5-fluorouracil administration or aging. These studies suggest that HIF-1α plays an essential role in the regulation of HSC quiescence and stress resistance *in vivo*. In addition to these HIF-1α loss-of-function studies, conditional deletion of the VHL gene in hematopoietic cells was performed as a HIF-1α gain-of-function experiment. Analysis of VHL mutant hematopoietic cells revealed that the functional properties of LT-HSCs and progenitors are differentially influenced by HIF-1α. HIF-1α protein levels are elevated in either biallelic (VHL$^{Δ/Δ}$) or monoallelic (VHL$^{+/Δ}$) conditional knockout hematopoietic cells. For example, only a minor population of normal hematopoietic progenitors (CD34$^+$ LSK cells) are in a quiescent state. In clear contrast, the proportion of VHL$^{+/Δ}$ hematopoietic progenitors in the quiescent phase is significantly higher. At steady state, HIF-1α protein levels are not high in hematopoietic progenitors, and forced stabilization of HIF-1α protein through monoallelic VHL deletion induces VHL$^{+/Δ}$ CD34$^+$ LSK progenitors to exit the cell cycle and maintains them in the G0 phase. Severe suppression of cell cycling and transplantation capacity is restored in HIF-1α$^{Δ/Δ}$:VHL$^{Δ/Δ}$ doubly mutated HSCs. The decreased frequency of LT-HSCs seen in VHL$^{Δ/Δ}$ mice is rescued by the co-deletion of the HIF-1α gene *in vivo*. Also, long-term *in vitro* exposure of LT-HSCs to a PHD inhibitor (dimethyloxalylglycine; DMOG), which stabilizes HIF-1α even under normoxic conditions, attenuates stem cell ability especially during BM transplantation (Eliasson P et al, 2010).

Collectively, these results provide evidence that there is an optimal HIF-1α protein level for HSC maintenance. HIF-1α is required for stress resistance and long-term maintenance of HSCs, and within an appropriate range, moderate increases of HIF-1α (to the level caused by VHL heterozygous deletion) are trophic for HSCs through the induction of quiescence. However, aberrantly high HIF-1α levels are also harmful to HSCs and lead to a loss of stem cell capacity and the exhaustion of the HSC pool. Homozygous deletion of VHL results in a severe suppression of the cell cycle and a homing defect during transplantation.

HIF-1α not only acts in the HSC system but also plays an important role in neural stem cells (NSCs) under hypoxic conditions. In this type of cell, HIF-1α induces the activation of the Wnt/β-catenin signalling pathway through the upregulation of β-catenin and the expression of the downstream transcription factors lymphoid enhancer-binding factor 1 and T-cell factor 1 (Mazumdar J et al, 2010). Wnt/β-catenin activity was closely correlated with hypoxic status in the subgranular zone of the hippocampus, which is one of the niches for NSCs. Loss of HIF-1α in NSCs resulted in a defective Wnt-dependent hippocampal neurogenic niche capacity. As a result, NSC proliferation and differentiation, and the production of new neurons, were attenuated. Interestingly, the biological effects of HIF-1α on NSCs (cell cycle promotion) are clearly different from those seen in HSCs (cell cycle quiescence). It will be important to dissect how these different lineage stem cell systems utilize the same protein (HIF-1α) to sustain themselves using different downstream molecular machinery and biological events. It is also of interest to investigate embryonic

HSCs, which actively proliferate in hypoxic conditions, because HIF-1α may support HSC proliferation in that stage. In addition, HIF-1α protein has been reported to inhibit Wnt/β-catenin activity in cancer cells (Kaidi A et al, 2007), suggesting that the interaction of the HIF-1α and Wnt/β-catenin pathway in stem/progenitor cells may differ from that of more differentiated or transformed cell types.

5. Conclusion

In this chapter, I have summarized our current knowledge regarding the hypoxia response and oxygen metabolism in HSCs at the BM niche. These studies open novel fields in stem cell biology. The invisible niche factor, oxygen, is usually essential because mitochondria utilize it for the energy production. However, molecular oxygen is a source of ROS during mitochondrial metabolism. Because an excessive dose of ROS can be damaging to HSC, escape from oxygen (in the hypoxic niche) is a reasonable strategy for the long-term maintenance of HSCs *in vivo*. Adult HSCs are quiescent and contain few mitochondria, whereas hematopoietic progenitor cells actively proliferate and contain many mitochondria. Thus, stem cells and progenitors have distinct metabolic states, and the transition from stem to progenitor cell may correspond to a critical metabolic change, namely from glycolysis to oxidative phosphorylation. Slow cell cycling or long-term quiescence is common in adult tissue stem cells. Dormancy in the cell cycle may be a crucial mechanism for the stress resistance of normal and leukemic stem cells.

Further investigation of oxygen metabolism in tissue stem cells will result in more effective maintenance, expansion, and manipulation of various somatic stem cells *ex vivo* and *in vivo*, maximizing the potential of therapeutic strategies using stem cells in regenerative medicine.   Also, an understanding of oxygen homeostasis in HSCs is essential for understanding senescence at the stem cell level as well as therapeutic targeting against leukemic stem cells.

6. Acknowledgments

I would like to thank to Drs. Atsushi Hirao, Makoto Suematsu, Nobuhito Goda, Tomoyoshi Soga, and Randall S. Johnson for providing thoughtful insights and collaborations for this review. Most of our work on hypoxia in HSCs was performed in Dr. Toshio Suda's laboratory at the Keio University School of Medicine, Tokyo, Japan under his careful management. I would like to acknowledge my deep appreciation of fruitful discussions with the previous and current members of the Stem Cell Metabolism group of the Suda lab, especially Dr. Hirono Iriuchishia, Dr. Chiharu Kobayashi, Dr. Hiroshi Kobayashi, Dr. June-Won Cheong, Dr. Ayako Ishizu, and Ms. Wakako Yamada. Also, I would like to thank Ms. Tomoko Muraki and Ms. Takako Hirose for the preparation of this manuscript. K.T. is supported by the Global COE Program for Human Metabolomic Systems Biology and for Stem Cell Medicine of the Japan Society for Promotion of Science, and also in part by a Ministry of Education, Culture, Sports, Science and Technology (MEXT) Grant-in-Aid for Young Scientists (A), a MEXT Grant-in-Aid for Scientific Research (A), and a MEXT Grant-in-Aid for Scientific Research on Innovative Areas. The author dedicates this paper to the memory of Masako Takubo, who passed away October 9, 2011.

7. References

Arai, F., Hirao, A., Ohmura, M., Sato, H., Matsuoka, S., Takubo, K., Ito, K., Koh, G.Y., Suda, T. (2004). Tie2/angiopoietin-1 signaling regulates hematopoietic stem cell quiescence in the bone marrow niche. *Cell.* 118, 149-161.

Calvi, L.M., Adams, G.B., Weibrecht, K.W., Weber, J.M., Olson, D.P., Knight, M.C., Martin, R.P., Schipani, E., Divieti, P., Bringhurst, F.R. et al. (2003). Osteoblastic cells regulate the haematopoietic stem cell niche. *Nature.* 425, 841-846.

Chow, D.C., Wenning, L.A., Miller, W.M., Papoutsakis, E.T. (2001). Modeling pO(2) distributions in the bone marrow hematopoietic compartment. II. Modified Kroghian models. *Biophys J.* 81, 685-696.

Cipolleschi, M.G., Dello, Sbarba P., Olivotto, M. (1993). The role of hypoxia in the maintenance of hematopoietic stem cells. *Blood.* 82, 2031-2037.

Danet, G.H., Pan, Y., Luongo, J.L., Bonnet, D.A., Simon, M.C. (2003). Expansion of human SCID-repopulating cells under hypoxic conditions. *J Clin Invest.* 112, 126-135.

Draenert, K., Draenert, Y. (1980). The vascular system of bone marrow. *Scan Electron Microsc* 113-122.

Eliasson, P., Rehn, M., Hammar, P., Larsson, P., Sirenko, O., Flippin, L.A., Cammenga, J., Jonsson, J.I. (2010). Hypoxia mediates low cell-cycle activity and increases the proportion of long-term-reconstituting hematopoietic stem cells during in vitro culture. *Exp Hematol.* 38, 301-310.

Epstein, A.C., Gleadle, J.M., McNeill, L.A., Hewitson, K.S., O'Rourke, J., Mole, D.R., Mukherji, M., Metzen, E., Wilson, M.I., Dhanda, A. et al. (2001). C. elegans EGL-9 and mammalian homologs define a family of dioxygenases that regulate HIF by prolyl hydroxylation. *Cell.* 107, 43-54.

Fuchs, E., Horsley, V. (2011). Ferreting out stem cells from their niches. *Nat Cell Biol.* 13, 513-518.

Goodell, M.A., Brose, K., Paradis, G., Conner, A.S., Mulligan, R.C. (1996). Isolation and functional properties of murine hematopoietic stem cells that are replicating in vivo. *J Exp Med.* 183, 1797-1806.

Harrison, J.S., Rameshwar, P., Chang, V., Bandari, P. (2002). Oxygen saturation in the bone marrow of healthy volunteers. *Blood.* 99, 394.

Hermitte, F., Brunet, de la Grange P., Belloc, F., Praloran, V., Ivanovic, Z. (2006). Very low O2 concentration (0.1%) favors G0 return of dividing CD34+ cells. *Stem Cells.* 24, 65-73.

Ivanovic, Z., Hermitte, F., Brunet, de la Grange P., Dazey, B., Belloc, F., Lacombe, F., Vezon, G., Praloran, V. (2004). Simultaneous maintenance of human cord blood SCID-repopulating cells and expansion of committed progenitors at low O2 concentration (3%). *Stem Cells.* 22, 716-724.

Jang, Y.Y., Sharkis, S.J. (2007). A low level of reactive oxygen species selects for primitive hematopoietic stem cells that may reside in the low-oxygenic niche. *Blood.* 110, 3056-3063.

Kaelin, W.G. Jr, Ratcliffe, P.J. (2008). Oxygen sensing by metazoans: the central role of the HIF hydroxylase pathway. *Mol Cell.* 30, 393-402.

Kaidi, A., Williams, A.C., Paraskeva, C. (2007). Interaction between beta-catenin and HIF-1 promotes cellular adaptation to hypoxia. *Nat Cell Biol.* 9, 210-217.

Kiel, M.J., Yilmaz, O.H., Iwashita, T., Yilmaz, O.H., Terhorst, C., Morrison, S.J. (2005). SLAM family receptors distinguish hematopoietic stem and progenitor cells and reveal endothelial niches for stem cells. *Cell.* 121, 1109-1121.

Kirito K, Fox N, Komatsu N, Kaushansky K. (2005) Thrombopoietin enhances expression of vascular endothelial growth factor (VEGF) in primitive hematopoietic cells through induction of HIF-1alpha. *Blood.* Jun 1;105(11):4258-63. Epub 2005 Feb 10.

Krishnamurthy, P., Ross, D.D., Nakanishi, T., Bailey-Dell, K., Zhou, S., Mercer, K.E., Sarkadi, B., Sorrentino, B.P., Schuetz, J.D. (2004). The stem cell marker Bcrp/ABCG2 enhances hypoxic cell survival through interactions with heme. *J Biol Chem.* 279, 24218-24225.

Lo, Celso C., Fleming, H.E., Wu, J.W., Zhao, C.X., Miake-Lye, S., Fujisaki, J., Cote, D., Rowe, D.W., Lin, C.P., Scadden, D.T. (2009). Live-animal tracking of individual haematopoietic stem/progenitor cells in their niche. *Nature.* 457, 92-96.

Mazumdar, J., O'Brien, W.T., Johnson, R.S., LaManna, J.C., Chavez, J.C., Klein, P.S., Simon, M.C. (2010). O2 regulates stem cells through Wnt/beta-catenin signalling. *Nat Cell Biol.* 12, 1007-1013.

Miharada K, Karlsson G, Rehn M, Rorby E, Siva K, Cammenga J, Karlsson S. (2011) Cripto regulates hematopoietic stem cells are a hypoxic niche related factor through cell surface receptor GRP78. (2011) *Cell Stem Cell,* Oct 4;9(4):330-44.

Mohyeldin A, Garzón-Muvdi T, Quiñones-Hinojosa A. (2010) Oxygen in stem cell biology: a critical component of the stem cell niche. *Cell Stem Cell.* Aug 6;7(2):150-61.

Naka K, Muraguchi T, Hoshii T, Hirao A. (2008) Regulation of reactive oxygen species and genomic stability in hematopoietic stem cells. *Antioxid Redox Signal.* Nov;10(11):1883-94.

Osawa, M., Hanada, K., Hamada, H., Nakauchi, H. (1996). Long-term lymphohematopoietic reconstitution by a single CD34-low/negative hematopoietic stem cell. *Science.* 273, 242-245.

Parmar, K., Mauch, P., Vergilio, J.A., Sackstein, R., Down, J.D. (2007). Distribution of hematopoietic stem cells in the bone marrow according to regional hypoxia. *Proc Natl Acad Sci U S A.* 104, 5431-5436.

Pedersen M, Löfstedt T, Sun J, Holmquist-Mengelbier L, Påhlman S, Rönnstrand L. (2008) Stem cell factor induces HIF-1alpha at normoxia in hematopoietic cells. *Biochem Biophys Res Commun.* Dec 5;377(1):98-103. Epub 2008 Oct 1.

Qian H, Buza-Vidas N, Hyland CD, Jensen CT, Antonchuk J, Månsson R, Thoren LA, Ekblom M, Alexander WS, Jacobsen SE. (2007) Critical role of thrombopoietin in maintaining adult quiescent hematopoietic stem cells. *Cell Stem Cell.* Dec 13;1(6):671-84. Epub 2007 Nov 20.

Rehn M, Olsson A, Reckzeh K, Diffner E, Carmeliet P, Landberg G, Cammenga J. (2011) Hypoxic induction of vascular endothelial growth factor regulates murine hematopoietic stem cell function in the low-oxygenic niche. *Blood.* 118(6):1534-43. Epub 2011 Jun 13.

Sattler M, Winkler T, Verma S, Byrne CH, Shrikhande G, Salgia R, Griffin JD. (1999) Hematopoietic growth factors signal through the formation of reactive oxygen species. *Blood.* May 1;93(9):2928-35.

Semenza, G.L. (2007). Oxygen-dependent regulation of mitochondrial respiration by hypoxia-inducible factor 1. *Biochem J. 405,* 1-9.

Semenza, G.L. (2009). Regulation of cancer cell metabolism by hypoxia-inducible factor 1. *Semin Cancer Biol. 19,* 12-16.

Semenza, G.L. (2010). Oxygen homeostasis. *Wiley Interdiscip Rev Syst Biol Med.* 2, 336-361.

Shima, H., Takubo, K., Tago, N., Iwasaki, H., Arai, F., Takahashi, T., Suda, T. (2010) Acquisition of G_0 state by CD34-positive cord blood cells after bone marrow transplantation. *Exp Hematol.* 38, 1231-1240.

Simsek, T., Kocabas, F., Zheng, J., Deberardinis, R.J., Mahmoud, A.I., Olson, E.N., Schneider, J.W., Zhang, C.C., Sadek, H.A. (2010). The distinct metabolic profile of hematopoietic stem cells reflects their location in a hypoxic niche. *Cell Stem Cell.* 7, 380-390.

Snippert, H.J., Clevers, H. (2011). Tracking adult stem cells. *EMBO Rep.* 12, 113-122.

Suda T, Takubo K, Semenza GL. (2011) Metabolic regulation of hematopoietic stem cells in the hypoxic niche. *Cell Stem Cell.* Oct 4;9(4):298-310.

Sugiyama, T., Kohara, H., Noda, M., Nagasawa, T. (2006). Maintenance of the hematopoietic stem cell pool by CXCL12-CXCR4 chemokine signaling in bone marrow stromal cell niches. *Immunity.* 25, 977-988.

Takubo, K., Goda, N., Yamada, W., Iriuchishima, H., Ikeda, E., Kubota, Y., Shima, H., Johnson, R.S., Hirao, A., Suematsu, M. et al. (2010). Regulation of the HIF-1alpha level is essential for hematopoietic stem cells. *Cell Stem Cell.* 7, 391-402.

Wang, G.L., Semenza, G.L. (1995). Purification and characterization of hypoxia-inducible factor 1. *J Biol Chem.* 270, 1230-1237.

Wilson, A., Laurenti, E., Oser, G., van, der Wath R.C., Blanco-Bose, W., Jaworski, M., Offner, S., Dunant, C.F., Eshkind, L., Bockamp, E. et al. (2008). Hematopoietic stem cells reversibly switch from dormancy to self-renewal during homeostasis and repair. *Cell.* 135, 1118-1129.

Xie, Y., Yin, T., Wiegraebe, W., He, X.C., Miller, D., Stark, D., Perko, K., Alexander, R., Schwartz, J., Grindley, J.C., Park J, Haug JS, Wunderlich JP, Li H, Zhang S, Johnson T, Feldman RA, Li L. (2009). Detection of functional haematopoietic stem cell niche using real-time imaging. *Nature.* 457, 97-101.

Yoshihara H, Arai F, Hosokawa K, Hagiwara T, Takubo K, Nakamura Y, Gomei Y, Iwasaki H, Matsuoka S, Miyamoto K, Miyazaki H, Takahashi T, Suda T. (2007) Thrombopoietin/MPL signaling regulates hematopoietic stem cell quiescence and interaction with the osteoblastic niche. *Cell Stem Cell.* Dec 13;1(6):685-97.

Zhang, J., Niu, C., Ye, L., Huang, H., He, X., Tong, W.G., Ross, J., Haug, J., Johnson, T., Feng, J.Q. Harris S, Wiedemann LM, Mishina Y, Li L. (2003). Identification of the haematopoietic stem cell niche and control of the niche size. *Nature.* 425, 836-841.

Zhou S, Schuetz JD, Bunting KD, Colapietro AM, Sampath J, Morris JJ, Lagutina I, Grosveld GC, Osawa M, Nakauchi H, Sorrentino BP. (2001) The ABC transporter Bcrp1/ABCG2 is expressed in a wide variety of stem cells and is a molecular determinant of the side-population phenotype. *Nat Med.* Sep;7(9):1028-34.

7

Regulation of Tyrosine Kinase Signaling by Cbl in Hematopoietic Stem Cells

Mayumi Naramura
University of Nebraska Medical Center
USA

1. Introduction

Phosphorylation of tyrosine residues is an essential biochemical reaction in many higher eukaryotes. One of the most important and well-studied functions of tyrosine phosphorylation is to convey extracellular signals to the cytoplasm and ultimately to the nucleus in order to control various cell functions such as proliferation, differentiation, migration and survival.

The first tyrosine kinase (TK) was discovered as the tumor-inducing activity from Rous sarcoma virus, which is now known as v-Src (Rous, 1911). Later studies revealed that the oncogenic properties of v-Src was due to the loss of the regulatory mechanisms to control its kinase activity (Martin, 2001). These findings clearly highlight the critical importance of precise regulation of TK activities in order to avoid detrimental consequences to the homeostasis of the organisms.

Various mechanisms are employed to control TK activities. In the Src family non-receptor tyrosine kinase (non-RTK), phosphorylation status of the tyrosine residue in the C-terminal regulatory region alters intramolecular interactions and therefore serves as a way to modulate kinase activity. The kinases and the phosphatases involved in this regulatory mechanism are, in turn, themselves under additional layers of regulation, thus, creating an intricate network of signal mediators to fine-tune cellular responses (Sen & Johnson, 2011). Incidentally, activity of a typical receptor tyrosine kinase (RTK) is regulated by ligand binding; RTKs alter conformation upon ligand binding and dimerize, which leads to transphosphorylation of critical tyrosine residues in the activation loop of the neighboring kinase in the cytoplasmic domain (He & Hristova). This initiates a cascade of biochemical reactions that activates downstream signaling pathways.

Subcellular localization of TKs is another important determinant of their activity (Murphy et al., 2009). There are now abundant evidence indicating that TKs can generate different signals dependent on their intracellular locations. Therefore, molecules that regulate protein trafficking and localization constitute a critical component of signal regulatory mechanism.

Covalent attachment of small proteins such as ubiquitin and small ubiquitin-like modifier (SUMO) to target proteins serves as a signal for various biological processing, including alteration of its localization and promotion of degradation (Schulman & Harper, 2009; van Wijk & Timmers, 2010). This reaction is mediated by a series of biochemical reactions involving the E1 or activating enzyme, the E2 or conjugating enzyme and the E3 ligase. Human genome encodes for two E1s, thirty E2 and over one thousand E3s for the ubiquitin system. This pathway architecture immediately implies that the substrate specificity of the ubiquitin system must be achieved largely at the level of E3s.

The Casitas B-lineage lymphoma (Cbl) family proteins are RING finger (RF)-containing multi-domain adaptors that function as E3 ubiquitin ligase primarily towards activated TKs (Thien & Langdon, 2001; Duan et al., 2004; Schmidt & Dikic, 2005). Using genetically-engineered mouse models, we and others showed that loss of Cbl, either singly or in combination with another family member Cbl-b, led to the enlargement of the hematopoietic stem cell (HSC) compartment (Naramura et al., 2011a). Additionally, mutations in the *CBL* gene have been identified in a small but significant number of hematological malignancies in human, and experimental evidence proved the oncogenicity of mutant *CBL* products (Naramura et al., 2011b). All together, these observations strongly support that the Cbl family proteins are critical regulators of hematopoietic homeostasis.

Here, we review functions of the Cbl family proteins and some of the candidate Cbl targets in the HSC compartment and discuss potential mechanisms of their regulation.

2. The Cbl family proteins

The Cbl family proteins are evolutionarily conserved signal regulators present through *C. elegans* to human (Figure 1). In mammals, this family includes Cbl (also known as c-Cbl, encoded by the *CBL* gene in human), Cbl-b (*CBLB* gene in human) and Cbl-c (also know as Cbl-3 or Cbl-SL, *CBLC* gene in human). Cbl was originally identified as a cellular homolog of a viral oncogene *v-Cbl* which caused leukemia and lymphoma in mice (Langdon et al., 1989). Cbl's involvement in signal transduction was suggested because it became prominently tyrosine-phosphorylated upon stimulation through various cell surface receptors (Donovan et al., 1994; Galisteo et al., 1995). But it was not until genetic studies in *C. elegans* identified the *sli-1* gene product as a Cbl homolog that Cbl was established as a negative regulator of RTK signaling.

2.1 Structure and biochemical functions of the Cbl family proteins

All Cbl family proteins share a high degree of homology in their N-terminal regions. These include the tyrosine kinase binding (TKB) domain, the RF domain and the short intervening linker region. X-ray crystallography studies revealed that the TKB domain comprised a four-helix bundle (4H), a calcium-binding EF hand and a variant Src homology region 2 (SH2) domain (Meng et al., 1999). The TKB domain mediates specific binding to cognate phosphotyrosine-containing motifs in activated TKs and select non-TK signal mediators (Lupher et al., 1996). The RF domain and the linker region together bind to E2 ubiquitin-conjugating enzymes and both of these motifs are essential for the E3 ubiquitin ligase activity of the Cbl family proteins (Joazeiro et al., 1999; Levkowitz et al., 1999; Yokouchi et al., 1999; Zheng et al., 2000).

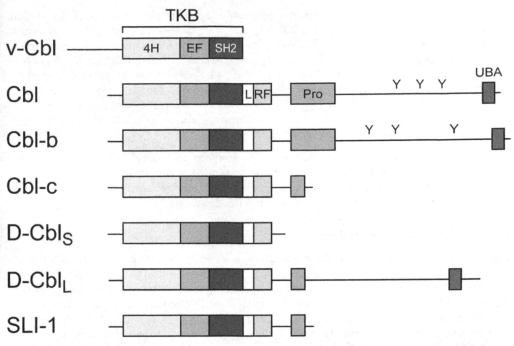

Fig. 1. Structure of the Cbl family proteins. The original oncogenic form of Cbl (v-Cbl), the three mammalian Cbl family proteins (Cbl, Cbl-b and Cbl-c), the short and long forms of *Drosophila* Cbl (D-Cbl$_S$ and D-Cbl$_L$) and the *C. elegans* homolog (SLI-1) are shown. TKB, tyrosine kinase binding; 4H, four-helix bundle; EF, EF hand; SH2, Src homology region 2; L, linker; RF, RING finger; Y, tyrosine; UBA, ubiquitin-associated.

Band and colleagues originally described that the Cbl TKB domain specifically recognized the phosphotyrosine-containing motif D(N/D)XpY, which was later refined as (N/D)XpY(S/T)XXP, found in several TKs such as ZAP70, epidermal growth factor receptor (EGFR), and Src (Lupher et al., 1997). Additional binding motifs, RA(V/I)XNQpY(S/T) and DpYR, were proposed in the adaptor protein APS (Hu & Hubbard, 2005) and the RTK c-Met (also known as hepatocyte growth factor receptor; Peschard et al., 2004), respectively. A recent comprehensive structural study showed that phosphopeptides with diverse sequences bound TKB at the same site, albeit in two different orientations (Ng et al., 2008). These studies collectively revealed the unique binding strategy for the specialized and biologically vital function of the Cbl family proteins and provided means to identify potential Cbl targets based on the amino acid sequences.

The C-terminal half of the Cbl family proteins are more divergent. A proline-rich region follows the RF domain in all mammalian Cbl family proteins, but this domain is more prominent in Cbl and Cbl-b than in Cbl-c. Biochemical studies have demonstrated that Cbl interacted with SH3-domain containing proteins such as Grb2 and Nck through the proline-rich region (Rivero-Lezcano et al., 1994; Fukazawa et al., 1995).

In addition to being a TK regulator, Cbl itself is subject to tyrosine phosphorylation. Phosphorylation at tyrosine residues 700, 731 and 774 have been extensively characterized; residues 700 and 774 provide docking sites for the SH2 domain-containing adaptor protein CrkL (Andoniou et al., 1996). Tyrosine 700 also mediates an interaction with the guanine nucleotide exchange factor Vav (Marengère et al., 1997). Tyrosine 731 provides a docking site of the p85 regulatory subunit of phosphatidylinositol 3-kinase (PI3K) (Hunter et al., 1999). Based on sequence homology and experimental data, tyrosine residues in the C-terminal domain of Cbl-b are thought to share many of the same functions as those in Cbl. Cbl-c does not possess comparable tyrosines.

The C-termini of Cbl and Cbl-b, but not Cbl-c, contain a conserved domain known as a ubiquitin-associated (UBA) domain, which is present in a variety of proteins involved in ubiquitin-mediated processes. Structural studies indicate that this domain is capable of binding ubiquitin and involved in dimerization (Kozlov et al., 2007; Peschard et al., 2007).

2.2 Insights from genetic models

The first critical clue into Cbl's functions came from genetic studies in *C. elegans* (Yoon et al., 1995). The vulval development in *C. elegans* is regulated by signals through the EGFR pathway. A reduction-of-function mutation in *let-23* (encodes the EGFR homolog) leads to death of most worms, and the vulval development is incomplete in surviving worms. However, when loss-of-function mutations in *sli-1* were introduced to this genetic background, worms survived and vulval development was restored. The sequence analysis of the *sli-1* gene revealed that it encoded a protein with a high similarity to Cbl, thus establishing Cbl as a negative regulator of the EGFR pathway.

Genetic studies in gene targeted mouse models provided further insights into the physiological roles of the Cbl family proteins in mammals. Cbl-deficient mice are viable, but they show recognizable changes in the hematopoietic, lymphoid, metabolic and reproductive systems. In contrast, effects of Cbl-b loss is mostly limited to the peripheral immune functions. Cbl-c expression appears to be restricted to the epithelial tissues, but no significant phenotypes were reported in mice deficient in Cbl-c (Table 1).

While mice deficient in either one of the Cbl family members are viable, simultaneous loss of Cbl and Cbl-b is not compatible with the survival of the organism and double-deficient mice do not survive beyond embryonic day 10 (Naramura et al., 2002). This indicates that Cbl and Cbl-b play redundant and overlapping functions in critical organ systems during fetal development. Using the Cre-loxP-mediated conditional gene deletion approach, effects of Cbl, Cbl-b loss have been analyzed in the T, B and HSC compartments (Naramura et al., 2002; Huang et al., 2006; Kitaura et al., 2007; Naramura et al., 2010). These studies demonstrated that, in the adaptive immune system, the Cbl family proteins are required to establish appropriate threshold for selection of T and B cells, and disruption of this process leads to autoimmune-like phenotypes in mice.

In the hematopoietic compartment, Cbl-deficiency leads to moderate splenomegaly and enhanced extramedullary hematopoiesis (Murphy et al., 1998). In the bone marrow, the lineage-negative, Sca-1-positive, c-Kit-positive (LSK) compartment, which is highly enriched for HSCs, is enlarged and Cbl-deficient HSCs showed enhanced capacity to reconstitute myeloabrated recipient's hematopoietic system (Rathinam et al., 2008). However, mice were outwardly normal and had a normal lifespan. When both Cbl and Cbl-b are deleted in the HSC, however, mice succumbed to aggressive myeloproliferative disease-like leukemia within two to three months after birth (Naramura et al., 2010).

Gene	Phenotype	Reference
Cbl	Altered T cell antigen receptor expression Increased tyrosine phosphorylation Enhanced thymic selection Splenomegaly and extramedullary hematopoiesis Decreased fertility Altered metabolism	(Murphy et al., 1998; Naramura et al., 1998; Thien et al., 1999; Molero et al., 2004; El Chami et al., 2005; Rathinam et al., 2008)
Cblb	Co-stiumlation-independent activation of peripheral T cells Predisposition to autoimmune diseases and inflammatory injury Resistance to spontaneous and transplanted tumors	(Bachmaier et al., 2000; Chiang et al., 2000; Krawczyk et al., 2000; Chiang et al., 2007; Loeser et al., 2007; Bachmaier et al., 2007)
Cblc	No apparent phenotypes	(Griffiths et al., 2003)

Table 1. Phenotypes of mice deficient in the Cbl family members

2.3 Cbl and hematological malignancies

Because of the involvement of various RTKs in cancer, it has long been speculated that the Cbl family proteins may play critical roles in the initiation and/or progression of cancer. Oncogenic mutations in RTKs that abrogate interaction with Cbl have been reported (Peschard & Park, 2003), but the direct evidence supporting Cbl's roles in cancer was not established until 2007.

The vast majority of CBL mutations reported so far are associated with myeloid disorders. Although the first human CBL mutations were described in acute myeloid leukemia (AML) samples (Sargin et al., 2007; Caligiuri et al., 2007; Abbas et al., 2008), later studies documented a significant number of cases in myelodysplastic syndromes-myeloproliferative neoplasms (MDS/MPN), a heterogeneous group of myeloid disorders including the chronic myelomonocytic leukemia (CMML), atypical chronic myeloid leukemia (aCML) and juvenile myelomonocytic leukemia (JMML) (Dunbar et al., 2008; Reindl et al., 2009; Grand et al., 2009; Loh et al., 2009; Sanada et al., 2009; Makishima et al., 2009; Muramatsu et al., 2010; Fernandes et al., 2010; Niemeyer et al., 2010). The association of CBL mutations with JMML is particularly thought-provoking because the pathogenesis of this rare pediatric hematological malignancy is closely associated with the activation of the Ras-MAPK signaling pathway (Loh, 2011). Among JMML patients, the activating mutations of PTPN11, NRAS and KRAS, and the loss of NF1, a gene encoding for a Ras GTPase-activator account for approximately 75 % of the total cases. Roughly half of the remainder of the cases are now attributed to CBL mutations. While in vitro experimental data indicate that the loss of the Cbl family proteins lead to prolonged Erk activation, it was never formally demonstrated whether Cbl can regulate Ras activity directly.

It is of note that most CBL mutations are either point mutation or internal deletion involving the linker and/or the RF regions rather than complete deletion at the CBL locus. As expected from domain-function analysis results, these mutant Cbl proteins lack E3 ubiquitin ligase activity. Interestingly, in patient samples with CBL mutations, the wild-type allele is often lost and replaced with the mutant allele by acquired uniparental isodisomy (aUPD). The CBLB, CBLC alleles are usually unaffected in these patients although mutations in these genes have been reported (Makishima et al., 2009; Makishima et al., 2011). All together, these clinical observations suggest that the presence of one wild-type copy of CBL is generally sufficient to maintain the functions of Cbl in the presence of normal Cbl-b and Cbl-c. These findings are consistent with the data in mice expressing a RF-mutant Cbl from the endogenous promoter on a Cblb, Cblc wild-type background (Thien et al., 2005; Rathinam et al., 2010); homozygous mutant mice are perinatally lethal, but hemizygous mutants over the wild-type Cbl allele develop normally. However, when the hemizygous mutant is expressed over the Cbl-null background, mice develop myeloproliferative disease-like leukemia within a year. This is a striking contrast when compared to the rapid progression and fatality of the HSC-specific Cbl, Cbl-b double-deficient mice (Naramura et al., 2010). These differences may reflect that the RF mutant and patient-derived oncogenic mutant Cbl proteins function as gain-of-function mutants rather than as dominant-negative inhibitors of Cbl-b (Cbl-c expression is minimal in the hematopoietic system). While these mutants lack E3 ubiquitin ligase activity and thus defective in promoting target degradation, they possess intact TKB and C-terminal protein-protein interaction motifs, which may enable them to form aberrant but stable multi-protein super-signaling complexes and activate unconventional signaling pathways.

2.4 Potential Cbl targets in the hematopoietic system

What, then, are the target of Cbl-dependent regulation in the HSC compartment? Because Cbl becomes phosphorylated upon stimulation with various cell surface receptors, it is conceivable that Cbl is involved in the regulation of signal transduction downstream of such pathways (Table 2). Among this diverse group of cell surface receptors, Kit and Flt3 are of particular interest because both of them are RTKs expressed in HSC and known to perform critical functions in the HSC compartment (Masson & Rönnstrand, 2009). Colony stimulating factor 1 receptor (CSF1R) is known to interact with Cbl (Lee et al., 1999), but it is expressed primarily in more differentiated myeloid/phagocytic cells than in HSCs. Endothelial-specific receptor tyrosine kinase (Tek, also known as Tie2) is another RTK expressed in the HSC compartment (Arai et al., 2004) and therefore may interact with Cbl. Thrombopoietin (TPO) is indispensable for the maintenance of HSC quiescence (Yoshihara et al., 2007; Qian et al., 2007). Although its receptor (TPO-R, also known as Mpl or c-Mpl) is not an RTK, stimulation with TPO induce phosphorylation of Cbl (Sasaki et al., 1995), Mpl have been shown to be ubiquitinylated (Saur et al., 2010) and Cbl loss alters the signal transduction downstream of TPO (Rathinam et al., 2008; Naramura et al., 2010). Therefore, Mpl may interact with Cbl indirectly. Other potential (direct as well as indirect) Cbl targets in the HSC compartment include the chemokine and integrin pathways.

In following sections, I will discuss how these pathways may be regulated by the Cbl family proteins in the HSCs.

Antigen and other immunological receptors
- T cell antigen receptor complex (Donovan et al., 1994; Meisner et al., 1995; Fukazawa et al., 1995)
- B cell antigen receptor complex (Cory et al., 1995; Tezuka et al., 1996; Panchamoorthy et al., 1996)
- Fcγ receptor (Marcilla et al., 1995)
- Fcε receptor (Matsuo et al., 1996; Suzuki et al., 1997)

RTKs
- Epidermal growth factor receptor (Galisteo et al., 1995)
- Insulin receptor (Ribon & Saltiel, 1997)
- Platelet-derived growth factor receptor (Bonita et al., 1997)
- Kit (Wisniewski et al., 1996; Brizzi et al., 1996)
- Flt3 (Lavagna-Sévenier et al., 1998)
- Fibroblast growth factor receptor (Wong et al., 2002)
- Colony stimulating factor 1 receptor (Wang et al., 1996)
- Met (Fixman et al., 1997; Garcia-Guzman et al., 2000)
- TrkB (McCarty & Feinstein, 1999)
- Tie2 (Wehrle et al., 2009)

Cytokine receptors
- Interleukin 2 receptor (Gesbert et al., 1998)
- Interleukin 3 receptor (Barber et al., 1997)
- Interleukin 4 receptor (Ueno et al., 1998)
- Erythropoietin receptor (Odai et al., 1995; Barber et al., 1997)
- Mpl (Sasaki et al., 1995; Brizzi et al., 1996)
- GM-CSF receptor (Odai et al., 1995)
- Prolactin receptor (Hunter et al., 1997)

Chemokine receptors (Chernock et al., 2001)

Integrins (Ojaniemi et al., 1997; Manié et al., 1997; Meng & Lowell, 1998)

Table 2. Partial list of potential upstream receptors for Cbl

3. Kit

The mouse dominant spotting mutation at the W locus was first described in the early 1900s (Durham, 1908). Mutations at this locus were studied extensively not only because they produced visible coat color changes, but also because mutant mice showed defects in hematopoiesis, mast cell development and gametogenesis (Russell, 1979). However, it was not until 1988 that the gene product at the W locus was found to encode for the cellular homolog of the *kit* oncogene which had been molecularly identified a few years earlier (Besmer et al., 1986; Chabot et al., 1988; Geissler et al., 1988).

Kit is a type III RTK that shares structural similarities with platelet-derived growth factor receptors (PDGFRs) α and β, Flt3 (also known as Flk-2, discussed below) and CSF1R. They are characterized by an extracellular domain with five immunoglobulin-like domains, a single transmembrane domain and an intracellular tyrosine kinase domain that is split into two by an intervening sequence.

HSCs are functionally defined as rare cells with the capacity to self-renew and give rise to all cell types of the hematopoietic lineage, including erythrocytes, granulocytes, monocytes, megakaryocytes and lymphocytes. No single marker specific for HSCs is known today. However, it is widely accepted that, in mice, most HSCs reside in a population of cells that express Kit and another cell surface protein Sca-1 and lack the expression of committed lineage markers (Ikuta & Weissman, 1992). Thus, Kit expression is intimately tied to HSCs.

The ligand for Kit is called stem cell factor (SCF) and encoded by the Steel (*Sl*) locus. The phenotypes of the *Sl* mutant mice are in most cases similar to those of *W* mutant mice, affecting hematopoiesis, mast cell development, fertility and coat colors (Galli et al., 1993). Collectively, these observations firmly established the essential roles of the SCF-Kit axis in these biological processes.

In the mouse embryo, hematopoietic cells are found in the blood islands in the yolk sac starting around embryonic day 7. Subsequently, at day 10-11 of gestation, HSCs migrate to the fetal liver and then to the spleen and the bone marrow, the primary hematopoietic organs in adult. The hematopoietic defect in *W* mice is detected throughout the course of development. Syngeneic transplantation experiments demonstrated that the defect exerted by *W* mutations was intrinsic to hematopoietic cells. The hematopoietic microenvironment in these animals are not affected and able to support hematopoiesis of normal donor-derived cells (Russell, 1979).

Kit activity is regulated at various levels. Ligand-receptor engagement of Kit initiates receptor dimerization and subsequent activation of its TK activity. Extensive biochemical studies have mapped intracellular phosphorylated tyrosine residues and their interacting proteins. These include Src family TKs, phosphatases such as SHP1 and SHP2, phospholipase Cγ, p85 subunit of phosphoinositide-3 kinase, (p85(PI3K)) and adaptor proteins such as Grb2 and APS (Lennartsson et al., 2005).

Cbl becomes phosphorylated when Kit-expressing cells are stimulated with SCF (Wisniewski et al., 1996). Earlier studies suggested that Cbl interacted with Kit indirectly through Grb2 (Brizzi et al., 1996), CrkL and p85(PI3K) (Sattler et al., 1997), and APS (Wollberg et al., 2003). More recent data suggest that Cbl binds to Kit directly at tyrosine 568, which is located in the juxtamembrane domain, and tyrosine 936, which is located in the carboxyterminal tail, ubiquitinylate Kit and target them for degradation (Masson et al., 2006). Both Cbl and Cbl-b function similarly towards Kit (Zeng et al., 2005). Hematopoietic cells deficient in Cbl functions are hypersensitive to stimulations through Kit (Naramura et al., 2010; Rathinam et al., 2010). These data all together strongly support that Kit may be one of the physiological targets of Cbl proteins in the HSC compartment.

Structurally, sequences surrounding tyrosine 568 partially conform to the canonical Cbl(TKB) recognition sequence while those around tyrosine 936 do not. Further analyses into the mechanisms of binding between Cbl and Kit may reveal novel molecular interactions that remained unknown so far.

4. Flt3

Flt3, another member of the type III RTKs, was originally identified by two separate groups through homology screening for TKs (Matthews et al., 1991; Rosnet et al., 1991). Its expression is detected in placenta, gonads, brain and hematopoietic cells, but its role outside of the hematopoietic system is not clear at present. Ligand for Flt3 (Flt3 ligand; FL) was identified a few years later and its transcript is expressed in wide range of both fetal and adult tissues (Lyman et al., 1993; Hannum et al., 1994).

Roles of Flt3 in HSCs appear to vary among species and also dependent upon developmental stages. The most primitive self-renewing HSCs with long-term reconstituting potential (LT-HSCs) are not found within Flt3$^+$ LSK cells in adult mouse bone marrow while the same biological activity was detected in both Flt3$^+$ and Flt3$^-$ populations in fetal liver (Adolfsson et al., 2001; Christensen & Weissman, 2001). Notably, human HSCs with multi-lineage reconstituting activity are Flt3$^+$ (Sitnicka et al., 2003). Flt3 deficient mice are viable and fertile, but show defects in B lymphocyte progenitors and dendritic cell generation (Mackarehtschian et al., 1995). The role of the FL-Flt3 axis in HSC maintenance and expansion remains controversial. Mackarehtschian et al. originally reported that Flt3-deficient bone marrow cells showed defects in lymphoid and myeloid reconstitution upon transplanting into myeloablated hosts (Mackarehtschian et al., 1995), while a more recent report by Buza-Vidas et al. concluded that Flt3 and FL were dispensable for maintenance and posttransplantation expansion of mouse HSCs (Buza-Vidas et al., 2009). Partly based on the phenotypes of Flt3 and FL deficient mice, models were proposed that Flt3 might function in the lineage restriction process from HSCs to lymphoid progenitors (Luc et al., 2007). However, in human, activating mutations in the *FLT3* gene, either in the form of internal tandem duplication (ITD) mutation in the juxtamembrane domain or point mutations in the kinase domain, are more frequently associated with myeloid malignancies rather than with lymphoid malignancies (Stirewalt & Radich, 2003). Clearly, the roles of Flt3 in the normal and pathological hematopoiesis need to be further delineated.

Cbl becomes tyrosine phosphorylated upon Flt3 engagement (Lavagna-Sévenier et al., 1998). It has been shown to physically interact with Flt3, and overexpression of an E3 ligase-defective mutant Cbl inhibited FL-induced Flt3 ubiquitylation and internalization, indicating involvement of Cbl in Flt3 signaling regulation (Sargin et al., 2007). Mice expressing a RF mutant Cbl from its endogenous locus are hypersensitive to FL stimulation (Rathinam et al., 2010), and we confirmed a similar phenotype in mouse bone marrow cells deficient in both Cbl and Cbl-b (Naramura, manuscript in preparation). Furthermore, deletion of FL blocks leukemia development in Cbl RING finger mutant mice (Rathinam et al., 2010).

Nevertheless, the mode of interaction between Cbl and Flt3 has not been clarified. Direct binding between Cbl and Flt3 has not been demonstrated. The sequences surrounding tyrosine 589 partially conform to the canonical Cbl(TKB) recognition sequence, and this region shares a very high homology to the sequences surrounding tyrosine 568 (a candidate Cbl binding site) in Kit. Notably, this is also the region frequently affected by ITD mutations. Alternatively, or in addition to the direct binding, because Flt3 is known to interact with Grb2 (Dosil et al., 1993; Zhang et al., 1999), a Cbl-binding adaptor protein, Cbl-Flt3 interaction may be mediated through this adaptor protein.

5. Other potential targets

As is clear from the list of potential Cbl upstream receptors, Kit and Flt3 may not be the only targets of Cbl-dependent regulation in HSCs. Although pathways other than Kit or Flt3 have not been as carefully examined in relation to Cbl, existing evidences suggest that following pathways may be regulated by the Cbl family proteins either directly or indirectly.

5.1 Tek

Tie2, encoded by the *TEK* gene, is an RTK expressed predominantly on endothelial cells, but they also provide crucial functions in the maintenance of quiescence and self-renewal capacity of the HSCs (Arai et al., 2004). The interaction between Tie2 and angiopoietin-1 (Ang-1), its ligand, has been shown to promote ubiquinylation of Tie2 by Cbl and receptor internalization (Wehrle et al., 2009). Structurally, the cytoplasmic domain of Tie2 does not contain any tyrosine residues that match the canonical Cbl(TKB) recognition sequence. However, activated Tie2 is known to bind Grb2 (Huang et al., 1995), thus may interact with Cbl indirectly through this adaptor.

5.2 Cytokine receptors

Cytokines such as hematopoietic growth factors and interleukins play essential roles in hematopoiesis. Cbl becomes tyrosine phosphorylated upon stimulation through various cytokine receptors (Table 2), and hematopoietic cells deficient in Cbl activity show enhanced sensitivity to cytokines (Rathinam et al., 2008; Sanada et al., 2009; Naramura et al., 2010). Receptors for these factors do not possess cytoplasmic tyrosine kinases but they activate the Janus kinase/Signal Transducers and Activators of Transcription (JAK/STAT) pathway (Yoshimura, 2009). Ligand binding induces receptor oligomerization, which activate associated JAK kinases and they, in turn, phosphorylate the receptor cytoplasmic domains and create binding sites for SH2-containing proteins.

There is no solid experimental evidence supporting the direct interaction between the JAK/STAT pathway and Cbl. Activation of the JAK/STAT pathway induces the expression of Suppressor of Cytokine Signaling (SOCS) family proteins, which function as E3 ubiquitin ligases for this pathway.

In addition to the JAK/STAT pathway, ligand binding to cytokine receptors activate the Ras-MAPK pathway through adaptor proteins such as APS and Grb2. Activation of this pathway is required for cell proliferation. As discussed above, these adaptor proteins are know to interact with Cbl, providing a potential link between the cytokine pathway and the Cbl family proteins.

6. Conclusion

In spite of its original identification as a cellular homolog of a viral oncogene, pathophysiological roles of the Cbl family proteins remained unclear for some time. Genetic studies in model organisms as well as identification of *CBL* mutations in patient-derived specimen played crucial roles in deciphering their essential functions as regulators of HSC homeostasis. Combined with molecular/biochemical information gathered over the last two decades, we now appreciate the complexity of the regulatory pathways surrounding the Cbl family proteins. While the primary focus of studies in the last ten years has been on Cbl's E3 ubiquitin ligase functions towards phosphotyrosine motif-containing targets, observations in cells expressing mutant Cbl proteins began to challenge this relatively-simplistic viewpoint. Further studies into this multifaceted protein family may uncover opportunities for novel diagnostics and therapeutics.

7. Acknowledgment

Works in the author's laboratory is supported by grants from the US Department of Defense Breast Cancer Research Program (W81XWH-10-1-0740) and the Nebraska Department of Health and Human Services (Stem Cell 2011-06).

8. References

Abbas, S., Rotmans, G., Löwenberg, B., & Valk, P. J. M. (2008). Exon 8 splice site mutations in the gene encoding the E3-ligase CBL are associated with core binding factor acute myeloid leukemias. *Haematologica*, Vol. 93, pp. 1595–1597.

Adolfsson, J., Borge, O. J., Bryder, D., Theilgaard-Mönch, K., Astrand-Grundström, I., Sitnicka, E., Sasaki, Y., & Jacobsen, S. E. (2001). Upregulation of Flt3 expression within the bone marrow Lin(-)Sca1(+)c-kit(+) stem cell compartment is accompanied by loss of self-renewal capacity. *Immunity*, Vol. 15, pp. 659–669.

Andoniou, C. E., Thien, C. B., & Langdon, W. Y. (1996). The two major sites of cbl tyrosine phosphorylation in abl-transformed cells select the crkL SH2 domain. *Oncogene*, Vol. 12, pp. 1981–1989.

Arai, F., Hirao, A., Ohmura, M., Sato, H., Matsuoka, S., Takubo, K., Ito, K., Koh, G. Y., & Suda, T. (2004). Tie2/angiopoietin-1 signaling regulates hematopoietic stem cell quiescence in the bone marrow niche. *Cell*, Vol. 118, pp. 149–161.

Bachmaier, K., Krawczyk, C., Kozieradzki, I., Kong, Y. Y., Sasaki, T., Oliveira-dos-Santos, A., Mariathasan, S., Bouchard, D., Wakeham, A., Itie, A., et al. (2000). Negative regulation of lymphocyte activation and autoimmunity by the molecular adaptor Cbl-b. *Nature*, Vol. 403, pp. 211–216.

Bachmaier, K., Toya, S., Gao, X., Triantafillou, T., Garrean, S., Park, G. Y., Frey, R. S., Vogel, S., Minshall, R., Christman, J. W., et al. (2007). E3 ubiquitin ligase Cblb regulates the acute inflammatory response underlying lung injury. *Nat. Med*, Vol. 13, pp. 920–926.

Barber, D. L., Mason, J. M., Fukazawa, T., Reedquist, K. A., Druker, B. J., Band, H., & D'Andrea, A. D. (1997). Erythropoietin and interleukin-3 activate tyrosine phosphorylation of CBL and association with CRK adaptor proteins. *Blood*, Vol. 89, pp. 3166–3174.

Besmer, P., Murphy, J. E., George, P. C., Qiu, F., Bergold, P. J., Lederman, L., Snyder, H. W., Brodeur, D., Zuckerman, E. E., & Hardy, W. D. (1986). A new acute transforming feline retrovirus and relationship of its oncogene v-kit with the protein kinase gene family. *Nature*, Vol. 320, pp. 415–421.

Bonita, D. P., Miyake, S., Lupher, M. L., Langdon, W. Y., & Band, H. (1997). Phosphotyrosine binding domain-dependent upregulation of the platelet-derived growth factor receptor α signaling cascade by transforming mutants of Cbl: implications for Cbl's function and oncogenicity. *Mol. Cell. Biol*, Vol. 17, pp. 4597–4610.

Brizzi, M. F., Dentelli, P., Lanfrancone, L., Rosso, A., Pelicci, P. G., & Pegoraro, L. (1996). Discrete protein interactions with the Grb2/c-Cbl complex in SCF- and TPO-mediated myeloid cell proliferation. *Oncogene*, Vol. 13, pp. 2067–2076.

Buza-Vidas, N., Cheng, M., Duarte, S., Nozad Charoudeh, H., Jacobsen, S. E. W., & Sitnicka, E. (2009). FLT3 receptor and ligand are dispensable for maintenance and posttransplantation expansion of mouse hematopoietic stem cells. *Blood*, Vol. 113, pp. 3453–3460.

Caligiuri, M. A., Briesewitz, R., Yu, J., Wang, L., Wei, M., Arnoczky, K. J., Marburger, T. B., Wen, J., Perrotti, D., Bloomfield, C. D., et al. (2007). Novel c-CBL and CBL-b ubiquitin ligase mutations in human acute myeloid leukemia. *Blood*, Vol. 110, pp. 1022–1024.

Chabot, B., Stephenson, D. A., Chapman, V. M., Besmer, P., & Bernstein, A. (1988). The proto-oncogene c-kit encoding a transmembrane tyrosine kinase receptor maps to the mouse W locus. *Nature*, Vol. 335, pp. 88–89.

Chernock, R. D., Cherla, R. P., & Ganju, R. K. (2001). SHP2 and cbl participate in α-chemokine receptor CXCR4-mediated signaling pathways. *Blood*, Vol. 97, pp. 608–615.

Chiang, J. Y., Jang, I. K., Hodes, R., & Gu, H. (2007). Ablation of Cbl-b provides protection against transplanted and spontaneous tumors. *J. Clin. Invest*, Vol. 117, pp. 1029–1036.

Chiang, Y. J., Kole, H. K., Brown, K., Naramura, M., Fukuhara, S., Hu, R. J., Jang, I. K., Gutkind, J. S., Shevach, E., & Gu, H. (2000). Cbl-b regulates the CD28 dependence of T-cell activation. *Nature*, Vol. 403, pp. 216–220.

Christensen, J. L., & Weissman, I. L. (2001). Flk-2 is a marker in hematopoietic stem cell differentiation: a simple method to isolate long-term stem cells. *Proc. Natl. Acad. Sci. U.S.A*, Vol. 98, pp. 14541–14546.

Cory, G. O., Lovering, R. C., Hinshelwood, S., MacCarthy-Morrogh, L., Levinsky, R. J., & Kinnon, C. (1995). The protein product of the c-cbl protooncogene is phosphorylated after B cell receptor stimulation and binds the SH3 domain of Bruton's tyrosine kinase. *J. Exp. Med.*, Vol. 182, pp. 611–615.

Donovan, J. A., Wange, R. L., Langdon, W. Y., & Samelson, L. E. (1994). The protein product of the c-cbl protooncogene is the 120-kDa tyrosine-phosphorylated protein in Jurkat cells activated via the T cell antigen receptor. *J. Biol. Chem*, Vol. 269, pp. 22921–22924.

Dosil, M., Wang, S., & Lemischka, I. R. (1993). Mitogenic signalling and substrate specificity of the Flk2/Flt3 receptor tyrosine kinase in fibroblasts and interleukin 3-dependent hematopoietic cells. *Mol. Cell. Biol.*, Vol. 13, pp. 6572–6585.

Duan, L., Reddi, A. L., Ghosh, A., Dimri, M., & Band, H. (2004). The Cbl family and other ubiquitin ligases: destructive forces in control of antigen receptor signaling. *Immunity*, Vol. 21, pp. 7–17.

Dunbar, A. J., Gondek, L. P., O'Keefe, C. L., Makishima, H., Rataul, M. S., Szpurka, H., Sekeres, M. A., Wang, X. F., McDevitt, M. A., & Maciejewski, J. P. (2008). 250K single nucleotide polymorphism array karyotyping identifies acquired uniparental disomy and homozygous mutations, including novel missense substitutions of c-Cbl, in myeloid malignancies. *Cancer Res*, Vol. 68, pp. 10349–10357.

Durham, F. M. (1908). A preliminary account of the inheritance of coat colour in mice. *Reports to the Evolution Committee of the Royal Society*, Vol. 4, pp. 41–53.

El Chami, N., Ikhlef, F., Kaszas, K., Yakoub, S., Tabone, E., Siddeek, B., Cunha, S., Beaudoin, C., Morel, L., Benahmed, M., et al. (2005). Androgen-dependent apoptosis in male germ cells is regulated through the proto-oncoprotein Cbl. *J. Cell Biol*, Vol. 171, pp. 651–661.

Fernandes, M. S., Reddy, M. M., Croteau, N. J., Walz, C., Weisbach, H., Podar, K., Band, H., Carroll, M., Reiter, A., Larson, R. A., et al. (2010). Novel oncogenic mutations of CBL in human acute myeloid leukemia that activate growth and survival pathways depend on increased metabolism. *J. Biol. Chem*, Vol. 285, pp. 32596–32605.

Fixman, E. D., Holgado-Madruga, M., Nguyen, L., Kamikura, D. M., Fournier, T. M., Wong, A. J., & Park, M. (1997). Efficient cellular transformation by the Met oncoprotein requires a functional Grb2 binding site and correlates with phosphorylation of the Grb2-associated proteins, Cbl and Gab1. *J. Biol. Chem*, Vol. 272, pp. 20167–20172.

Fukazawa, T., Reedquist, K. A., Trub, T., Soltoff, S., Panchamoorthy, G., Druker, B., Cantley, L., Shoelson, S. E., & Band, H. (1995). The SH3 domain-binding T cell tyrosyl phosphoprotein p120. Demonstration of its identity with the c-cbl protooncogene product and in vivo complexes with Fyn, Grb2, and phosphatidylinositol 3-kinase. *J. Biol. Chem*, Vol. 270, pp. 19141–19150.

Galisteo, M. L., Dikic, I., Batzer, A. G., Langdon, W. Y., & Schlessinger, J. (1995). Tyrosine phosphorylation of the c-cbl proto-oncogene protein product and association with epidermal growth factor (EGF) receptor upon EGF stimulation. *J. Biol. Chem*, Vol. 270, pp. 20242–20245.

Galli, S. J., Tsai, M., & Wershil, B. K. (1993). The c-kit receptor, stem cell factor, and mast cells. What each is teaching us about the others. *Am. J. Pathol.*, Vol. 142, pp. 965–974.

Garcia-Guzman, M., Larsen, E., & Vuori, K. (2000). The proto-oncogene c-Cbl is a positive regulator of Met-induced MAP kinase activation: a role for the adaptor protein Crk. *Oncogene*, Vol. 19, pp. 4058–4065.

Geissler, E. N., Ryan, M. A., & Housman, D. E. (1988). The dominant-white spotting (W) locus of the mouse encodes the c-kit proto-oncogene. *Cell*, Vol. 55, pp. 185–192.

Gesbert, F., Garbay, C., & Bertoglio, J. (1998). Interleukin-2 stimulation induces tyrosine phosphorylation of p120-Cbl and CrkL and formation of multimolecular signaling complexes in T lymphocytes and natural killer cells. *J. Biol. Chem.*, Vol. 273, pp. 3986–3993.

Grand, F. H., Hidalgo-Curtis, C. E., Ernst, T., Zoi, K., Zoi, C., McGuire, C., Kreil, S., Jones, A., Score, J., Metzgeroth, G., et al. (2009). Frequent CBL mutations associated with 11q acquired uniparental disomy in myeloproliferative neoplasms. *Blood*, Vol. 113, pp. 6182–6192.

Griffiths, E. K., Sanchez, O., Mill, P., Krawczyk, C., Hojilla, C. V., Rubin, E., Nau, M. M., Khokha, R., Lipkowitz, S., Hui, C.-C., et al. (2003). Cbl-3-deficient mice exhibit normal epithelial development. *Mol. Cell. Biol*, Vol. 23, pp. 7708–7718.

Hannum, C., Culpepper, J., Campbell, D., McClanahan, T., Zurawski, S., Kastelein, R., Bazan, J. F., Hudak, S., Wagner, J., Mattson, J., et al. (1994). Ligand for FLT3/FLK2 receptor tyrosine kinase regulates growth of haematopoietic stem cells and is encoded by variant RNAs. *Nature*, Vol. 368, pp. 643–648.

He, L., & Hristova, K. Physical-chemical principles underlying RTK activation, and their implications for human disease. *Biochimica et Biophysica Acta (BBA) - Biomembranes*, Vol. In Press, Uncorrected Proof. Available at: http://www.sciencedirect.com/science/article/pii/S0005273611002495 [Accessed September 1, 2011].

Hu, J., & Hubbard, S. R. (2005). Structural Characterization of a Novel Cbl Phosphotyrosine Recognition Motif in the APS Family of Adapter Proteins. *Journal of Biological Chemistry*, Vol. 280, pp. 18943–18949.

Huang, F., Kitaura, Y., Jang, I., Naramura, M., Kole, H. H., Liu, L., Qin, H., Schlissel, M. S., & Gu, H. (2006). Establishment of the major compatibility complex-dependent development of CD4+ and CD8+ T cells by the Cbl family proteins. *Immunity*, Vol. 25, pp. 571–581.

Huang, L., Turck, C. W., Rao, P., & Peters, K. G. (1995). GRB2 and SH-PTP2: potentially important endothelial signaling molecules downstream of the TEK/TIE2 receptor tyrosine kinase. *Oncogene*, Vol. 11, pp. 2097–2103.

Hunter, S., Burton, E. A., Wu, S. C., & Anderson, S. M. (1999). Fyn Associates with Cbl and Phosphorylates Tyrosine 731 in Cbl, A Binding Site for Phosphatidylinositol 3-Kinase. *Journal of Biological Chemistry*, Vol. 274, pp. 2097–2106.

Hunter, S., Koch, B. L., & Anderson, S. M. (1997). Phosphorylation of cbl after stimulation of Nb2 cells with prolactin and its association with phosphatidylinositol 3-kinase. *Mol. Endocrinol*, Vol. 11, pp. 1213–1222.

Ikuta, K., & Weissman, I. L. (1992). Evidence that hematopoietic stem cells express mouse c-kit but do not depend on steel factor for their generation. *Proceedings of the National Academy of Sciences*, Vol. 89, pp. 1502–1506.

Joazeiro, C. A., Wing, S. S., Huang, H., Leverson, J. D., Hunter, T., & Liu, Y. C. (1999). The tyrosine kinase negative regulator c-Cbl as a RING-type, E2-dependent ubiquitin-protein ligase. *Science*, Vol. 286, pp. 309–312.

Kitaura, Y., Jang, I. K., Wang, Y., Han, Y.-C., Inazu, T., Cadera, E. J., Schlissel, M., Hardy, R. R., & Gu, H. (2007). Control of the B cell-intrinsic tolerance programs by ubiquitin ligases Cbl and Cbl-b. *Immunity*, Vol. 26, pp. 567–578.

Kozlov, G., Peschard, P., Zimmerman, B., Lin, T., Moldoveanu, T., Mansur-Azzam, N., Gehring, K., & Park, M. (2007). Structural basis for UBA-mediated dimerization of c-Cbl ubiquitin ligase. *J. Biol. Chem*, Vol. 282, pp. 27547–27555.

Krawczyk, C., Bachmaier, K., Sasaki, T., Jones, R. G., Snapper, S. B., Bouchard, D., Kozieradzki, I., Ohashi, P. S., Alt, F. W., & Penninger, J. M. (2000). Cbl-b is a negative regulator of receptor clustering and raft aggregation in T cells. *Immunity*, Vol. 13, pp. 463–473.

Langdon, W. Y., Hartley, J. W., Klinken, S. P., Ruscetti, S. K., & Morse, H. C. (1989). v-cbl, an oncogene from a dual-recombinant murine retrovirus that induces early B-lineage lymphomas. *Proc. Natl. Acad. Sci. U.S.A*, Vol. 86, pp. 1168–1172.

Lavagna-Sévenier, C., Marchetto, S., Birnbaum, D., & Rosnet, O. (1998). FLT3 signaling in hematopoietic cells involves CBL, SHC and an unknown P115 as prominent tyrosine-phosphorylated substrates. *Leukemia*, Vol. 12, pp. 301–310.

Lee, P. S., Wang, Y., Dominguez, M. G., Yeung, Y. G., Murphy, M. A., Bowtell, D. D., & Stanley, E. R. (1999). The Cbl protooncoprotein stimulates CSF-1 receptor multiubiquitination and endocytosis, and attenuates macrophage proliferation. *EMBO J*, Vol. 18, pp. 3616–3628.

Lennartsson, J., Jelacic, T., Linnekin, D., & Shivakrupa, R. (2005). Normal and Oncogenic Forms of the Receptor Tyrosine Kinase Kit. *STEM CELLS*, Vol. 23, pp. 16–43.

Levkowitz, G., Waterman, H., Ettenberg, S. A., Katz, M., Tsygankov, A. Y., Alroy, I., Lavi, S., Iwai, K., Reiss, Y., Ciechanover, A., et al. (1999). Ubiquitin ligase activity and tyrosine phosphorylation underlie suppression of growth factor signaling by c-Cbl/Sli-1. *Mol. Cell*, Vol. 4, pp. 1029–1040.

Loeser, S., Loser, K., Bijker, M. S., Rangachari, M., van der Burg, S. H., Wada, T., Beissert, S., Melief, C. J. M., & Penninger, J. M. (2007). Spontaneous tumor rejection by cbl-b-deficient CD8+ T cells. *J. Exp. Med*, Vol. 204, pp. 879–891.

Loh, M. L. (2011). Recent advances in the pathogenesis and treatment of juvenile myelomonocytic leukaemia. *Br. J. Haematol.*, Vol. 152, pp. 677–687.

Loh, M. L., Sakai, D. S., Flotho, C., Kang, M., Fliegauf, M., Archambeault, S., Mullighan, C. G., Chen, L., Bergstraesser, E., Bueso-Ramos, C. E., et al. (2009). Mutations in CBL occur frequently in juvenile myelomonocytic leukemia. *Blood*, Vol. 114, pp. 1859–1863.

Luc, S., Buza-Vidas, N., & Jacobsen, S. E. W. (2007). Biological and molecular evidence for existence of lymphoid-primed multipotent progenitors. *Ann. N. Y. Acad. Sci.*, Vol. 1106, pp. 89–94.

Lupher, M. L., Reedquist, K. A., Miyake, S., Langdon, W. Y., & Band, H. (1996). A novel phosphotyrosine-binding domain in the N-terminal transforming region of Cbl interacts directly and selectively with ZAP-70 in T cells. *J. Biol. Chem*, Vol. 271, pp. 24063–24068.

Lupher, M. L., Songyang, Z., Shoelson, S. E., Cantley, L. C., & Band, H. (1997). The Cbl phosphotyrosine-binding domain selects a D(N/D)XpY motif and binds to the Tyr292 negative regulatory phosphorylation site of ZAP-70. *J. Biol. Chem*, Vol. 272, pp. 33140–33144.

Lyman, S. D., James, L., Vanden Bos, T., de Vries, P., Brasel, K., Gliniak, B., Hollingsworth, L. T., Picha, K. S., McKenna, H. J., & Splett, R. R. (1993). Molecular cloning of a ligand for the flt3/flk-2 tyrosine kinase receptor: a proliferative factor for primitive hematopoietic cells. *Cell*, Vol. 75, pp. 1157–1167.

Mackarehtschian, K., Hardin, J. D., Moore, K. A., Boast, S., Goff, S. P., & Lemischka, I. R. (1995). Targeted disruption of the flk2/flt3 gene leads to deficiencies in primitive hematopoietic progenitors. *Immunity*, Vol. 3, pp. 147–161.

Makishima, H., Cazzolli, H., Szpurka, H., Dunbar, A., Tiu, R., Huh, J., Muramatsu, H., O'Keefe, C., Hsi, E., Paquette, R. L., et al. (2009). Mutations of e3 ubiquitin ligase cbl family members constitute a novel common pathogenic lesion in myeloid malignancies. *J. Clin. Oncol*, Vol. 27, pp. 6109–6116.

Makishima, H., Jankowska, A. M., McDevitt, M. A., O'Keefe, C., Dujardin, S., Cazzolli, H., Przychodzen, B., Prince, C., Nicoll, J., Siddaiah, H., et al. (2011). CBL, CBLB, TET2, ASXL1, and IDH1/2 mutations and additional chromosomal aberrations constitute molecular events in chronic myelogenous leukemia. *Blood*, Vol. 117, pp. e198–e206.

Manié, S. N., Sattler, M., Astier, A., Phifer, J. S., Canty, T., Morimoto, C., Druker, B. J., Salgia, R., Griffin, J. D., & Freedman, A. S. (1997). Tyrosine phosphorylation of the product of the c-cbl protooncogene is [corrected] induced after integrin stimulation. *Exp. Hematol.*, Vol. 25, pp. 45–50.

Marcilla, A., Rivero-Lezcano, O. M., Agarwal, A., & Robbins, K. C. (1995). Identification of the major tyrosine kinase substrate in signaling complexes formed after engagement of Fcγ receptors. *J. Biol. Chem.*, Vol. 270, pp. 9115–9120.

Marengère, L. E., Mirtsos, C., Kozieradzki, I., Veillette, A., Mak, T. W., & Penninger, J. M. (1997). Proto-oncoprotein Vav interacts with c-Cbl in activated thymocytes and peripheral T cells. *J. Immunol*, Vol. 159, pp. 70–76.

Martin, G. S. (2001). The hunting of the Src. *Nat Rev Mol Cell Biol*, Vol. 2, pp. 467–475.

Masson, K., Heiss, E., Band, H., & Rönnstrand, L. (2006). Direct binding of Cbl to Tyr568 and Tyr936 of the stem cell factor receptor/c-Kit is required for ligand-induced ubiquitination, internalization and degradation. *Biochem. J.*, Vol. 399, pp. 59.

Masson, K., & Rönnstrand, L. (2009). Oncogenic signaling from the hematopoietic growth factor receptors c-Kit and Flt3. *Cellular Signalling*, Vol. 21, pp. 1717–1726.

Matsuo, T., Hazeki, K., Hazeki, O., Katada, T., & Ui, M. (1996). Specific association of phosphatidylinositol 3-kinase with the protooncogene product Cbl in Fcγ receptor signaling. *FEBS Lett.*, Vol. 382, pp. 11–14.

Matthews, W., Jordan, C. T., Wiegand, G. W., Pardoll, D., & Lemischka, I. R. (1991). A receptor tyrosine kinase specific to hematopoietic stem and progenitor cell-enriched populations. *Cell*, Vol. 65, pp. 1143–1152.

McCarty, J. H., & Feinstein, S. C. (1999). The TrkB receptor tyrosine kinase regulates cellular proliferation via signal transduction pathways involving SHC, PLCγ, and CBL. *J. Recept. Signal Transduct. Res.*, Vol. 19, pp. 953–974.

Meisner, H., Conway, B. R., Hartley, D., & Czech, M. P. (1995). Interactions of Cbl with Grb2 and phosphatidylinositol 3′-kinase in activated Jurkat cells. *Mol. Cell. Biol.*, Vol. 15, pp. 3571–3578.

Meng, F., & Lowell, C. A. (1998). A β1 integrin signaling pathway involving Src-family kinases, Cbl and PI-3 kinase is required for macrophage spreading and migration. *EMBO J.*, Vol. 17, pp. 4391–4403.

Meng, W., Sawasdikosol, S., Burakoff, S. J., & Eck, M. J. (1999). Structure of the amino-terminal domain of Cbl complexed to its binding site on ZAP-70 kinase. *Nature*, Vol. 398, pp. 84–90.

Molero, J. C., Jensen, T. E., Withers, P. C., Couzens, M., Herzog, H., Thien, C. B. F., Langdon, W. Y., Walder, K., Murphy, M. A., Bowtell, D. D. L., et al. (2004). c-Cbl-deficient mice have reduced adiposity, higher energy expenditure, and improved peripheral insulin action. *J. Clin. Invest*, Vol. 114, pp. 1326–1333.

Muramatsu, H., Makishima, H., Jankowska, A. M., Cazzolli, H., O'Keefe, C., Yoshida, N., Xu, Y., Nishio, N., Hama, A., Yagasaki, H., et al. (2010). Mutations of an E3 ubiquitin ligase c-Cbl but not TET2 mutations are pathogenic in juvenile myelomonocytic leukemia. *Blood*, Vol. 115, pp. 1969–1975.

Murphy, J. E., Padilla, B. E., Hasdemir, B., Cottrell, G. S., & Bunnett, N. W. (2009). Endosomes: A legitimate platform for the signaling train. *Proceedings of the National Academy of Sciences*, Vol. 106, pp. 17615–17622.

Murphy, M. A., Schnall, R. G., Venter, D. J., Barnett, L., Bertoncello, I., Thien, C. B., Langdon, W. Y., & Bowtell, D. D. (1998). Tissue hyperplasia and enhanced T-cell signalling via ZAP-70 in c-Cbl-deficient mice. *Mol. Cell. Biol*, Vol. 18, pp. 4872–4882.

Naramura, M., Band, V., & Band, H. (2011a). Indispensable roles of mammalian Cbl family proteins as negative regulators of protein tyrosine kinase signaling: Insights from in vivo models. *Commun Integr Biol*, Vol. 4, pp. 159–162.

Naramura, M., Jang, I.-K., Kole, H., Huang, F., Haines, D., & Gu, H. (2002). c-Cbl and Cbl-b regulate T cell responsiveness by promoting ligand-induced TCR down-modulation. *Nat. Immunol*, Vol. 3, pp. 1192–1199.

Naramura, M., Kole, H. K., Hu, R. J., & Gu, H. (1998). Altered thymic positive selection and intracellular signals in Cbl-deficient mice. *Proc. Natl. Acad. Sci. U.S.A*, Vol. 95, pp. 15547–15552.

Naramura, M., Nadeau, S., Mohapatra, B., Ahmad, G., Mukhopadhyay, C., Sattler, M., Raja, S. M., Natarajan, A., Band, V., & Band, H. (2011b). Mutant Cbl proteins as oncogenic drivers in myeloproliferative disorders. *Oncotarget*. Available at: http://www.ncbi.nlm.nih.gov/pubmed/21422499 [Accessed March 27, 2011].

Naramura, M., Nandwani, N., Gu, H., Band, V., & Band, H. (2010). Rapidly fatal myeloproliferative disorders in mice with deletion of Casitas B-cell lymphoma (Cbl) and Cbl-b in hematopoietic stem cells. *Proc. Natl. Acad. Sci. U.S.A*, Vol. 107, pp. 16274–16279.

Ng, C., Jackson, R. A., Buschdorf, J. P., Sun, Q., Guy, G. R., & Sivaraman, J. (2008). Structural basis for a novel intrapeptidyl H-bond and reverse binding of c-Cbl-TKB domain substrates. *EMBO J*, Vol. 27, pp. 804–816.

Niemeyer, C. M., Kang, M. W., Shin, D. H., Furlan, I., Erlacher, M., Bunin, N. J., Bunda, S., Finklestein, J. Z., Sakamoto, K. M., Gorr, T. A., et al. (2010). Germline CBL mutations cause developmental abnormalities and predispose to juvenile myelomonocytic leukemia. *Nat. Genet*, Vol. 42, pp. 794–800.

Odai, H., Sasaki, K., Iwamatsu, A., Hanazono, Y., Tanaka, T., Mitani, K., Yazaki, Y., & Hirai, H. (1995). The proto-oncogene product c-Cbl becomes tyrosine phosphorylated by stimulation with GM-CSF or Epo and constitutively binds to the SH3 domain of Grb2/Ash in human hematopoietic cells. *J. Biol. Chem.*, Vol. 270, pp. 10800–10805.

Ojaniemi, M., Martin, S. S., Dolfi, F., Olefsky, J. M., & Vuori, K. (1997). The proto-oncogene product p120(cbl) links c-Src and phosphatidylinositol 3'-kinase to the integrin signaling pathway. *J. Biol. Chem*, Vol. 272, pp. 3780–3787.

Panchamoorthy, G., Fukazawa, T., Miyake, S., Soltoff, S., Reedquist, K., Druker, B., Shoelson, S., Cantley, L., & Band, H. (1996). p120cbl is a major substrate of tyrosine phosphorylation upon B cell antigen receptor stimulation and interacts in vivo with Fyn and Syk tyrosine kinases, Grb2 and Shc adaptors, and the p85 subunit of phosphatidylinositol 3-kinase. *J. Biol. Chem*, Vol. 271, pp. 3187–3194.

Peschard, P., Ishiyama, N., Lin, T., Lipkowitz, S., & Park, M. (2004). A conserved DpYR motif in the juxtamembrane domain of the Met receptor family forms an atypical c-Cbl/Cbl-b tyrosine kinase binding domain binding site required for suppression of oncogenic activation. *J. Biol. Chem*, Vol. 279, pp. 29565–29571.

Peschard, P., Kozlov, G., Lin, T., Mirza, I. A., Berghuis, A. M., Lipkowitz, S., Park, M., & Gehring, K. (2007). Structural basis for ubiquitin-mediated dimerization and activation of the ubiquitin protein ligase Cbl-b. *Mol. Cell*, Vol. 27, pp. 474–485.

Peschard, P., & Park, M. (2003). Escape from Cbl-mediated downregulation: a recurrent theme for oncogenic deregulation of receptor tyrosine kinases. *Cancer Cell*, Vol. 3, pp. 519–523.

Qian, H., Buza-Vidas, N., Hyland, C. D., Jensen, C. T., Antonchuk, J., Månsson, R., Thoren, L. A., Ekblom, M., Alexander, W. S., & Jacobsen, S. E. W. (2007). Critical role of thrombopoietin in maintaining adult quiescent hematopoietic stem cells. *Cell Stem Cell*, Vol. 1, pp. 671-684.

Rathinam, C., Thien, C. B. F., Flavell, R. A., & Langdon, W. Y. (2010). Myeloid leukemia development in c-Cbl RING finger mutant mice is dependent on FLT3 signaling. *Cancer Cell*, Vol. 18, pp. 341-352.

Rathinam, C., Thien, C. B. F., Langdon, W. Y., Gu, H., & Flavell, R. A. (2008). The E3 ubiquitin ligase c-Cbl restricts development and functions of hematopoietic stem cells. *Genes Dev*, Vol. 22, pp. 992-997.

Reindl, C., Quentmeier, H., Petropoulos, K., Greif, P. A., Benthaus, T., Argiropoulos, B., Mellert, G., Vempati, S., Duyster, J., Buske, C., et al. (2009). CBL exon 8/9 mutants activate the FLT3 pathway and cluster in core binding factor/11q deletion acute myeloid leukemia/myelodysplastic syndrome subtypes. *Clin. Cancer Res*, Vol. 15, pp. 2238-2247.

Ribon, V., & Saltiel, A. R. (1997). Insulin stimulates tyrosine phosphorylation of the proto-oncogene product of c-Cbl in 3T3-L1 adipocytes. *Biochem. J.*, Vol. 324 (Pt 3), pp. 839-845.

Rivero-Lezcano, O. M., Sameshima, J. H., Marcilla, A., & Robbins, K. C. (1994). Physical association between Src homology 3 elements and the protein product of the c-cbl proto-oncogene. *J. Biol. Chem.*, Vol. 269, pp. 17363-17366.

Rosnet, O., Marchetto, S., deLapeyriere, O., & Birnbaum, D. (1991). Murine Flt3, a gene encoding a novel tyrosine kinase receptor of the PDGFR/CSF1R family. *Oncogene*, Vol. 6, pp. 1641-1650.

Rous, P. (1911). A SARCOMA OF THE FOWL TRANSMISSIBLE BY AN AGENT SEPARABLE FROM THE TUMOR CELLS. *The Journal of Experimental Medicine*, Vol. 13, pp. 397-411.

Russell, E. S. (1979). Hereditary anemias of the mouse: a review for geneticists. *Adv. Genet.*, Vol. 20, pp. 357-459.

Sanada, M., Suzuki, T., Shih, L.-Y., Otsu, M., Kato, M., Yamazaki, S., Tamura, A., Honda, H., Sakata-Yanagimoto, M., Kumano, K., et al. (2009). Gain-of-function of mutated C-CBL tumour suppressor in myeloid neoplasms. *Nature*, Vol. 460, pp. 904-908.

Sargin, B., Choudhary, C., Crosetto, N., Schmidt, M. H. H., Grundler, R., Rensinghoff, M., Thiessen, C., Tickenbrock, L., Schwäble, J., Brandts, C., et al. (2007). Flt3-dependent transformation by inactivating c-Cbl mutations in AML. *Blood*, Vol. 110, pp. 1004-1012.

Sasaki, K., Odai, H., Hanazono, Y., Ueno, H., Ogawa, S., Langdon, W. Y., Tanaka, T., Miyagawa, K., Mitani, K., & Yazaki, Y. (1995). TPO/c-mpl ligand induces tyrosine phosphorylation of multiple cellular proteins including proto-oncogene products, Vav and c-Cbl, and Ras signaling molecules. *Biochem. Biophys. Res. Commun*, Vol. 216, pp. 338-347.

Sattler, M., Salgia, R., Shrikhande, G., Verma, S., Pisick, E., Prasad, K. V., & Griffin, J. D. (1997). Steel factor induces tyrosine phosphorylation of CRKL and binding of CRKL to a complex containing c-kit, phosphatidylinositol 3-kinase, and p120(CBL). *J. Biol. Chem*, Vol. 272, pp. 10248-10253.

Saur, S. J., Sangkhae, V., Geddis, A. E., Kaushansky, K., & Hitchcock, I. S. (2010). Ubiquitination and degradation of the thrombopoietin receptor c-Mpl. *Blood*, Vol. 115, pp. 1254–1263.

Schmidt, M. H. H., & Dikic, I. (2005). The Cbl interactome and its functions. *Nat. Rev. Mol. Cell Biol*, Vol. 6, pp. 907–918.

Schulman, B. A., & Harper, J. W. (2009). Ubiquitin-like protein activation by E1 enzymes: the apex for downstream signalling pathways. *Nat Rev Mol Cell Biol*, Vol. 10, pp. 319–331.

Sen, B., & Johnson, F. M. (2011). Regulation of Src Family Kinases in Human Cancers. *J Signal Transduct*, Vol. 2011.

Sitnicka, E., Buza-Vidas, N., Larsson, S., Nygren, J. M., Liuba, K., & Jacobsen, S. E. W. (2003). Human CD34+ hematopoietic stem cells capable of multilineage engrafting NOD/SCID mice express flt3: distinct flt3 and c-kit expression and response patterns on mouse and candidate human hematopoietic stem cells. *Blood*, Vol. 102, pp. 881–886.

Stirewalt, D. L., & Radich, J. P. (2003). The role of FLT3 in haematopoietic malignancies. *Nat. Rev. Cancer*, Vol. 3, pp. 650–665.

Suzuki, H., Takei, M., Yanagida, M., Nakahata, T., Kawakami, T., & Fukamachi, H. (1997). Early and late events in Fcε RI signal transduction in human cultured mast cells. *J. Immunol.*, Vol. 159, pp. 5881–5888.

Tezuka, T., Umemori, H., Fusaki, N., Yagi, T., Takata, M., Kurosaki, T., & Yamamoto, T. (1996). Physical and functional association of the cbl protooncogen product with an src-family protein tyrosine kinase, p53/56lyn, in the B cell antigen receptor-mediated signaling. *J. Exp. Med.*, Vol. 183, pp. 675–680.

Thien, C. B. F., Blystad, F. D., Zhan, Y., Lew, A. M., Voigt, V., Andoniou, C. E., & Langdon, W. Y. (2005). Loss of c-Cbl RING finger function results in high-intensity TCR signaling and thymic deletion. *EMBO J*, Vol. 24, pp. 3807–3819.

Thien, C. B., Bowtell, D. D., & Langdon, W. Y. (1999). Perturbed regulation of ZAP-70 and sustained tyrosine phosphorylation of LAT and SLP-76 in c-Cbl-deficient thymocytes. *J. Immunol*, Vol. 162, pp. 7133–7139.

Thien, C. B., & Langdon, W. Y. (2001). Cbl: many adaptations to regulate protein tyrosine kinases. *Nat. Rev. Mol. Cell Biol*, Vol. 2, pp. 294–307.

Ueno, H., Sasaki, K., Honda, H., Nakamoto, T., Yamagata, T., Miyagawa, K., Mitani, K., Yazaki, Y., & Hirai, H. (1998). c-Cbl is tyrosine-phosphorylated by interleukin-4 and enhances mitogenic and survival signals of interleukin-4 receptor by linking with the phosphatidylinositol 3'-kinase pathway. *Blood*, Vol. 91, pp. 46–53.

Wang, Y., Yeung, Y. G., Langdon, W. Y., & Stanley, E. R. (1996). c-Cbl is transiently tyrosine-phosphorylated, ubiquitinated, and membrane-targeted following CSF-1 stimulation of macrophages. *J. Biol. Chem*, Vol. 271, pp. 17–20.

Wehrle, C., Van Slyke, P., & Dumont, D. J. (2009). Angiopoietin-1-induced ubiquitylation of Tie2 by c-Cbl is required for internalization and degradation. *Biochem. J.*, Vol. 423, pp. 375–380.

van Wijk, S. J. L., & Timmers, H. T. M. (2010). The family of ubiquitin-conjugating enzymes (E2s): deciding between life and death of proteins. *The FASEB Journal*, Vol. 24, pp. 981–993.

Wisniewski, D., Strife, A., & Clarkson, B. (1996). c-kit ligand stimulates tyrosine phosphorylation of the c-Cbl protein in human hematopoietic cells. *Leukemia*, Vol. 10, pp. 1436–1442.

Wollberg, P., Lennartsson, J., Gottfridsson, E., Yoshimura, A., & Rönnstrand, L. (2003). The adapter protein APS associates with the multifunctional docking sites Tyr-568 and Tyr-936 in c-Kit. *Biochem. J*, Vol. 370, pp. 1033–1038.

Wong, A., Lamothe, B., Lee, A., Schlessinger, J., Lax, I., & Li, A. (2002). FRS2 α attenuates FGF receptor signaling by Grb2-mediated recruitment of the ubiquitin ligase Cbl. *Proc. Natl. Acad. Sci. U.S.A.*, Vol. 99, pp. 6684–6689.

Yokouchi, M., Kondo, T., Houghton, A., Bartkiewicz, M., Horne, W. C., Zhang, H., Yoshimura, A., & Baron, R. (1999). Ligand-induced ubiquitination of the epidermal growth factor receptor involves the interaction of the c-Cbl RING finger and UbcH7. *J. Biol. Chem*, Vol. 274, pp. 31707–31712.

Yoon, C. H., Lee, J., Jongeward, G. D., & Sternberg, P. W. (1995). Similarity of sli-1, a regulator of vulval development in C. elegans, to the mammalian proto-oncogene c-cbl. *Science*, Vol. 269, pp. 1102–1105.

Yoshihara, H., Arai, F., Hosokawa, K., Hagiwara, T., Takubo, K., Nakamura, Y., Gomei, Y., Iwasaki, H., Matsuoka, S., Miyamoto, K., et al. (2007). Thrombopoietin/MPL signaling regulates hematopoietic stem cell quiescence and interaction with the osteoblastic niche. *Cell Stem Cell*, Vol. 1, pp. 685–697.

Yoshimura, A. (2009). Regulation of cytokine signaling by the SOCS and Spred family proteins. *Keio J Med*, Vol. 58, pp. 73–83.

Zeng, S., Xu, Z., Lipkowitz, S., & Longley, J. B. (2005). Regulation of stem cell factor receptor signaling by Cbl family proteins (Cbl-b/c-Cbl). *Blood*, Vol. 105, pp. 226–232.

Zhang, S., Mantel, C., & Broxmeyer, H. E. (1999). Flt3 signaling involves tyrosyl-phosphorylation of SHP-2 and SHIP and their association with Grb2 and Shc in Baf3/Flt3 cells. *J. Leukoc. Biol.*, Vol. 65, pp. 372–380.

Zheng, N., Wang, P., Jeffrey, P. D., & Pavletich, N. P. (2000). Structure of a c-Cbl-UbcH7 complex: RING domain function in ubiquitin-protein ligases. *Cell*, Vol. 102, pp. 533–539.

8

Skeletogenesis and the Hematopoietic Niche

Elizabeth Sweeney and Olena Jacenko
University of Pennsylvania
USA

1. Introduction

The reciprocal regulation of the skeletal and the immune systems has been clinically appreciated for years. In particular, factors produced by immune cells during homeostasis and activation markedly affect the skeleton, which in turn affects the marrow niche environments (as reviewed in (Compston 2002). This relationship also extends to an interdependence between bone and hematopoiesis during immune cell development, however the critical cell types and extracellular matrix components involved in establishing and maintaining hematopoietic niches within the bone marrow are only recently beginning to be defined. Indeed, some immuno-osseous disorders with hematopoietic defects such as bone marrow failure and immune dysfunction, as well as certain cancers, may result from a defective hematopoietic niche (Spranger et al. 1991; Kuijpers et al. 2004; Hermanns et al. 2005; Walkley et al. 2007; Walkley et al. 2007; Raaijmakers et al. 2010). Likewise during aging, a progressive decline in cell replacement and repair manifests in both the skeletal and hematopoietic systems with reduced bone mass and diminished blood cell formation respectively (as reviewed in (Rossi et al. 2008) and (Gruver et al. 2007). Further, this altered hematopoiesis due to aging leads to deficient immune function and increased incidence of malignancies (Rossi et al. 2005; Janzen et al. 2006; Mayack et al. 2010). Thus, the dynamic relationship between skeletal and hematopoietic maintenance throughout life suggests that these clinical outcomes may ensue from cell signaling deficiencies or from defects in the structural environment supporting hematopoiesis. This chapter provides an overview of our current understanding of how hematopoietic niches may be established, how they promote hematopoiesis, and how the skeletal status may modulate niche function.

2. Coordinate skeletal and hematopoietic development

The vertebrate skeleton develops by one of two essential processes, endochondral (EO) and intramembranous (IO) ossification mechanisms (as reviewed in (Chan, D. and Jacenko 1998). The direct differentiation of ectomesenchymal cells to osteoblasts in IO represents the rudimentary mechanism through which many skull bones and all periosteal bones form. The IO-derived bone is referred to as "dense", "compact" or "cortical", and as the names imply, is a solid bone with primary functions relating to weight bearing and protection (**Fig. 1C**). In contrast, EO relies on the generation of a cartilaginous skeletal blueprint that is gradually replaced by a "trabecular", "spongy", "cancellous" bone and a marrow capable of sustaining hematopoiesis (Chan, D. and Jacenko 1998; Mackie et al. 2008) (**Fig. 1C**). This replacement mechanism of EO is responsible for the formation of the vertebrate axial and appendicular skeleton, as well as certain cranial bones (Jacenko et al. 1991; Chan, D. and Jacenko 1998).

As EO initiates during embryogenesis, its distinctive feature is the emergence of hypertrophic cartilage, which is present in all skeletal elements that will develop a marrow cavity, e.g. long bones, hips, vertebrae, ribs, certain skull bones. The eventual replacement of cartilage by bone and marrow via EO relies on the sequential maturation of chondrocytes from resting, to proliferating, to hypertrophic (**Fig. 1A**). Chondrocyte hypertrophy manifests with a dramatic increase in cell size, cessation of proliferation, and synthesis of a new repertoire of differentiation-specific gene products (Godman and Porter 1960; Chan, D. and Jacenko 1998; Alvarez et al. 2001; James et al. 2010). Among these is the matrix protein collagen X, which represents the predominant biosynthetic product of hypertrophic cartilage (Gibson and Flint 1985; Schmid and Linsenmayer 1985). Concomitant with hypertrophy is a transformation from a non-calcified avascular cartilage matrix, to a calcifiable one that is permissive to vascular invasion. Morphometric analysis suggests that before vascular invasion, the terminal hypertrophic chondrocytes undergo either autophagy (Srinivas and Shapiro 2006; Bohensky et al. 2007) or apoptosis (Farnum and Wilsman 1989), the rate of which controls longitudinal growth of the skeletal element, as well as the transition from cartilage to trabecular bone and marrow (Farnum and Wilsman 1989).

Subsequent vascular entry into hypertrophic cartilage is critical to skeleto-hematopoietic development, since it leads to an influx of mesenchymal cells, hematopoietic precursors, and chondro/osteoclasts. This influx of cells, together with growth factors, cytokines and hormones, establishes the primary center of ossification and the marrow environment where hematopoiesis ensues (**Fig. 1**). Specifically, while chondro/osteoclasts degrade hypertrophic cartilage, multipotent stromal cells, including mesenchymal and perivascular reticular cells, form the marrow stroma, a meshwork of non-hematopoietic cells supporting hematopoiesis by providing structural scaffolding and producing hematopoietic factors (Taichman et al. 1996; Bianco et al. 1999). As hypertrophic cartilage continues to be degraded, matrix remnants serve as scaffolds upon which differentiating osteoblasts deposit bone matrix, thus forming trabecular bony spicules with hypertrophic cartilage cores (**Fig. 1B**) (Chan, D. and Jacenko 1998). Of note, the origin of the trabecular bone osteoblasts at the junction between marrow and the hypertrophic cartilage, termed the chondro-osseous junction, is still debated (Roach 1992; Roach et al. 1995; Roach and Erenpreisa 1996; Nakamura et al. 2006; Hilton et al. 2007; Maes et al. 2010). Following the formation of the primary ossification zones in the central or diaphyseal regions of skeletal elements, the establishment of secondary ossification centers at outer epiphyseal ends of bones defines the growth plate regions at the metaphysis (**Fig. 1A**). The growth plates occupy the narrow space that separates the marrow of the primary and secondary ossification centers, and are composed of a gradient of differentiating chondrocytes culminating in a zone of hypertrophic chondrocytes (**Fig. 1A & B**) (as reviewed in (Lefebvre and Smits 2005). The continual replacement of the hypertrophic chondrocytes by trabecular bone and marrow allows for longitudinal skeletal growth, robust hematopoiesis, and the progression of EO without consumption of the skeletal model until maturity, when in most non-rodent vertebrates EO ceases and growth plates close (**Fig. 1C**) (Kilborn et al. 2002). Thus, the end result of EO is a porous network of primary trabecular bone, consisting of a hybrid hyptertrophic cartilage-bone matrix, and engulfed by a hematopoietic marrow (**Fig. 1B & C**). Subsequent bone remodeling gradually leads to a complete replacement of the hybrid primary bone by mature secondary bone, and is coincident with a gradual decline in lymphopoiesis and the onset of immunosenescence (**Fig. 1C**) (as reviewed in (Compston 2002; Gruver et al. 2007).

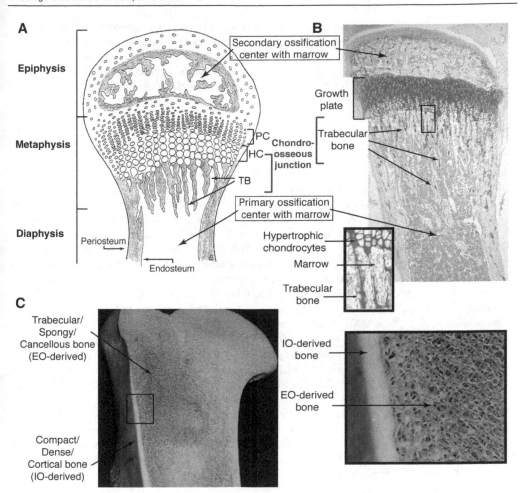

Fig. 1. Architecture of the endochondral bone. A) A schematic of a developing long bone illustrating its architecture. The epiphysis, or the bulbous end, lined by articular cartilage and containing the secondary ossification center with marrow, is supported by the flared metaphysis, which in turn rests upon the slender cylindrical shaft of the diaphysis. The growth plate separates the primary and secondary ossification centers, and consists of a gradient of differentiating chondrocyte zones; the proliferative cartilage (PC) and hypertrophic cartilage (HC) zones are marked, as well as the hybrid trabecular bone (TB) protruding into the marrow. The locations of the two-layered periosteal membrane surrounding the diaphysis and the inner endosteal network are marked. B) A longitudinal tibial section from a week-3 wild type mouse stained with safranin-orange, hematoxylin & eosin (H&E) and counterstained with fast green. Using these stains, the negatively charged cartilaginous matrix appears orange while the bone stains light blue-green; mature erythrocytes stain green, while other marrow elements stain pink-purple with H&E. The boxed inset is a high magnification of the chondro-osseous junction containing hypertrophic chondrocytes, bone and marrow with vascular. The hybrid nature of the trabecular bone can

be appreciated by the orange staining of the cartilaginous core, with green-blue bone matrix deposited on the surface (magnification, 10x). C) The inorganic mineralized matrix of a mature zebra bone illustrates the structural differences between the EO-derived trabecular /spongy/cancellous bone and the IO-derived compact/dense/cortical bone. Boxed is a high magnification of the EO- and IO-derived bone tissues. Note the mesh-like structure of trabecular bone for hematopoietic cell support.

Taken together, the proper differentiation of chondrocytes, vascular invasion and the gradual replacement of the cartilaginous anlagen by trabecular bone and marrow through EO, underscore the intricate orchestration of skeleto-hematopoiteic development. Moreover, the coincident establishment and localization of trabecular bone within the site of active hematopoiesis likely reflects a critical hematopoietic niche in the chondro-osseous region (**Fig. 1B boxed**) (Jacenko et al. 1993; Nilsson et al. 1997; Gress and Jacenko 2000; Nilsson et al. 2001; Jacenko et al. 2002; Yoshimoto et al. 2003; Arai, F. et al. 2004; Balduino et al. 2005; Sweeney et al. 2008; Kohler et al. 2009; Lo Celso et al. 2009; Xie et al. 2009; Sweeney et al. 2010). This skeleto-hematopoietic link is strongly supported by several animal models where alterations in process of EO leads to hematopoietic defects (**Table 1**), including mouse models with altered: collagen X (Jacenko et al. 1993; Gress and Jacenko 2000; Jacenko et al. 2002; Sweeney et al. 2008; Sweeney et al. 2010), parathyroid hormone related protein (PTHrP) receptor in osteoblasts (Calvi et al. 2001; Calvi et al. 2003; Kuznetsov et al. 2004; Wu et al. 2008), osteoblast numbers (Visnjic et al. 2001; Visnjic et al. 2004; Zhu et al. 2007), bone morphogenic protein (BMP) receptor type 1A in marrow cells (Zhang, J. et al. 2003), osteoclast function (Blin-Wakkach et al. 2004; Mansour et al. 2011), retinoic acid receptor gamma (Purton et al. 2006; Walkley et al. 2007), $G_s\alpha$ in ostoblasts (Wu et al. 2008), Dicer in ostoblasts (Raaijmakers et al. 2010), glypican-3 (Viviano et al. 2005), and perlecan (Rodgers et al. 2008). **Table 1** presents a list of mouse models with defects in hematopoiesis due to alterations in a component within the niche environment. Only those mouse models are summarized that were proven, by and large, via bone marrow transplantation experiments to have an aberrant niche environment, since wild type marrow cells could not rescue the disease phenotype of the host.

3. Overview of the hematopoietic niche

Hematopoiesis is the process by which hematopoietic stem cells (HSCs) generate and replenish progenitors that develop into fully mature blood and immune cells, and populate the periphery. During vertebrate ontogeny, hematopoiesis is established sequentially in several different anatomic sites (see Development of Hematopoietic Stem Cells chapter in this book for review). Coincident with the onset of EO (approximately the last third of embryonic development), hematopoiesis shifts from the fetal liver and spleen to the EO-derived marrow, which represents the predominant site of blood cell production after birth (Aguila and Rowe 2005; Cumano and Godin 2007). Therefore, the marrow has become a tissue of study for hematopoietic cell biology post parturition. Additionally, due to the ease of marrow cell isolation in combination with the extensive list of cell markers identifying HSCs at different stages of differentiation (as summarized in (Morrison and Spradling 2008), stem cell niche biology has also utilized the marrow environment for study.

Year	Protein/ cell	Description	Hematopoietic highlights	References
1993	Collagen X	Collagen X is a short chain collagen secreted by hypertrophic chondrocytes in the growth plate of endochondrally develop-ing bones. In these mice, collagen X is either knocked-out or mutated to cause dominant interfer-ence.	-Altered chondro-osseous junction -Decreased trabecular bone, -No change in HSPCs, -Decreased B lymphocytes through-out life, -Diminished immunity in vitro and in vivo, -Altered hematopoietic/lymphopoietic cytokines, e.g. decreased SCF, CXCL-12, IL-7, -Disease phenotype retained after transfer of wild type HSPCs into collagen X mice	Jacenko, 1993; Jacenko, 1996; Gress, 2000; Jacenko 2001; Jacenko 2002; Sweeney, 2008; Sweeney, 2010
2001	PTH/PTHrP receptor	Parathyroid hormone (PTH) and the PTH related protein (PTHrP) receptor (PPR) are involved in calcium homeostasis and activation of osteoblasts, thus indirectly osteoclasts. In these mice, a constitu-tively active form of PPR is expressed in mesenchymal cells under the 2.3kb promotor of collagen I.	-Delayed hematopoiesis due to delay in the bone to marrow transition, -With aging, increased trabecular bone and osteoblast numbers, -Increased HSPCs, -Increase in Notch signaling, -Increase in IL-6, CXCL-12, SCF, -Decrease in B cells at all stages	Calvi, 2001; Calvi, 2003; Kuznetsov, 2004; Wu 2008
2001	Osteoblast deletion	Osteoblasts have been implicated as a niche cell where increased in osteoblasts resulted in increases in HSPCs. These mice were generated with the herpes thymidine kinase gene under the 2.3kb promotor of collagen for deletion of collagen I expressing mesenchymal cells after ganciclovir treatment.	-Loss of bone lining cells and trabecular bone elements, -Decrease in marrow cellularity, -Decreases in HSPCs, -Decreases in lymphoid, erythroid, and myeloid progenitor cells, -Decrease in osteoclasts, -Increased extramedullary hemato-poiesis, -Recovery from disease phenotype after ganciclovire removed	Visnjic, 2001; Visnjic, 2004; Zhu, 2007
2003	BMPR1A	The bone morphogenic protein receptor, type 1A (BMPR1A) is a receptor for BMPs, which have been shown to influence hematopoiesis. These mice were generated with a PolyI:C-inducible Mx-1-Cre to delete BMPR1A in hematopoietic and stromal cells.	-Increases in spindle-shaped N-cadherin+ CD45- osteoblasts (SNO), -Increases in HSPCs, -LT-HSC observed attached to SNO cells, -No block in HPC differentiation to the lymphoid or myeloid lineages	Zhang, 2003
				Continued on facing page

Table 1. Mouse models with altered hematopoetic niche enviroments.

Year	Protein/ cell	Description	Hematopoietic highlights	References
2004	Tcirg 1	The T cell immune regulator 1 (Tcirg1) is a subunit of the vacuolar protein pump (V-ATPase) involved in osteoclast resorption of bone. In these mice there is a mutation of Tcrig1 rendering osteoclasts ineffective at bone resorption.	-Increases in myelomonocytic differentiation, -Reduced medullary cavity size, -Defective B cell differentiation leading to reduced numbers, -Reduced interferon-γ secretion from T cells, -Decreased IL-7 secretion from bone marrow cells, -Rescue of phenotype with restoration of marrow environment after wild type cell transfer	Blin-Wakkach, 2004; Mansour, 2011
2005	Osteopontin	Osteopontin is an extracellular matrix glycoprotein made by several cell types, including osteoblasts, fibroblasts, chondrocytes, etc. In these mice, osteopontin is knocked-out, and in 1998 Rittling et.al. showed no alterations to bone mophology, but increased osteoclastogenesis.	-Increased number of HSPCs, -No change in lymphoid or myeloid cell production, -Decreased HSPC apoptosis, -Increased Jagged 1 and Angiopoietin 1 stromal expression, -Disease phenotype retained after transfer of wild type HSPCs to Opn-/- mice	Rittling, 1998; Stier, 2005; Nilsson, 2005
2005	p27Kip1 and MAD1	Cyclin-dependent kinase inhibitors MAD1 and p27Kip1 are negative regulators of cell cycle. In these two studies, mice had either p27Kip1 knocked-out (Chien, 2006) or p27Kip1 and MAD1 knocked-out (Walkley, 2005).	-Hyperplasia of hematopoietic organs, -Increased myeloid and erythroid colony forming cells, -Increase in LT-HSCs, -Disease phenotype retained after transfer of wild type HSPCs into p27Kip1-/- mice	Walkley, 2005; Chien, 2006
2005	gp130	Glycoprotein 103 (gp130) is a subunit of the cytokine receptors for the IL-6 family. These mice were generated with the Tcre mouse for excision of gp103 in hematopoietic and endothelial cells.	-Hypocellular marrow, -Impairment in erythro-and thrombopoiesis, -Reduction in T lymphocytes in the thymus, -Reduction of B lymphopoiesis in the marrow, -Extramedullary hematopoiesis, -Disease phenotype retained after transplant of wild type HSPCs into gp130 mice	Yao, 2005

Continued on facing page

Table 1. continued

Year	Protein/cell	Description	Hematopoietic highlights	References
2006	RAR gamma	Retinoic acid receptors (RAR) are nuclear hormone receptors that act as ligand-dependent transcriptional regulators. In these mice the RARgamma is knocked-out.	-Decrease in HSPCs, -Increased granulopoiesis, -Myloproliferative-like disease with excessive extramedullary hemato-poiesis, -Loss of trabecular bone by 12 weeks of age, -Disease phenotype retained after transfer of wild type HSPCs into RARγ-/- mice	Purton, 2006; Walkley, 2007
2007	Rb	Retinoblastoma protein (Rb) is a central regulator of the cell cycle and several downstream regulators have been shown to have affects on hematopoiesis. These mice were generated using an inducible deletion construct in conjunction with Mx-1 Cre for deletion of Rb in hematopoietic and stromal cells.	-Myloproliferative disease pheno-type, -Increased HSPC differentiation, -Egress of HSPCs from marrow to extramedullary sites, -Loss of Rb was found to be necessary from both the myeloid-derived cells and the environment for presentation of the disease phenotype	Walkley, 2007
2008	Gsα	Gsa is a heterotrimeric G protein subunit that activates the cAMP-dependent pathway by activating adenylate cyclase and is part of the parathyroid hormone (PTH) and the PTH related protein (PTHrP) receptor. In these mice, Gsa was ablated in cells expressing ostrix, e.g. early osteopro-genitors and chondro-cytes.	-Decreases in B cell precursors in the marrow and in the periphery, -No negative affect on other hematopoietic lineages, -Decreases in IL-7 expression from osteoblasts, -Decreases in trabecular bone, -Disease phenotype not transferable to wild type mice with marrow transplant	Wu, 2008
2008	Bis (BAG-3 or CAIR-1)	Bcl-2 interacting cell death suppressor (Bis) is a protein involved in antiapoptotic and antistress pathways. In this mouse, Bis was truncated for loss of function.	-Reduced lymphoid tissues, -Perturbed vasculature with defects in endothelial cells, -Loss of HSPCs, -Defect in B lymphopoiesis, -Decreased splenic hematopoietic cell numbers, -Defects in stromal progenitor cells, -Loss of stromal cells expressing CXCL-12 and IL-7, -Osteoblast lineage unaffected, -Disease phenotype retained after transplant of wild type cells into Bis-/- mice	Youn, 2008; Kwon, 2010

Continued on facing page

Table 1. continued

Year	Protein/cell	Description	Hematopoietic highlights	References
2008	Hf2/merlin	Neurofibromin 2 (Nf2)/moesin-ezrin-radixin-like (merlin) is a cytoskeletal scaffolding protein involved in cell-cell communications. These mice were generated with a PolyI:C-inducible Mx-1-Cre to delete Nf2/merlin in hematopoietic and stromal cells.	-Egress of HSPCs, -Hypocellular marrow, -Increases in marrow vascularity, -Hematopoietic lineages unaffected, -After time, increases in trabecular bone and osteoblast numbers accompanied by restoration in marrow cellularity, -Disease phenotype retained after transplant of wild type cells into Nf2/merlin mice	Larsson, 2008
2010	Dicer	Dicer is an endoribonuclease that cleaves double-stranded RNA and pre-mircoRNA into small interfering RNA. In these mice, Dicer was ablated in cells expressing ostrix, e.g. early osteoprogenitors and chondrocytes.	-Decreases in leukocytes, platelets and red blood cells, -Decreases in B cell number with increases in myeloid cells, -No change in HSPC number, -Extramedullary hematopoiesis, -Slight decrease in osteoblast number with impaired differentiation, -Bone volume unchanged, but altered bone texture, -Disease phenotype retained after transplant of wild type cells into Dicer mice	Raaijmakers, 2010
2010	CAR cells	CXC chemokine ligand (CXCL) 12 abundant reticular (CAR) cells have been implicated as a hematopoietic niche cell in the marrow. These mice were designed to have inducible selective ablation of CAR cells with the diptheria toxin receptor.	-Reduced cycling of lymphoid and erythroid progenitor cells, -Reduced HSPC numbers, -HSPCs more quiescent, -HSPCs express more myeloid genes, -No changes in osteoblasts or endothelial cells, -Impaired production of SCF and CXCL-12	Omatsu, 2010
2010	Nestin+ cells	Nestin is an intermediate filament protein expressed in nerve cells and reported here in rare non-hematopoietic cells with mesencymal progenitor cell qualities. These mice were generated using the inducible diphtheria toxin with Nes-creERT2 for selective depletion of nestin expressing cells.	-Rapid reduction of HSPCs in marrow and increase in HSPCs in spleen, -Reduction of adrenergic nerve fibers, -Reduction of wild type HSPC homing to marrow of Nestin mice	Mendez-Ferrer, 2010

Continued on facing page

Table 1. continued

Year	Protein/cell	Description	Hematopoietic highlights	References
2010	Ebf2	Early B cell factor 2 (Ebf2) is a transcription factor expressed in neurons, immature osteoblsts and adipocytes. In these mice, Ebf2 is knocked-out.	-Impaired lymphopoiesis, -Reduced numbers of HSPCs, -Mice were smaller then wild type cohorts, -Disease phenotype rescued after transplant of Ebf2-/- cells into wild type mice	Corradi, 2003; Kieslinger, 2010
2011	Agrin	Agrin is a heparan sulfate proteoglycan matrix protein expressed on MSCs and trabecular osteoblasts in the niche. In these mice, agrin expression is deficient with low levels of muscle specific kinase (MuSK) expression for postnatal survival.	-Marrow hypoplasia with decreases in myeloid and lymphoid cells, -Reduced CD45+ cell numbers in marrow, spleen and marrow, -Decreases in thymus T-lineage populations, -Decreases in ST-HSC in marrow, but normal levels in fetal liver, -Disease phenotype is not transfered to wild type mice after transplant with MuSK-L:Agrin-/- hematopoietic cells	Mazzon, 2011

Table 1. continued

The idea of a unique tissue environment, or stem cell niche, as a tissue setting that can direct progenitor cell behavior, e.g. quiescence, proliferation, differentiation, etc. was proposed over four decades ago (Wolf and Trentin 1968; Trentin 1971; Schofield 1978; Wolf 1979). Hematopoietic niches, or hematopoietic microenvironments (HME), are defined by the association of particular cell types, their secreted matrix products and their soluble hematopoietic factors (Yin and Li 2006; Rodgers et al. 2008). The identity of the cellular, matrix and soluble components that influence HSCs, including the long-term populating (LT-HSC), short-term populating (ST-HSC), or the more differentiated hematopoietic progenitor cells (HPC), as well as the lymphoid and myeloid lineages, remains an active topic of investigation. However, at least two hematopoietic niches have been described, an osteoblastic (or endosteal) niche, ascribed to osteoblasts residing on bone surfaces, and a vascular niche, ascribed to endothelial cells and subendothelial MSCs or pericytes lining marrow sinusoids. Many have argued that more quiescent LT-HSCs and ST-HSCs are located in the osteoblast niche, while differentiating HPCs are located in the vascular niche for mobilization to the periphery (Lord et al. 1975; Shackney et al. 1975; Gong 1978; Nilsson et al. 2001; Heissig et al. 2002; Arai, F. et al. 2004; Balduino et al. 2005; Jang and Sharkis 2007; Bourke et al. 2009). However, these regions in the marrow are so close in proximity (Arai, F. et al. 2004; Kiel et al. 2005; Lo Celso et al. 2009; Xie et al. 2009), that the osteoblast and vascular niches may be the same, or perhaps interchangeable to some degree. Additionally, recent work has identified other cells involved in hematopoiesis that do not fully comply with these proposed niche regions, such as CXC chemokine ligand (CXCL)-12 expressing reticular cells that are scattered throughout the marrow (Tokoyoda et al. 2004; Sugiyama et al. 2006; Omatsu et al. 2010). Below we will discuss the different cellular, matrix and soluble components within the marrow that have been shown to influence hematopoiesis.

3.1 Cells of the niche

Experiments designed to identify the cells of the HME date back over fifty years (Pfeiffer 1948; Tavassoli and Crosby 1968; Tavassoli and Weiss 1971; Meck et al. 1973; Friedenstein et al. 1974; Tavassoli and Khademi 1980; Friedenstein et al. 1982; Patt et al. 1982; Tavassoli 1984; Friedenstein et al. 1987; Gurevitch and Fabian 1993; Kawai et al. 1994; Kuznetsov et al. 1997; Hara et al. 2003; Akintoye et al. 2006; Mankani et al. 2007; Sacchetti et al. 2007; Chan, C.K. et al. 2008; Mankani et al. 2008; Song et al. 2010). In these studies, ectopic bone with a functional HME was generated in host mice using various bone marrow derived osteoprogenitor seed cells. More recently, different osteoprogenitor pools have been isolated that can either generate EO-like bone with active hematopoiesis or compact IO-like bone without an HME (Akintoye et al. 2006; Chan, C.K. et al. 2008). Collectively, these studies have shown that functional HMEs form through the progression of EO with contributions from cartilage, bone, vasculature, and marrow stromal cells. Further, similar conclusions about the necessity of EO-derived components, e.g. cells and matrix molecules, were obtained through analyses of several mouse models with skeleto-hematopoietic defects (**Table 1**), including mice with disrupted collagen X function in the HME (Jacenko et al. 1993; Gress and Jacenko 2000; Jacenko et al. 2002; Sweeney et al. 2008; Sweeney et al. 2010). Discussed below are the data describing which cell type(s), associated matrix and soluble factors are necessary for blood cell development in the marrow, including: multipotent stromal cells (fibroblasts, pericytes, reticular cells, and adipocytes), osteoblasts, chondrocytes, endothelial cells, and cells of hematopoietic origin (hematopoietic stem/progenitor cells (HSPC), osteoclasts and macrophages).

3.1.1 Fibroblasts and perivascular cells

As early as the 1970's, in vitro studies with marrow stromal adherent colonies showed that this pool of cells is able to support hematopoiesis (Friedenstein et al. 1970; Dexter et al. 1973; Friedenstein et al. 1974; Friedenstein et al. 1976; Dexter et al. 1977). These plastic adherent colonies have been thought to contain mesenchymal progenitor cells, and likely mesodermal progenitor cells as well (Petrini et al. 2009). This would account for recent data indicating that marrow derived progenitor cells generate adipocytes, chondrocytes and osteoblasts, traditional mesenchymal cell types, as well as fibroblasts, smooth muscle cells, endothelial cells, and pericytes/subendothelial cells (Bentley and Foidart 1980; Muguruma et al. 2006; Sacchetti et al. 2007; Crisan et al. 2008; Kalajzic et al. 2008; Augello et al. 2010; Mendez-Ferrer et al. 2010). Thus, isolated marrow stromal cells will be referred to as multipotent stromal cells (MSC) throughout (Horwitz et al. 2005). The MSCs isolated for ectopic bone assays have been described as osteoprogenitor cells that generate bone with a HME able to support host-derived hematopoiesis (Kuznetsov et al. 1997; Akintoye et al. 2006; Sacchetti et al. 2007; Chan, C.K. et al. 2008; Morikawa et al. 2009). Of note, many of these osteoprogenitor cells have been shown to have stem-like qualities, such as self-replication and the ability to differentiate into several different cell types. For example, Sacchetti et al. isolated human-derived MCAM/CD146-expressing subendothelial cells, which can self-replicate as well as give rise to osteoblasts, chondrocytes and reticular cells in ectopic HMEs (Sacchetti et al. 2007). More recently, these data were replicated in the mouse by Morikawa et al. who also identified a perivascular cell type that has the ability to self-replicate and give rise to adipocytes, osteoblasts, chondrocytes and endothelial cells (Morikawa et al. 2009). An additional perivascular cell has also been identified as a HME cell type, the nestin-expressing MSCs (Mendez-Ferrer et al. 2010). These, nestin+ MSCs have been shown to be spatially associate with HSPCs in the marrow and to express several HSPC maintenance genes, e.g. CXCL-12, stem cell factor (SCF)/kit ligand, angiopoietin (Ang)-1, interlukin (IL)-7, vascular cell adhesion molecule (VCAM)-1, and osteopontin (Mendez-Ferrer et al. 2010). Further, numbers of HSPC were rapidly reduced in the marrow of mice that were selectively depleted of nestin+ MSCs (**Table 1**) (Mendez-Ferrer et al. 2010). These mouse models also revealed a necessity for marrow nestin+ MSCs for homing of transferred HSPCs (Mendez-Ferrer et al. 2010). Together, these data suggest that MSCs and associated daughter cells not only make up the physical structure of the HME, but also provide maintenance and differentiation signals to HSPCs.

3.1.2 CXCL-12 abundant reticular cells

Reticular cells are of mesodermal origin and are a type of fibroblast cell localized to the intertrabecular region of the marrow near both the osteoblast and vascular niches (Weiss 1976; Rouleau et al. 1990). Recently, a sub-set of marrow reticular cells has been shown to express high levels of CXCL-12 (or stromal derived factor (SDF)-1) and have been termed CXCL-12 abundant reticular (CAR) cells (Tokoyoda et al. 2004; Sugiyama et al. 2006). CXCL-12 is reportedly involved in several aspects of hematopoiesis, including HSPC homing and maintenance, as well as B cell development (Nagasawa et al. 1994; Nagasawa et al. 1996; Ara et al. 2003; Broxmeyer et al. 2005; Jung et al. 2006; Sugiyama et al. 2006). Using CXCL-12/GFP knock-in mice, HSPCs, early lineage B cells and plasma B cells have been shown to spatially associate with CAR cells (Tokoyoda et al. 2004), suggesting CAR cells are a HME cell type. To address the importance of CXCL-12 expressing cells in the HME, Omatsu et al. designed a mouse model with selective ablation of CAR cells (**Table 1**) (Omatsu et al. 2010). These assays showed no change in the osteoblast or vascular niches, but impaired production of SCF and CXCL-12, combined with marked reduction in cycling lymphoid and erythroid progenitors. Further, the HSPC population in these mice was more quiescent, diminished in numbers and expressed myeloid selector genes. Finally, CAR cells can give rise to adipocytes and osteoblasts (Bianco et al. 1988; Balduino et al. 2005; Sipkins et al. 2005; Omatsu et al. 2010). Thus, these data combined with the ectopic bone assays and the nestin+ reticular cell studies discussed above, raise the possibility that the CAR, osteoprogenitor and nestin+ cells are from a similar cell pool, sharing differentiation capabilities and roles in hematopoiteitc support.

3.1.3 Adipocytes

Within the young marrow there are few adipocytes, however this phenomenon is reversed with aging and after marrow insult, such as post irradiation (Burkhardt et al. 1987; Verma et al. 2002). Although adipocytes have been described as having a positive influence on hematopoiesis via growth factors secretion (Lanotte et al. 1982), other studies have reported that these growth factors are in too low a concentration to influence HSPCs and that adipocytes secrete anti-hematopoietic factors as well (Hotamisligil et al. 1993; Zhang, Y. et al. 1995; Yokota et al. 2000; Corre et al. 2006; Belaid-Choucair et al. 2008; Miharada et al. 2008). Further, an increase in marrow adiposity has been negatively correlated with hematopoiesis in vivo (Touw and Lowenberg 1983; Naveiras et al. 2009). Interestingly,

Naveiras et al. have shown that in the adult mouse spine there is a proximal to distal gradient of marrow adipocity, with thoracic vertebrae being virtually free of adipocytes. This provides an in vivo model to study the affects of adipocytes on hematopoietic cells under homeostatic conditions. These studies showed that the number, frequency and cycling capacity of HSPCs was reduced as the number of adipocytes was increased (Naveiras et al. 2009). In support, after irradiation and marrow transplantation of mice genetically incapable of forming adipocytes, or in wild type mice treated with an inhibitor of adipogenesis, there was enhanced HSPC expansion compared to non-treated wild type cohorts (Naveiras et al. 2009). Of note, in these models of reduced/abrogated adipogenesis, as well as in a model where the fatty marrow is surgically removed, the increase in hematopoiesis is concomitant with an increase in bone formation (Tavassoli et al. 1974; Naveiras et al. 2009). These data suggest that after marrow insult and in the absence of adipocytes, there are signals enhancing osteoblast activity and bone formation, which may contribute to the enhanced hematopoiesis measured, as discussed below. This is supported by the clinical observations that aged patients have an increase in adiposity in the marrow, which is correlated with a decrease in bone formation and decreased hematopoiesis (Verma et al. 2002; Rossi et al. 2005; Mayack et al. 2010).

3.1.4 Osteoblasts

With the identification of osteoblast-like cells in stromal cultures (Friedenstein et al. 1987; Benayahu et al. 1991; Benayahu et al. 1992) and osteoprogenitors within marrow preparations for ectopic bone assays (Kuznetsov et al. 1997; Akintoye et al. 2006; Sacchetti et al. 2007; Chan, C.K. et al. 2008; Morikawa et al. 2009), Emerson and Taichman designed in vitro assays to assess the ability of isolated osteoblasts to support hematopoiesis (Taichman and Emerson 1994; Taichman et al. 1996; Taichman et al. 1997; Jung et al. 2005; Jung et al. 2006; Zhu et al. 2007). These assays showed that osteoblasts can support hematopoiesis through the secretion of pro-hematopoietic cytokines, e.g. granulocyte colony-stimulating factor (G-CSF), granulocyte-macrophage colony-stimulating factor (GM-CSF), CXCL-12, IL-6, and IL-7, and that cell-cell contact is necessary for support via integrin binding (very late antigen (VLA)-4/5 and VCAM/ICAM). Further, these assays confirmed a connection between osteoblasts and B cell development. To assess the contribution of osteoblasts to hematopoiesis in vivo, several different mouse models have been generated that either increase osteoblasts (Calvi et al. 2001; Calvi et al. 2003; Zhang, J. et al. 2003), decrease osteoblasts (Visnjic et al. 2001; Visnjic et al. 2004), disrupt EO-based trabecular bone formation (Jacenko et al. 1993; Gress and Jacenko 2000; Jacenko et al. 2001; Jacenko et al. 2002; Sweeney et al. 2008; Sweeney et al. 2010), alter osteoblast signaling (Wu et al. 2008), or modify osteoblast RNA processing (**Table 1**) (Raaijmakers et al. 2010). These in vivo models have confirmed that osteoblasts can support hematopoiesis, are involved in B lymphopoiesis, make pro-hematopoietic cytokines, make cell-cell contact with HSPCs, and moreover, have implicated osterix expressing osteoprogenitors as mediators of hematopoiesis.

The above studies, as well as many imaging studies of HSPC in bone, support the osteoblast hematopoietic niche theory and suggest that the osteoblast niche may additionally encompass the B lymphopoietic niche (Nilsson et al. 1997; Nilsson et al. 2001; Yoshimoto et al. 2003; Arai, F. et al. 2004; Balduino et al. 2005; Kohler et al. 2009; Lo Celso et al. 2009; Xie et al. 2009). For instance, Xie et al. showed that GFP+ HSPCs home to the trabecular bone surface in the marrow, and others have reported early developing B lymphocytes at the endosteal region of the marrow (Hermans et al. 1989; Jacobsen and Osmond 1990; Osmond 1990; Xie et al. 2009). This zone is the chondro-osseous region where hypertrophic chondrocytes, trabecular osteoblasts and marrow cells are juxtaposed (**Fig. 1**). Hypertrophic chondrocytes and their matrix components are also essential for trabecular bone formation, and are proposed to be part of the osteoblast/lymphopoietic niche (Jacenko et al. 2002; Rodgers et al. 2008; Sweeney et al. 2008; Sweeney et al. 2010). Interestingly, hypertrophic chondrocytes have been described to trans-differentiate into osteoblasts (Roach 1992; Galotto et al. 1994; Roach et al. 1995; Roach and Erenpreisa 1996), and express osteoblast-like markers, e.g. osterix, osteocalcin, osteonectin, osteopontin and collagen I (Roach 1992; Yagi et al. 2003), suggesting similarities in the cells of the chondro-osseous niche. Indeed, it has been suggested that chondro-osteoprogenitor cells that expresses the chondrocyte-like marker collagen II contribute to both the perichondrial and trabecular osteoblast populations (Nakamura et al. 2006; Hilton et al. 2007). In contrast, however Maes et al. do not report any contribution from the collagen II labeled hypertrophic chondrocytes to trabecular bone (Maes et al. 2010). Taken together, these finding are reminiscent of the reports indicating that progenitor cells in the marrow can give rise to different cell types with many similarities, e.g. osteoprogenitors, CAR and nestin+ cells not only share gene expression profiles, but are all located in the chondro-osseous environment (Weiss 1976; Rouleau et al. 1990; Sugiyama et al. 2006). The possible overlap between the cells of the chondro-osseous region can also be appreciated when comparing osteoblasts and reticular cells that can support B lymphopoiesis and both express VCAM-1 and IL-7 (Ryan et al. 1991; Funk et al. 1995; Zhu et al. 2007). Moreover, using an osteoblast lineage tracer mouse generated with an osterix-LacZ construct, cells of the perichondrium, trabecular bone, cartilage and marrow stroma, some intimately associated with blood vessels in a pericyte-like fashion, were all positive for osterix expression (Maes et al. 2010), again confirming an overlap of cell phenotypes in the chondro-osseous HME.

3.1.5 Chondrocytes

As previously discussed, chondrocytes provide the blueprint for future bone with a marrow cavity during EO, and are adjacent to the postulated osteoblast and vascular niches (**Fig. 1B boxed**) (Arai, F. et al. 2004; Kiel et al. 2005; Kohler et al. 2009; Xie et al. 2009). Indeed, growth plate chondrocytes, as well as osteoblasts and vascular cells, express leukemia inhibitory factor (LIF), which can synergize with growth factors to promote the proliferation of HSPCs (Keller et al. 1996; Grimaud et al. 2002). Additionally, Wei et al. recently showed that hypertrophic chondrocytes express CXCR-4, the receptor for CXCL-12 made by stromal cells and osteoblasts (Peled et al. 1999; Kortesidis et al. 2005; Dar et al. 2006; Jung et al. 2006; Sacchetti et al. 2007; Wei et al. 2010). These data begin to reveal the cross talk between the hypertrophic chondrocytes and the cells of the chondro-osseous environment that are players within the hematopoietic niche, e.g. osteoblasts, stromal and hematopoietic cells.

To date, no imaging studies have attempted to localize HSPCs to hypertrophic chondrocytes. However, the contribution of various matrix components, in particular the heparan sulfate proteoglycans (HSPG), in establishing reservoirs of soluble factors for cell signaling and/or retention of HSPCs has been well established (as reviewed in (Rodgers et al. 2008) also see (Gordon et al. 1988; Roberts et al. 1988; Siczkowski et al. 1992; Verfaillie 1993; Allouche and Bikfalvi 1995; Bruno et al. 1995; Klein et al. 1995; Gupta et al. 1996; Gupta et al. 1998; Borghesi et al. 1999; Siebertz et al. 1999; Zweegman et al. 2004; Rodgers et al. 2008; Spiegel et al. 2008). In support, our laboratory has shown altered localization of both hyaluronan and HSPGs within the hypertrophic cartilage zone of the growth plates in the collagen X mouse models that display altered hematopoiesis (Jacenko et al. 2001), which directly links EO and the hypertrophic cartilage matrix to hematopoiesis (Jacenko et al. 1993; Gress and Jacenko 2000; Jacenko et al. 2001; Jacenko et al. 2002; Sweeney et al. 2008; Sweeney et al. 2010). Briefly, collagen X is a short chain, network forming collagen that is the major secreted matrix protein of hypertrophic chondrocytes and is localized to the hypertrophic cartilage/chondro-osseous region (Campbell et al. 2004), where it is proposed to form a hexagonal lattice-like network in the matrix (Jacenko et al. 1991; Chan, D. and Jacenko 1998). Affinity co-electrophoresis studies demonstrated that collagen X and heparin, a structural analog of heparan sulfate, can endogenously bind (Sweeney, unpublished). We thus proposed that the hypertrophic chondrocyte derived matrix, made up of the collagen X network that is likely stabilized by associating with the HSPGs, is enriched with hematopoietic factors and is a vital component of the HME (Jacenko et al. 2001; Rodgers et al. 2008). In accord, mouse models where the function of collagen X was altered via transgenesis or targeted gene knock-out have both an altered HME structure, as well as aberrant hematopoiesis. Specifically, alterations within the EO-derived chondro-osseous junction include aberrant growth plate histomorphometry, collapsed hypertrophic chondrocyte matrix network, diminished and altered localization for HSPG within hypertrophic cartilage and trabecular bone, and decreased trabecular bone. The hematopoietic changes include diminished B lymphopoiesis throughout life, perinatal lethality within a sub-set of mice due to opportunistic infections by the third week of life, decreased responses to concanavalin A by splenocytes from mice at all ages, and the succumbing of all collagen X mice to non-virulent pathogen challenge (**Table 1**) (Jacenko et al. 1993; Rosati et al. 1994; Jacenko et al. 1996; Kwan et al. 1997; Gress and Jacenko 2000; Jacenko et al. 2001; Jacenko et al. 2002; Sweeney et al. 2008; Sweeney et al. 2010). Additionally, altered levels of hematopoietic cytokines have been measured from the collagen X mouse derived hypertrophic chondrocytes and trabecular osteoblasts when compared to wild type cohorts (Sweeney, 2011 Ann N Y Acad. Sci. in press). The altered cytokine availability may negatively affect hematopoiesis, which may be even further amplified by the altered chondro-osseous matrix in the collagen X mice, e.g. loss of functional collagen X and diminished HSPGs at the chondro-ossous HME (Jacenko et al. 2001). In support of the notion that matrix/cytokine signaling can affect cell differentiation in the HME, fate switching was sited as the cause of decreased osteoblast progenitors and bone formation in a knock-out mouse for the critical transforming growth factor (TGF)-β binding proteoglycans, biglycan and decorin (Bi et al. 2005). Overall, the collagen X mouse models have highlighted the contribution of EO-derived cells and matrix components to HMEs and to hematopoietic cell development.

3.1.6 Endothelial cells

Marrow arterioles and capillaries supply the sinusoids, which in turn supply the marrow with cells and nutrients (reviewed in (Kopp et al. 2005). These are the sites of the vascular niche, and examples of active vascular niches can be appreciated during development when hematopoiesis takes place in the yolk sac, aorta-gonad-mesonephros region and placenta perivascularly (Cumano et al. 1996; Medvinsky and Dzierzak 1996; Sanchez et al. 1996; de Bruijn et al. 2002; North et al. 2002; Gekas et al. 2005; Ottersbach and Dzierzak 2005). Additionally, throughout life in some species, such as the zebra fish, hematopoiesis is not coincident with bone (Murayama et al. 2006). Further, the characteristics of the marrow sinusoids, e.g. chemokine and adhesion molecule expression, not only allow them to be conduits for hematopoietic cells to and from the circulation, but also to serve as an area for HSPC differentiation (Rafii et al. 1994; Rafii et al. 1995; Schweitzer et al. 1996; Naiyer et al. 1999; Abkowitz et al. 2003; Avecilla et al. 2004). In agreement, endothelial cells from several sources are able to support HSPC maintenance and differentiation toward lymphoid and myeloid lineages in culture (Rafii et al. 1995; Ohneda et al. 1998; Li et al. 2004; Wittig et al. 2009; Butler et al. 2010). Visualizing the vascular niche in vivo with a pure sub-set of HSCs also provided support for the vascular niche theory. These studies revealed approximately 60% of HSC residing in the chondro-osseous HME, and of that population, approximately 60% were proximal to the vasculature, where as 15% were near bone (Kiel et al. 2005). Moreover, one aspect of the osteoblast niche theory maintains that HSCs are bound to osteoblasts by a N-cadherin-mediated homophilic adhesion, however in a mouse model where HSC specific N-cadherin was depleted, hematopoiesis was fully functional (Zhang, J. et al. 2003; Kiel et al. 2009). More in vivo support is provided by the biglycan deficient mice, which present with decreased trabecular osteoblasts and bone formation, however show no defects in hematopoiesis, HSC frequency or function, and show HSC localization to the vasculature (Kiel et al. 2007). These data suggest an overlap in niche location with perhaps some ability for compensation between the osteoblast and vascular niches, albeit limited. In support, via histochemistry of the long bone, one can appreciate the spatial proximity of osteoblasts to the vasculature (**Fig. 1B boxed**).

3.1.7 Hematopoietic derived cells influence the niche

Discussed above are the data linking non-hematopoietic cells with hematopoiesis, however there are also data supporting reciprocal affects of hematopoietic derived cells influencing non-hematopoietic lineages. For example, HSPCs regulate MSC differentiation toward the osteoblast lineage via expression of BMP-2 and -6, suggesting that the HSPCs can actively maintain the osteoblast niche (Jung et al. 2008). Additionally, macrophages intercalated throughout bone have been described as osteoblast helper cells since they promote osteoblast mineralization in vitro and form a canopy over osteoblasts generating bone in vivo (Chang et al. 2008). An additional player in osteoblastogenesis is the megakaryocyte. In mouse models with increased numbers of megakaryocytes due to maturation arrest, increased osteoblast proliferation and bone mass were measured (Kacena et al. 2004). Additionally, megakaryocytes have been described as niche restoring cells post-irradiation since they migrate to the damaged bone surfaces and increase local concentrations of CXCL-12, platelet-derived growth factor (PDGF)-β and basic fibroblast growth factor (bFGF), which are associated with osteoblast proliferation (Kacena et al. 2006; Dominici et al. 2009).

A reciprocal balance between bone deposition by osteoblasts, bone resorption by osteoclasts and signaling by osteocytes is extensively noted in the literature, and is appreciated clinically. These coupled interactions will not be discussed here other than to acknowledge that the function of one cell type highly depends upon and is affected by the actions of the other (Khosla 2003). Thereby, the continual signaling between cells of the mesenchymal and hematopoietic lineages underlies the tightly coupled process of bone remodeling, and its uncoupling can lead to skeletal disorders such as osteoporosis, osteopetrosis, as well as calcium homeostasis imbalances. Such examples are also seen in mouse models; for example, in one model where osteoclasts are depleted, instead of having increased bone mass due to lack of resorption, there is decreased bone mass compared to wild type cohorts (Kong et al. 1999). Collectively, the intricate cross talk between cells within the HME can both positively and negatively affect the niche environment as well as hematopoiesis, and is a vast area if research that remains to be adequately explored.

3.2 Soluble factors and the extracellular matrix in the niche

3.2.1 Cytokines, chemokines, growth factors, and neurotransmitters

As referred to above, the hematopoietic and non-hematopoietic cells within the HME are surrounded in all dimensions by matrix components and soluble factors. The building blocks of the extracellular matrices found within the chondro-osseous environment can include collagens, proteoglycans (PGs; including the HSPGs) and their glycosaminoglycan (GAG) constituents and glycoproteins. Collagens generally provide structural support for cells in the niche by forming supramolecular aggregates around cells (Jacenko et al. 1991), while the PGs, such as the HSPGs, can trap and store soluble factors for presentation to local cells (as reviewed in (Rodgers et al. 2008). The amount and ratio of these molecules in the matrix also dictates the mechanical properties of the HME, which has recently become a topic of investigation in the stem cell field. For instance, matrix elasticity in the HME can influence fate choices of HSPCs (Holst et al. 2010), a phenomenon also reported with MSCs (as reviewed in (Discher et al. 2009). Thus, the matrix provides structural integrity to the HME, acts as a substrate for cell migration and anchorage, and actively regulates cell morphology, development and metabolic function (Peerani and Zandstra 2010). The cells in the HME receive information for maintenance, development, differentiation, etc. via cell-cell interactions, cell-matrix interactions, and exposure to variable concentrations and combinations of soluble factors, e.g. cytokines, chemokines, hormones, and growth factors. Many soluble factors have been implicated in hematopoiesis, such as CXCL-12, SCF, Fms-related tyrosine kinase 3 ligand (Flt-3L), thrombopoietin (TPO), FGF, G-CSF, GM-CSF, LIF, Wnt, BMP-4, IL-3, 6, 7, 8, 11, 12, 14, 15 (Guba et al. 1992; Heinrich et al. 1993; Verfaillie 1993; Funk et al. 1995; Rafii et al. 1997; Taichman et al. 1997; Peled et al. 1999; Majumdar et al. 2000; Ponomaryov et al. 2000; Petit et al. 2002; Avecilla et al. 2004; Kortesidis et al. 2005; Dar et al. 2006; Jung et al. 2006; Spiegel et al. 2007; Wittig et al. 2009), or in maintenance and quiescence of HSCs, e.g. Ang-1 and TGF (Eaves et al. 1991; Fortunel et al. 2000; Arai, F. et al. 2004) (cytokine functions reviewed in (Zhang, C.C. and Lodish 2008). The HME cell types discussed above are the primary sources of these soluble factors, however lymphocytes have also been shown to stimulate and suppress hematopoiesis through the release of different factors during both homeostasis and immune activation (Nathan et al. 1978; Bacigalupo et al. 1980; Mangan et al. 1982; Harada et al. 1985; Trinchieri et al. 1987; Crawford et al. 2010). Interestingly, many of these soluble factors are sequestered and presented by the matrix, specifically HSPGs, which have been described as key orchestrators of hematopoiesis (Bruno et al. 1995; Gupta et al. 1996; Gupta et al. 1998; Borghesi et al. 1999). This is particularly relevant to the collagen X mouse models that present with a disrupted collagen X network coupled with a decreased HSPG staining intensity at the chondro-osseous HME and diminished cytokine levels, leading to diminished B lymphopoiesis (Gress and Jacenko 2000; Jacenko et al. 2001; Jacenko et al. 2002; Sweeney et al. 2008; Sweeney et al. 2010). These findings imply that the structural defects in the matrix may lead to changes in the cytokine reservoirs, which in turn would negatively affect hematopoietic cell development. By extension, human diseases associated with altered matrix components at the HME may have altered hematopoiesis due to changes in cytokine availability, such as with Simpson-Golabi Behmel syndrome where alterations in the HSPG glypican-3 results in skeletal and hematopoietic abnormalities (Pilia et al. 1996; Viviano et al. 2005).

There is increasing evidence that the nervous system can also affect the immune system through neurotransmitter signaling. The bone and marrow are supplied with autonomic efferent and afferent sensory innervations, specifically at the epiphysis and metaphysis of long bone, which includes the chondro-osseous HME (**Fig. 1A**) (reviewed in (Mignini et al. 2003). Catecholamines, acetylcholine and peptide transmitters of neural and non-neural origin are released in the HME, which contribute to neuro-immune modulations. For example, signaling from the nervous system can regulate HSPC egress and repopulation of the marrow (Katayama et al. 2006; Spiegel et al. 2007), which has been shown to be coupled to the circadian rhythm (Mendez-Ferrer et al. 2008). Indeed, HSPCs have receptors for several neurotransmitters, which can stimulate cell proliferation (Spiegel et al. 2008; Kalinkovich et al. 2009). Of note, beta-adrenergic agonists have been shown to stimulate osteoclast activity (Arai, M. et al. 2003), which could have an effect on the osteoblast niche via two methods, a) physically by decreasing bone lining cells and releasing HSPCs, and b) chemically via the release of soluble factor (Kollet et al. 2006; Mansour et al. 2011). Calcium is an example of one such soluble factor, which serves as an attractant to HSPCs encouraging homing to the osteoblast niche (Adams et al. 2006). Hematopoietic cell egress from the marrow has also been linked to many systemic causes, including exercise, inflammation, bleeding, cytotoxic drugs, and psychological anxiety (reviewed in (Lapid et al. 2008). These data serve as reminders that hematopoiesis and the HME can be influenced by factors outside of the local environment.

3.2.2 Cell and matrix influence

In the HME, cell-cell interactions influence cell fate decisions and mobility/homing; examples of such interactions include: Notch-1/Jagged-1, N-cadherin/N-cadherin and VLA-4/VCAM-1 (reviewed in (Coskun and Hirschi 2010). On the other hand, cell-matrix interactions influence not only cell behavior, but also cell anchorage to the niche. To date, the matrix proteins within the HME include: collagens (Types I, II, III, IV and X), glycoproteins (fibronectin, lamanin, nidogen, tenasin C, thrombospondin, vitronectin), PGs (perlecan, decorin, agrin) and the GAG hyaluronan (Bentley and Foidart 1980; Bentley 1982; Spooncer et al. 1983; Zuckerman and Wicha 1983; Zuckerman et al. 1985; Klein 1995; Ohta et al. 1998; Campbell et al. 2004; Mazzon et al. 2011). These matrix constituents can signal to hematopoietic cells through cell receptors such as: integrins, immunoglobulin-like molecules, cadherins, selectins, and mucins (Teixido et al. 1992; Coulombel et al. 1997; Levesque and Simmons 1999; Zhang, J. et al. 2003; Merzaban et al. 2011). Notably, the HME matrix network is not static, but is continually remodeled by different enzymes including metalloproteinases, neutrophil elastase and hepranase. Matrix turnover can thus assist in the release of hematopoietic cells from the niche (Levesque et al. 2001; Heissig et al. 2002; Petit et al. 2002; Spiegel et al. 2008), as well as liberate bound soluble hematopoietic factors (Heissig et al. 2002; Spiegel et al. 2008). An example of one such cell-matrix interaction in the HME is the VLA-4/fibronectin binding between HSPCs and the matrix, which provides the hematopoietic cell with anchorage as well as proliferation stimuli (Weinstein et al. 1989; Klein et al. 1998; Sagar et al. 2006). Hyaluronan also impacts HSPC maintenance, propagation, homing and homeostasis via CD44 binding (Avigdor et al. 2004; Matrosova et al. 2004; Haylock and Nilsson 2006). Most recently, Mazzon et al. have found the binding between agrin, expressed by trabecular osteoblasts and MSCs in the niche, and HSPCs leads to survival and proliferation signals (Mazzon et al. 2011). Finally, mature plasma B cells homing back to the marrow via CXCL-12 signals are anchored to their marrow niche via matrix-bound ligands produced by local myeloid cells (O'Connor et al. 2004; Crowley et al. 2005; Ingold et al. 2005; Moreaux et al. 2005; Nagasawa 2006; Schwaller et al. 2007; Huard et al. 2008; Moreaux et al. 2009). In fact, it has been shown that this interaction maintains long-lived antibody producing plasma B cells in the marrow by stimulating expression of anti-apoptotic genes in the lymphocytes (O'Connor et al. 2004; Huard et al. 2008). Thus, the cell-matrix interactions in the marrow serve to support hematopoietic maintenance and development, as well as support the persistence of mature hematopoietic cells that have returned to the marrow.

4. Summary and perspectives

All the specialized cells of the blood are generated through hematopoiesis via the directed differentiation of HSCs. The bone marrow, which is the predominant hematopoietic tissue after birth (Aguila and Rowe 2005; Cumano and Godin 2007), is formed through EO, where the cartilage anlage serves as a transient template for trabecular bone, and defines the environment of the marrow stroma. Thereby, either directly or indirectly, the process of EO establishes the hematopoietic niche by providing the niche with both the structure matrix constituents and the cellular components (Jacenko et al. 1993; Taichman and Emerson 1994; Taichman et al. 1996; Taichman et al. 1997; Gress and Jacenko 2000; Calvi et al. 2001; Visnjic et al. 2001; Jacenko et al. 2002; Calvi et al. 2003; Zhang, J. et al. 2003; Visnjic et al. 2004; Jung et al. 2005; Jung et al. 2006; Zhu et al. 2007; Chan, C.K. et al. 2008; Sweeney et al. 2008; Wu et al. 2008; Raaijmakers et al. 2010; Sweeney et al. 2010). Many cell types, matrix components and soluble factors contribute to the HME (**Fig. 2**). Through several different methods, HSPCs have been visualized in the chondro-osseous HME (Nilsson et al. 1997; Nilsson et al. 2001; Yoshimoto et al. 2003; Arai, F. et al. 2004; Balduino et al. 2005; Kiel et al. 2005; Kohler et al. 2009; Xie et al. 2009), which is comprised of vasculature sinusoids, sympathetic nerves, complex and diverse matrix regions, as well as osteoblasts, hypertrophic chondrocytes, endothelial cells, pericytes, CXCL-12 expressing cells, adipocytes, nestin+ cells, MSCs, macrophages intercalated in the endosteum, and cells of the immune system, both developing and recirculating. The cells of the HME express the cytokines, growth factors and chemokines utilized throughout hematopoiesis, as well as the matrix molecules that provides structural support, cell-matrix signaling and reservoirs of soluble factors (**Fig. 2**). We propose that the chondro-osseous HME is not static, but is continuously changing in response to various systemic influences (Lapid et al. 2008), as well as to remodeling of the hybrid trabecular bone-hypertrophic cartilage spicules into mature secondary bone (**Fig. 1C & 2**). During remodeling of the HME, both cells and

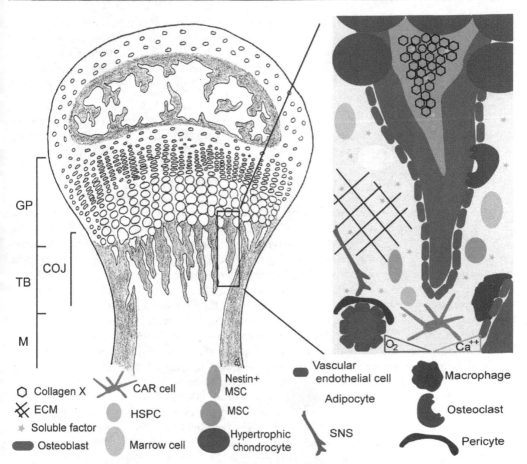

Fig. 2. The cells, matrix components and soluble factors within the chondro-osseous hematopoietic microenvironment. The putative hematopoietic niche has been localized to the chondro-osseous junction (COJ) of endochondrally developing bones, e.g. the juncture of the growth plate (GP) hypertrophic chondrocytes and the trabecular bone (TB) and marrow (M). Boxed, a cartoon in higher magnification represents the chondro-osseous hematopoietic environment, which includes: osteoblasts, hypertrophic chondrocytes, endothelial cells, pericytes, CXCL-12 abundant cells (CAR), adipocytes, endosteal intercalating macrophages, and other marrow cells, such as lymphocytes. Additionally, progenitor cells such as hematopoietic stem/progenitor cells (HSPC), multipotent stromal cells (MSC) and nestin expressing (nestin +) MSC are represented. All of these cells serve as a source of secreted factors, including cytokines, chemokines and growth factors, as well as neurotransmitters from the sympathetic nervous system (SNS). Also note the gradients of oxygen (O_2) and calcium (Ca^{++}) released from the vasculature or remodeled bone respectively. Finally, the extracellular matrix (ECM) in the marrow and in the core of trabecular bone, consisting of hypertrophic cartilage derived lattice-like collagen X and HSPGs, can serve as a substrate for cell anchorage, migration, and/or signaling through cell-ECM binding and as a reservoirs of secreted factors.

soluble factors are released into the milieu; for example matrix degrading enzymes release HSPCs for egress, and the combined activity of osteoclasts and enzymes release soluble factors from bone, including the trabecular bone with a collagen X/HSPG core (**Fig. 2**). Thus, the chondro-osseous HME is a continually active site with intrinsic and systemic signals influencing the cellular cross talk that ensures proper quiescence, maintenance, and differentiation of the HSPCs.

As itemized in **Table 1** and discussed above, various mouse models have revealed important cell and matrix players in the HME, while others have implicated the importance of proper cell cycle (Walkley et al. 2005; Walkley et al. 2007), transcription (Corradi et al. 2003; Purton et al. 2006; Walkley et al. 2007; Kieslinger et al. 2010), cell-cell communication (Larsson et al. 2008), and survival signals (Youn et al. 2008; Kwon et al. 2010) in the HME (**Table 1**). Still, the exact cellular make up and location of the HME is continually under debate, though most agree the cells of the osteoblast and vascular niches are important players in hematopoiesis. The possibility of osteoblast and vascular niches spatially overlapping or having the ability to provide some compensation for each other to some extent, is another intriguing theory. Evidence for this is observed with the biglycan deficient mouse model that presents with reduced bone, yet intact hematopoiesis (Kiel et al. 2007), as well as with the recently identified CAR cells that unite the osteoblast and vascular niches in the chondro-osseous HME by the observation that they are in contact with 90% of HSPCs throughout the trabecular bone region and the marrow sinusoidal region (Sugiyama et al. 2006; Omatsu et al. 2010). Additionally, there is similarity in the expression of hematopoietic soluble factors between the osteoblasts, endothelial cells, and CAR cells, such as CXCL-12 implicated in the homing, growth, development and maintenance of hematopoietic cells (Peled et al. 1999; Ponomaryov et al. 2000; Tokoyoda et al. 2004; Broxmeyer et al. 2005; Kortesidis et al. 2005; Dar et al. 2006; Sugiyama et al. 2006). Moreover, Medici et al. have confirmed an endothelial to osteoblast and chondrocyte transition in vivo, further supporting a cell interchange and overlap theory (Medici et al. 2010). In contrast, there is also evidence that the osteoblast and vascular niches provide different roles in hematopoiesis, e.g. a quiescence and maintenance role verses a differentiation and egress role (Lord et al. 1975; Shackney et al. 1975; Gong 1978; Nilsson et al. 2001; Heissig et al. 2002; Arai, F. et al. 2004; Balduino et al. 2005; Jang and Sharkis 2007; Bourke et al. 2009). Further, although these niches are proximal in the chondro-oseous region, mathematical modeling has predicted a layer of only two myeloid cells is sufficient to deplete most oxygen provided by a near by sinusoid (Chow et al. 2001). Thus, the local environment within each niche may differ significantly in chemical signals, such as with oxygen and calcium (**Fig. 2**).

Overall, the research generated in the hematopoietic niche field is beginning to shed light on many hematologic disorders, such as myelodysplasia, myeloproliferative syndromes and leukemias that seem to be influenced by the quality of the marrow environment (Walkley et al. 2007; Walkley et al. 2007; Raaijmakers et al. 2010). Further information on niche components, specifically the matrix molecules, will assist in generating bio-mimicking composites necessary for in vitro culture and expansion of patient specific hematopoietic tissues, for such clinical applications as autologous marrow transfers. The past sixty years of hematopoietic biology research has increased our understanding of marrow stromal cell types, as well as the three-dimensional regions that provide structure and organization of cell signaling for the maintenance and propagation of HSPCs. The study of the hematopoietic niche will continue to provide details on necessary niche components, which may assist in the understanding of other stem cell niches, including the vascular, skin, hair, and neural niches, and provide therapeutic cues for immuno-osseous diseases that present with skeletal defects and altered hematopoiesis, such as McKusick type metaphyseal chondrodysplasia (cartilage-hair hypoplasia; CHH), Shwachmen-Diamond syndrome, Schimke dysplasia (Spranger et al. 1991; Kuijpers et al. 2004; Hermanns et al. 2005), and others.

5. References

Abkowitz, J. L., A. E. Robinson, S. Kale, M. W. Long & J. Chen (2003). "Mobilization of hematopoietic stem cells during homeostasis and after cytokine exposure." *Blood* 102(4): 1249-1253

Adams, G. B., K. T. Chabner, I. R. Alley, D. P. Olson, Z. M. Szczepiorkowski, M. C. Poznansky, C. H. Kos, M. R. Pollak, E. M. Brown & D. T. Scadden (2006). "Stem cell engraftment at the endosteal niche is specified by the calcium-sensing receptor." *Nature* 439(7076): 599-603

Aguila, H. L. & D. W. Rowe (2005). "Skeletal development, bone remodeling, and hematopoiesis." *Immunol Rev* 208: 7-18

Akintoye, S. O., T. Lam, S. Shi, J. Brahim, M. T. Collins & P. G. Robey (2006). "Skeletal site-specific characterization of orofacial and iliac crest human bone marrow stromal cells in same individuals." *Bone* 38(6): 758-768

Allouche, M. & A. Bikfalvi (1995). "The role of fibroblast growth factor-2 (FGF-2) in hematopoiesis." *Prog Growth Factor Res* 6(1): 35-48

Alvarez, J., M. Balbin, M. Fernandez & J. M. Lopez (2001). "Collagen metabolism is markedly altered in the hypertrophic cartilage of growth plates from rats with growth impairment secondary to chronic renal failure." *J Bone Miner Res* 16(3): 511-524

Ara, T., K. Tokoyoda, T. Sugiyama, T. Egawa, K. Kawabata & T. Nagasawa (2003). "Long-term hematopoietic stem cells require stromal cell-derived factor-1 for colonizing bone marrow during ontogeny." *Immunity* 19(2): 257-267

Arai, F., A. Hirao, M. Ohmura, H. Sato, S. Matsuoka, K. Takubo, K. Ito, G. Y. Koh & T. Suda (2004). "Tie2/angiopoietin-1 signaling regulates hematopoietic stem cell quiescence in the bone marrow niche." *Cell* 118(2): 149-161

Arai, M., T. Nagasawa, Y. Koshihara, S. Yamamoto & A. Togari (2003). "Effects of beta-adrenergic agonists on bone-resorbing activity in human osteoclast-like cells." *Biochim Biophys Acta* 1640(2-3): 137-142

Augello, A., T. B. Kurth & C. De Bari (2010). "Mesenchymal stem cells: a perspective from in vitro cultures to in vivo migration and niches." *Eur Cell Mater* 20: 121-133

Avecilla, S. T., K. Hattori, B. Heissig, R. Tejada, F. Liao, K. Shido, D. K. Jin, S. Dias, F. Zhang, T. E. Hartman, N. R. Hackett, R. G. Crystal, L. Witte, D. J. Hicklin, P. Bohlen, D. Eaton, D. Lyden, F. de Sauvage & S. Rafii (2004). "Chemokine-mediated interaction of hematopoietic progenitors with the bone marrow vascular niche is required for thrombopoiesis." *Nat Med* 10(1): 64-71

Avigdor, A., P. Goichberg, S. Shivtiel, A. Dar, A. Peled, S. Samira, O. Kollet, R. Hershkoviz, R. Alon, I. Hardan, H. Ben-Hur, D. Naor, A. Nagler & T. Lapidot (2004). "CD44 and hyaluronic acid cooperate with SDF-1 in the trafficking of human CD34+ stem/progenitor cells to bone marrow." *Blood* 103(8): 2981-2989

Bacigalupo, A., M. Podesta, M. C. Mingari, L. Moretta, M. T. Van Lint & A. Marmont (1980). "Immune suppression of hematopoiesis in aplastic anemia: activity of T-gamma lymphocytes." *J Immunol* 125(4): 1449-1453

Balduino, A., S. P. Hurtado, P. Frazao, C. M. Takiya, L. M. Alves, L. E. Nasciutti, M. C. El-Cheikh & R. Borojevic (2005). "Bone marrow subendosteal microenvironment harbours functionally distinct haemosupportive stromal cell populations." *Cell Tissue Res* 319(2): 255-266

Belaid-Choucair, Z., Y. Lepelletier, G. Poncin, A. Thiry, C. Humblet, M. Maachi, A. Beaulieu, E. Schneider, A. Briquet, P. Mineur, C. Lambert, D. Mendes-Da-Cruz, M. L. Ahui, V. Asnafi, M. Dy, J. Boniver, B. V. Nusgens, O. Hermine & M. P. Defresne (2008). "Human bone marrow adipocytes block granulopoiesis through neuropilin-1-induced granulocyte colony-stimulating factor inhibition." *Stem Cells* 26(6): 1556-1564

Benayahu, D., A. Fried, D. Zipori & S. Wientroub (1991). "Subpopulations of marrow stromal cells share a variety of osteoblastic markers." *Calcif Tissue Int* 49(3): 202-207

Benayahu, D., M. Horowitz, D. Zipori & S. Wientroub (1992). "Hemopoietic functions of marrow-derived osteogenic cells." *Calcif Tissue Int* 51(3): 195-201

Bentley, S. A. (1982). "Collagen synthesis by bone marrow stromal cells: a quantitative study." *Br J Haematol* 50(3): 491-497

Bentley, S. A. & J. M. Foidart (1980). "Some properties of marrow derived adherent cells in tissue culture." *Blood* 56(6): 1006-1012

Bi, Y., C. H. Stuelten, T. Kilts, S. Wadhwa, R. V. Iozzo, P. G. Robey, X. D. Chen & M. F. Young (2005). "Extracellular matrix proteoglycans control the fate of bone marrow stromal cells." *J Biol Chem* 280(34): 30481-30489

Bianco, P., M. Costantini, L. C. Dearden & E. Bonucci (1988). "Alkaline phosphatase positive precursors of adipocytes in the human bone marrow." *Br J Haematol* 68(4): 401-403

Bianco, P., M. Riminucci, S. Kuznetsov & P. G. Robey (1999). "Multipotential cells in the bone marrow stroma: regulation in the context of organ physiology." *Crit Rev Eukaryot Gene Expr* 9(2): 159-173

Blin-Wakkach, C., A. Wakkach, P. M. Sexton, N. Rochet & G. F. Carle (2004). "Hematological defects in the oc/oc mouse, a model of infantile malignant osteopetrosis." *Leukemia* 18(9): 1505-1511

Bohensky, J., I. M. Shapiro, S. Leshinsky, S. P. Terkhorn, C. S. Adams & V. Srinivas (2007). "HIF-1 regulation of chondrocyte apoptosis: induction of the autophagic pathway." *Autophagy* 3(3): 207-214

Borghesi, L. A., Y. Yamashita & P. W. Kincade (1999). "Heparan sulfate proteoglycans mediate interleukin-7-dependent B lymphopoiesis." *Blood* 93(1): 140-148

Bourke, V. A., C. J. Watchman, J. D. Reith, M. L. Jorgensen, A. Dieudonne & W. E. Bolch (2009). "Spatial gradients of blood vessels and hematopoietic stem and progenitor cells within the marrow cavities of the human skeleton." *Blood* 114(19): 4077-4080

Broxmeyer, H. E., C. M. Orschell, D. W. Clapp, G. Hangoc, S. Cooper, P. A. Plett, W. C. Liles, X. Li, B. Graham-Evans, T. B. Campbell, G. Calandra, G. Bridger, D. C. Dale & E. F. Srour (2005). "Rapid mobilization of murine and human hematopoietic stem and progenitor cells with AMD3100, a CXCR4 antagonist." *J Exp Med* 201(8): 1307-1318

Bruno, E., S. D. Luikart, M. W. Long & R. Hoffman (1995). "Marrow-derived heparan sulfate proteoglycan mediates the adhesion of hematopoietic progenitor cells to cytokines." *Exp Hematol* 23(11): 1212-1217

Burkhardt, R., G. Kettner, W. Bohm, M. Schmidmeier, R. Schlag, B. Frisch, B. Mallmann, W. Eisenmenger & T. Gilg (1987). "Changes in trabecular bone, hematopoiesis and bone marrow vessels in aplastic anemia, primary osteoporosis, and old age: a comparative histomorphometric study." *Bone* 8(3): 157-164

Butler, J. M., D. J. Nolan, E. L. Vertes, B. Varnum-Finney, H. Kobayashi, A. T. Hooper, M. Seandel, K. Shido, I. A. White, M. Kobayashi, L. Witte, C. May, C. Shawber, Y. Kimura, J. Kitajewski, Z. Rosenwaks, I. D. Bernstein & S. Rafii (2010). "Endothelial cells are essential for the self-renewal and repopulation of Notch-dependent hematopoietic stem cells." *Cell Stem Cell* 6(3): 251-264

Calvi, L. M., G. B. Adams, K. W. Weibrecht, J. M. Weber, D. P. Olson, M. C. Knight, R. P. Martin, E. Schipani, P. Divieti, F. R. Bringhurst, L. A. Milner, H. M. Kronenberg & D. T. Scadden (2003). "Osteoblastic cells regulate the haematopoietic stem cell niche." *Nature* 425(6960): 841-846

Calvi, L. M., N. A. Sims, J. L. Hunzelman, M. C. Knight, A. Giovannetti, J. M. Saxton, H. M. Kronenberg, R. Baron & E. Schipani (2001). "Activated parathyroid hormone/parathyroid hormone-related protein receptor in osteoblastic cells differentially affects cortical and trabecular bone." *J Clin Invest* 107(3): 277-286

Campbell, M. R., C. J. Gress, E. H. Appleman & O. Jacenko (2004). "Chicken collagen X regulatory sequences restrict transgene expression to hypertrophic cartilage in mice." *Am J Pathol* 164(2): 487-499

Chan, C. K., C. C. Chen, C. A. Luppen, J. B. Kim, A. T. Deboer, K. Wei, J. A. Helms, C. J. Kuo, D. L. Kraft & I. L. Weissman (2008). "Endochondral ossification is required for haematopoietic stem-cell niche formation." *Nature*

Chan, D. & O. Jacenko (1998). "Phenotypic and biochemical consequences of collagen X mutations in mice and humans." *Matrix Biol* 17(3): 169-184

Chang, M. K., L. J. Raggatt, K. A. Alexander, J. S. Kuliwaba, N. L. Fazzalari, K. Schroder, E. R. Maylin, V. M. Ripoll, D. A. Hume & A. R. Pettit (2008). "Osteal tissue macrophages are intercalated throughout human and mouse bone lining tissues and regulate osteoblast function in vitro and in vivo." *J Immunol* 181(2): 1232-1244

Chow, D. C., L. A. Wenning, W. M. Miller & E. T. Papoutsakis (2001). "Modeling pO(2) distributions in the bone marrow hematopoietic compartment. I. Krogh's model." *Biophys J* 81(2): 675-684

Compston, J. E. (2002). "Bone marrow and bone: a functional unit." *J Endocrinol* 173(3): 387-394

Corradi, A., L. Croci, V. Broccoli, S. Zecchini, S. Previtali, W. Wurst, S. Amadio, R. Maggi, A. Quattrini & G. G. Consalez (2003). "Hypogonadotropic hypogonadism and peripheral neuropathy in Ebf2-null mice." *Development* 130(2): 401-410

Corre, J., C. Barreau, B. Cousin, J. P. Chavoin, D. Caton, G. Fournial, L. Penicaud, L. Casteilla & P. Laharrague (2006). "Human subcutaneous adipose cells support complete differentiation but not self-renewal of hematopoietic progenitors." *J Cell Physiol* 208(2): 282-288

Coskun, S. & K. K. Hirschi (2010). "Establishment and regulation of the HSC niche: Roles of osteoblastic and vascular compartments." *Birth Defects Res C Embryo Today* 90(4): 229-242

Coulombel, L., I. Auffray, M. H. Gaugler & M. Rosemblatt (1997). "Expression and function of integrins on hematopoietic progenitor cells." *Acta Haematol* 97(1-2): 13-21

Crawford, L. J., R. Peake, S. Price, T. C. Morris & A. E. Irvine (2010). "Adiponectin is produced by lymphocytes and is a negative regulator of granulopoiesis." *J Leukoc Biol* 88(4): 807-811

Crisan, M., S. Yap, L. Casteilla, C. W. Chen, M. Corselli, T. S. Park, G. Andriolo, B. Sun, B. Zheng, L. Zhang, C. Norotte, P. N. Teng, J. Traas, R. Schugar, B. M. Deasy, S. Badylak, H. J. Buhring, J. P. Giacobino, L. Lazzari, J. Huard & B. Peault (2008). "A perivascular origin for mesenchymal stem cells in multiple human organs." *Cell Stem Cell* 3(3): 301-313

Crowley, J. E., L. S. Treml, J. E. Stadanlick, E. Carpenter & M. P. Cancro (2005). "Homeostatic niche specification among naive and activated B cells: a growing role for the BLyS family of receptors and ligands." *Semin Immunol* 17(3): 193-199

Cumano, A., F. Dieterlen-Lievre & I. Godin (1996). "Lymphoid potential, probed before circulation in mouse, is restricted to caudal intraembryonic splanchnopleura." *Cell* 86(6): 907-916

Cumano, A. & I. Godin (2007). "Ontogeny of the hematopoietic system." *Annu Rev Immunol* 25: 745-785

Dar, A., O. Kollet & T. Lapidot (2006). "Mutual, reciprocal SDF-1/CXCR4 interactions between hematopoietic and bone marrow stromal cells regulate human stem cell migration and development in NOD/SCID chimeric mice." *Exp Hematol* 34(8): 967-975

de Bruijn, M. F., X. Ma, C. Robin, K. Ottersbach, M. J. Sanchez & E. Dzierzak (2002). "Hematopoietic stem cells localize to the endothelial cell layer in the midgestation mouse aorta." *Immunity* 16(5): 673-683

Dexter, T. M., T. D. Allen & L. G. Lajtha (1977). "Conditions controlling the proliferation of haemopoietic stem cells in vitro." *J Cell Physiol* 91(3): 335-344

Dexter, T. M., T. D. Allen, L. G. Lajtha, R. Schofield & B. I. Lord (1973). "Stimulation of differentiation and proliferation of haemopoietic cells in vitro." *J Cell Physiol* 82(3): 461-473

Discher, D. E., D. J. Mooney & P. W. Zandstra (2009). "Growth factors, matrices, and forces combine and control stem cells." *Science* 324(5935): 1673-1677

Dominici, M., V. Rasini, R. Bussolari, X. Chen, T. J. Hofmann, C. Spano, D. Bernabei, E. Veronesi, F. Bertoni, P. Paolucci, P. Conte & E. M. Horwitz (2009). "Restoration and reversible expansion of the osteoblastic hematopoietic stem cell niche after marrow radioablation." *Blood* 114(11): 2333-2343

Eaves, C. J., J. D. Cashman, R. J. Kay, G. J. Dougherty, T. Otsuka, L. A. Gaboury, D. E. Hogge, P. M. Lansdorp, A. C. Eaves & R. K. Humphries (1991). "Mechanisms that regulate the cell cycle status of very primitive hematopoietic cells in long-term human marrow cultures. II. Analysis of positive and negative regulators produced by stromal cells within the adherent layer." *Blood* 78(1): 110-117

Farnum, C. E. & N. J. Wilsman (1989). "Cellular turnover at the chondro-osseous junction of growth plate cartilage: analysis by serial sections at the light microscopical level." *J Orthop Res* 7(5): 654-666

Fortunel, N., J. Hatzfeld, L. Aoustin, P. Batard, K. Ducos, M. N. Monier, A. Charpentier & A. Hatzfeld (2000). "Specific dose-response effects of TGF-beta1 on developmentally distinct hematopoietic stem/progenitor cells from human umbilical cord blood." *Hematol J* 1(2): 126-135

Friedenstein, A. J., R. K. Chailakhjan & K. S. Lalykina (1970). "The development of fibroblast colonies in monolayer cultures of guinea-pig bone marrow and spleen cells." *Cell Tissue Kinet* 3(4): 393-403

Friedenstein, A. J., R. K. Chailakhyan & U. V. Gerasimov (1987). "Bone marrow osteogenic stem cells: in vitro cultivation and transplantation in diffusion chambers." *Cell Tissue Kinet* 20(3): 263-272

Friedenstein, A. J., R. K. Chailakhyan, N. V. Latsinik, A. F. Panasyuk & I. V. Keiliss-Borok (1974). "Stromal cells responsible for transferring the microenvironment of the hemopoietic tissues. Cloning in vitro and retransplantation in vivo." *Transplantation* 17(4): 331-340

Friedenstein, A. J., J. F. Gorskaja & N. N. Kulagina (1976). "Fibroblast precursors in normal and irradiated mouse hematopoietic organs." *Exp Hematol* 4(5): 267-274

Friedenstein, A. J., N. W. Latzinik, A. G. Grosheva & U. F. Gorskaya (1982). "Marrow microenvironment transfer by heterotopic transplantation of freshly isolated and cultured cells in porous sponges." *Exp Hematol* 10(2): 217-227

Funk, P. E., R. P. Stephan & P. L. Witte (1995). "Vascular cell adhesion molecule 1-positive reticular cells express interleukin-7 and stem cell factor in the bone marrow." *Blood* 86(7): 2661-2671

Galotto, M., G. Campanile, G. Robino, F. D. Cancedda, P. Bianco & R. Cancedda (1994). "Hypertrophic chondrocytes undergo further differentiation to osteoblast-like cells and participate in the initial bone formation in developing chick embryo." *J Bone Miner Res* 9(8): 1239-1249

Gekas, C., F. Dieterlen-Lievre, S. H. Orkin & H. K. Mikkola (2005). "The placenta is a niche for hematopoietic stem cells." *Dev Cell* 8(3): 365-375

Gibson, G. J. & M. H. Flint (1985). "Type X collagen synthesis by chick sternal cartilage and its relationship to endochondral development." *J Cell Biol* 101(1): 277-284

Godman, G. C. & K. R. Porter (1960). "Chondrogenesis, studied with the electron microscope." *J Biophys Biochem Cytol* 8: 719-760

Gong, J. K. (1978). "Endosteal marrow: a rich source of hematopoietic stem cells." *Science* 199(4336): 1443-1445

Gordon, M. Y., G. P. Riley & D. Clarke (1988). "Heparan sulfate is necessary for adhesive interactions between human early hemopoietic progenitor cells and the extracellular matrix of the marrow microenvironment." *Leukemia* 2(12): 804-809

Gress, C. J. & O. Jacenko (2000). "Growth plate compressions and altered hematopoiesis in collagen X null mice." *J Cell Biol* 149(4): 983-993

Grimaud, E., F. Blanchard, C. Charrier, F. Gouin, F. Redini & D. Heymann (2002). "Leukaemia inhibitory factor (lif) is expressed in hypertrophic chondrocytes and vascular sprouts during osteogenesis." *Cytokine* 20(5): 224-230

Gruver, A. L., L. L. Hudson & G. D. Sempowski (2007). "Immunosenescence of ageing." *J Pathol* 211(2): 144-156

Guba, S. C., C. I. Sartor, L. R. Gottschalk, Y. H. Jing, T. Mulligan & S. G. Emerson (1992). "Bone marrow stromal fibroblasts secrete interleukin-6 and granulocyte-macrophage colony-stimulating factor in the absence of inflammatory stimulation: demonstration by serum-free bioassay, enzyme-linked immunosorbent assay, and reverse transcriptase polymerase chain reaction." *Blood* 80(5): 1190-1198

Gupta, P., J. B. McCarthy & C. M. Verfaillie (1996). "Stromal fibroblast heparan sulfate is required for cytokine-mediated ex vivo maintenance of human long-term culture-initiating cells." *Blood* 87(8): 3229-3236

Gupta, P., T. R. Oegema, Jr., J. J. Brazil, A. Z. Dudek, A. Slungaard & C. M. Verfaillie (1998). "Structurally specific heparan sulfates support primitive human hematopoiesis by formation of a multimolecular stem cell niche." *Blood* 92(12): 4641-4651

Gurevitch, O. & I. Fabian (1993). "Ability of the hemopoietic microenvironment in the induced bone to maintain the proliferative potential of early hemopoietic precursors." *Stem Cells* 11(1): 56-61

Hara, H., H. Ohdan, D. Tokita, T. Onoe, W. Zhou & T. Asahara (2003). "Construction of ectopic xenogeneic bone marrow structure associated with persistent multi-lineage mixed chimerism by engraftment of rat bone marrow plugs into mouse kidney capsules." *Xenotransplantation* 10(3): 259-266

Harada, M., K. Odaka, K. Kondo, S. Nakao, M. Ueda, K. Matsue, T. Mori & T. Matsuda (1985). "Effect of activated lymphocytes on the regulation of hematopoiesis: suppression of in vitro granulopoiesis and erythropoiesis by OKT8+ Ia- T cells induced by concanavalin-A stimulation." *Exp Hematol* 13(9): 963-967

Haylock, D. N. & S. K. Nilsson (2006). "The role of hyaluronic acid in hemopoietic stem cell biology." *Regen Med* 1(4): 437-445

Heinrich, M. C., D. C. Dooley, A. C. Freed, L. Band, M. E. Hoatlin, W. W. Keeble, S. T. Peters, K. V. Silvey, F. S. Ey, D. Kabat & et al. (1993). "Constitutive expression of steel factor gene by human stromal cells." *Blood* 82(3): 771-783

Heissig, B., K. Hattori, S. Dias, M. Friedrich, B. Ferris, N. R. Hackett, R. G. Crystal, P. Besmer, D. Lyden, M. A. Moore, Z. Werb & S. Rafii (2002). "Recruitment of stem and progenitor cells from the bone marrow niche requires MMP-9 mediated release of kit-ligand." *Cell* 109(5): 625-637

Hermanns, P., A. A. Bertuch, T. K. Bertin, B. Dawson, M. E. Schmitt, C. Shaw, B. Zabel & B. Lee (2005). "Consequences of mutations in the non-coding RMRP RNA in cartilage-hair hypoplasia." *Hum Mol Genet* 14(23): 3723-3740

Hermans, M. H., H. Hartsuiker & D. Opstelten (1989). "An in situ study of B-lymphocytopoiesis in rat bone marrow. Topographical arrangement of terminal deoxynucleotidyl transferase-positive cells and pre-B cells." *J Immunol* 142(1): 67-73

Hilton, M. J., X. Tu & F. Long (2007). "Tamoxifen-inducible gene deletion reveals a distinct cell type associated with trabecular bone, and direct regulation of PTHrP expression and chondrocyte morphology by Ihh in growth region cartilage." *Dev Biol* 308(1): 93-105

Holst, J., S. Watson, M. S. Lord, S. S. Eamegdool, D. V. Bax, L. B. Nivison-Smith, A. Kondyurin, L. Ma, A. F. Oberhauser, A. S. Weiss & J. E. Rasko (2010). "Substrate elasticity provides mechanical signals for the expansion of hemopoietic stem and progenitor cells." *Nat Biotechnol* 28(10): 1123-1128

Horwitz, E. M., K. Le Blanc, M. Dominici, I. Mueller, I. Slaper-Cortenbach, F. C. Marini, R. J. Deans, D. S. Krause & A. Keating (2005). "Clarification of the nomenclature for MSC: The International Society for Cellular Therapy position statement." *Cytotherapy* 7(5): 393-395

Hotamisligil, G. S., N. S. Shargill & B. M. Spiegelman (1993). "Adipose expression of tumor necrosis factor-alpha: direct role in obesity-linked insulin resistance." *Science* 259(5091): 87-91

Huard, B., T. McKee, C. Bosshard, S. Durual, T. Matthes, S. Myit, O. Donze, C. Frossard, C. Chizzolini, C. Favre, R. Zubler, J. P. Guyot, P. Schneider & E. Roosnek (2008). "APRIL secreted by neutrophils binds to heparan sulfate proteoglycans to create plasma cell niches in human mucosa." *J Clin Invest* 118(8): 2887-2895

Ingold, K., A. Zumsteg, A. Tardivel, B. Huard, Q. G. Steiner, T. G. Cachero, F. Qiang, L. Gorelik, S. L. Kalled, H. Acha-Orbea, P. D. Rennert, J. Tschopp & P. Schneider (2005). "Identification of proteoglycans as the APRIL-specific binding partners." *J Exp Med* 201(9): 1375-1383

Jacenko, O., D. Chan, A. Franklin, S. Ito, C. B. Underhill, J. F. Bateman & M. R. Campbell (2001). "A dominant interference collagen X mutation disrupts hypertrophic chondrocyte pericellular matrix and glycosaminoglycan and proteoglycan distribution in transgenic mice." *Am J Pathol* 159(6): 2257-2269

Jacenko, O., S. Ito & B. R. Olsen (1996). "Skeletal and hematopoietic defects in mice transgenic for collagen X." *Ann N Y Acad Sci* 785: 278-280

Jacenko, O., P. A. LuValle & B. R. Olsen (1993). "Spondylometaphyseal dysplasia in mice carrying a dominant negative mutation in a matrix protein specific for cartilage-to-bone transition." *Nature* 365(6441): 56-61

Jacenko, O., B. R. Olsen & P. LuValle (1991). "Organization and regulation of collagen genes." *Crit Rev Eukaryot Gene Expr* 1(4): 327-353

Jacenko, O., D. W. Roberts, M. R. Campbell, P. M. McManus, C. J. Gress & Z. Tao (2002). "Linking hematopoiesis to endochondral skeletogenesis through analysis of mice transgenic for collagen X." *Am J Pathol* 160(6): 2019-2034

Jacobsen, K. & D. G. Osmond (1990). "Microenvironmental organization and stromal cell associations of B lymphocyte precursor cells in mouse bone marrow." *Eur J Immunol* 20(11): 2395-2404

James, C. G., L. A. Stanton, H. Agoston, V. Ulici, T. M. Underhill & F. Beier (2010). "Genome-wide analyses of gene expression during mouse endochondral ossification." *PLoS One* 5(1): e8693

Jang, Y. Y. & S. J. Sharkis (2007). "A low level of reactive oxygen species selects for primitive hematopoietic stem cells that may reside in the low-oxygenic niche." *Blood* 110(8): 3056-3063

Janzen, V., R. Forkert, H. E. Fleming, Y. Saito, M. T. Waring, D. M. Dombkowski, T. Cheng, R. A. DePinho, N. E. Sharpless & D. T. Scadden (2006). "Stem-cell ageing modified by the cyclin-dependent kinase inhibitor p16INK4a." *Nature* 443(7110): 421-426

Jung, Y., J. Song, Y. Shiozawa, J. Wang, Z. Wang, B. Williams, A. Havens, A. Schneider, C. Ge, R. T. Franceschi, L. K. McCauley, P. H. Krebsbach & R. S. Taichman (2008). "Hematopoietic stem cells regulate mesenchymal stromal cell induction into osteoblasts thereby participating in the formation of the stem cell niche." *Stem Cells* 26(8): 2042-2051

Jung, Y., J. Wang, A. Havens, Y. Sun, J. Wang, T. Jin & R. S. Taichman (2005). "Cell-to-cell contact is critical for the survival of hematopoietic progenitor cells on osteoblasts." *Cytokine* 32(3-4): 155-162

Jung, Y., J. Wang, A. Schneider, Y. X. Sun, A. J. Koh-Paige, N. I. Osman, L. K. McCauley & R. S. Taichman (2006). "Regulation of SDF-1 (CXCL12) production by osteoblasts; a possible mechanism for stem cell homing." *Bone* 38(4): 497-508

Kacena, M. A., C. M. Gundberg & M. C. Horowitz (2006). "A reciprocal regulatory interaction between megakaryocytes, bone cells, and hematopoietic stem cells." *Bone* 39(5): 978-984

Kacena, M. A., R. A. Shivdasani, K. Wilson, Y. Xi, N. Troiano, A. Nazarian, C. M. Gundberg, M. L. Bouxsein, J. A. Lorenzo & M. C. Horowitz (2004). "Megakaryocyte-osteoblast interaction revealed in mice deficient in transcription factors GATA-1 and NF-E2." *J Bone Miner Res* 19(4): 652-660

Kalajzic, Z., H. Li, L. P. Wang, X. Jiang, K. Lamothe, D. J. Adams, H. L. Aguila, D. W. Rowe & I. Kalajzic (2008). "Use of an alpha-smooth muscle actin GFP reporter to identify an osteoprogenitor population." *Bone* 43(3): 501-510

Kalinkovich, A., A. Spiegel, S. Shivtiel, O. Kollet, N. Jordaney, W. Piacibello & T. Lapidot (2009). "Blood-forming stem cells are nervous: direct and indirect regulation of immature human CD34+ cells by the nervous system." *Brain Behav Immun* 23(8): 1059-1065

Katayama, Y., M. Battista, W. M. Kao, A. Hidalgo, A. J. Peired, S. A. Thomas & P. S. Frenette (2006). "Signals from the sympathetic nervous system regulate hematopoietic stem cell egress from bone marrow." *Cell* 124(2): 407-421

Kawai, M., H. Hattori, K. Yasue, H. Mizutani, M. Ueda, T. Kaneda & T. Hoshino (1994). "Development of hemopoietic bone marrow within the ectopic bone induced by bone morphogenetic protein." *Blood Cells* 20(1): 191-199; discussion 200-191

Keller, J. R., J. M. Gooya & F. W. Ruscetti (1996). "Direct synergistic effects of leukemia inhibitory factor on hematopoietic progenitor cell growth: comparison with other hematopoietins that use the gp130 receptor subunit." *Blood* 88(3): 863-869

Khosla, S. (2003). "Parathyroid hormone plus alendronate--a combination that does not add up." *N Engl J Med* 349(13): 1277-1279

Kiel, M. J., M. Acar, G. L. Radice & S. J. Morrison (2009). "Hematopoietic stem cells do not depend on N-cadherin to regulate their maintenance." *Cell Stem Cell* 4(2): 170-179

Kiel, M. J., G. L. Radice & S. J. Morrison (2007). "Lack of evidence that hematopoietic stem cells depend on N-cadherin-mediated adhesion to osteoblasts for their maintenance." *Cell Stem Cell* 1(2): 204-217

Kiel, M. J., O. H. Yilmaz, T. Iwashita, O. H. Yilmaz, C. Terhorst & S. J. Morrison (2005). "SLAM family receptors distinguish hematopoietic stem and progenitor cells and reveal endothelial niches for stem cells." *Cell* 121(7): 1109-1121

Kieslinger, M., S. Hiechinger, G. Dobreva, G. G. Consalez & R. Grosschedl (2010). "Early B cell factor 2 regulates hematopoietic stem cell homeostasis in a cell-nonautonomous manner." *Cell Stem Cell* 7(4): 496-507

Kilborn, S. H., G. Trudel & H. Uhthoff (2002). "Review of growth plate closure compared with age at sexual maturity and lifespan in laboratory animals." *Contemp Top Lab Anim Sci* 41(5): 21-26

Klein, G. (1995). "The extracellular matrix of the hematopoietic microenvironment." *Experientia* 51(9-10): 914-926

Klein, G., S. Conzelmann, S. Beck, R. Timpl & C. A. Muller (1995). "Perlecan in human bone marrow: a growth-factor-presenting, but anti-adhesive, extracellular matrix component for hematopoietic cells." *Matrix Biol* 14(6): 457-465

Klein, G., C. Kibler, F. Schermutzki, J. Brown, C. A. Muller & R. Timpl (1998). "Cell binding properties of collagen type XIV for human hematopoietic cells." *Matrix Biol* 16(6): 307-317

Kohler, A., V. Schmithorst, M. D. Filippi, M. A. Ryan, D. Daria, M. Gunzer & H. Geiger (2009). "Altered cellular dynamics and endosteal location of aged early hematopoietic progenitor cells revealed by time-lapse intravital imaging in long bones." *Blood* 114(2): 290-298

Kollet, O., A. Dar, S. Shivtiel, A. Kalinkovich, K. Lapid, Y. Sztainberg, M. Tesio, R. M. Samstein, P. Goichberg, A. Spiegel, A. Elson & T. Lapidot (2006). "Osteoclasts degrade endosteal components and promote mobilization of hematopoietic progenitor cells." *Nat Med* 12(6): 657-664

Kong, Y. Y., H. Yoshida, I. Sarosi, H. L. Tan, E. Timms, C. Capparelli, S. Morony, A. J. Oliveira-dos-Santos, G. Van, A. Itie, W. Khoo, A. Wakeham, C. R. Dunstan, D. L. Lacey, T. W. Mak, W. J. Boyle & J. M. Penninger (1999). "OPGL is a key regulator of osteoclastogenesis, lymphocyte development and lymph-node organogenesis." *Nature* 397(6717): 315-323

Kopp, H. G., S. T. Avecilla, A. T. Hooper & S. Rafii (2005). "The bone marrow vascular niche: home of HSC differentiation and mobilization." *Physiology (Bethesda)* 20: 349-356

Kortesidis, A., A. Zannettino, S. Isenmann, S. Shi, T. Lapidot & S. Gronthos (2005). "Stromal-derived factor-1 promotes the growth, survival, and development of human bone marrow stromal stem cells." *Blood* 105(10): 3793-3801

Kuijpers, T. W., E. Nannenberg, M. Alders, R. Bredius & R. C. Hennekam (2004). "Congenital aplastic anemia caused by mutations in the SBDS gene: a rare presentation of Shwachman-Diamond syndrome." *Pediatrics* 114(3): e387-391

Kuznetsov, S. A., P. H. Krebsbach, K. Satomura, J. Kerr, M. Riminucci, D. Benayahu & P. G. Robey (1997). "Single-colony derived strains of human marrow stromal fibroblasts form bone after transplantation in vivo." *J Bone Miner Res* 12(9): 1335-1347

Kuznetsov, S. A., M. Riminucci, N. Ziran, T. W. Tsutsui, A. Corsi, L. Calvi, H. M. Kronenberg, E. Schipani, P. G. Robey & P. Bianco (2004). "The interplay of osteogenesis and hematopoiesis: expression of a constitutively active PTH/PTHrP receptor in osteogenic cells perturbs the establishment of hematopoiesis in bone and of skeletal stem cells in the bone marrow." *J Cell Biol* 167(6): 1113-1122

Kwan, K. M., M. K. Pang, S. Zhou, S. K. Cowan, R. Y. Kong, T. Pfordte, B. R. Olsen, D. O. Sillence, P. P. Tam & K. S. Cheah (1997). "Abnormal compartmentalization of cartilage matrix components in mice lacking collagen X: implications for function." *J Cell Biol* 136(2): 459-471

Kwon, K. R., J. Y. Ahn, M. S. Kim, J. Y. Jung, J. H. Lee & I. H. Oh (2010). "Disruption of bis leads to the deterioration of the vascular niche for hematopoietic stem cells." *Stem Cells* 28(2): 268-278

Lanotte, M., D. Metcalf & T. M. Dexter (1982). "Production of monocyte/macrophage colony-stimulating factor by preadipocyte cell lines derived from murine marrow stroma." *J Cell Physiol* 112(1): 123-127

Lapid, K., Y. Vagima, O. Kollet & T. Lapidot (2008). "Egress and mobilization of hematopoietic stem and progenitor cells."

Larsson, J., M. Ohishi, B. Garrison, M. Aspling, V. Janzen, G. B. Adams, M. Curto, A. I. McClatchey, E. Schipani & D. T. Scadden (2008). "Nf2/merlin regulates hematopoietic stem cell behavior by altering microenvironmental architecture." *Cell Stem Cell* 3(2): 221-227

Lefebvre, V. & P. Smits (2005). "Transcriptional control of chondrocyte fate and differentiation." *Birth Defects Res Part C: Embryo Today: Reviews* 75(3): 200-212

Levesque, J. P. & P. J. Simmons (1999). "Cytoskeleton and integrin-mediated adhesion signaling in human CD34+ hemopoietic progenitor cells." *Exp Hematol* 27(4): 579-586

Levesque, J. P., Y. Takamatsu, S. K. Nilsson, D. N. Haylock & P. J. Simmons (2001). "Vascular cell adhesion molecule-1 (CD106) is cleaved by neutrophil proteases in the bone marrow following hematopoietic progenitor cell mobilization by granulocyte colony-stimulating factor." *Blood* 98(5): 1289-1297

Li, W., S. A. Johnson, W. C. Shelley & M. C. Yoder (2004). "Hematopoietic stem cell repopulating ability can be maintained in vitro by some primary endothelial cells." *Exp Hematol* 32(12): 1226-1237

Lo Celso, C., H. E. Fleming, J. W. Wu, C. X. Zhao, S. Miake-Lye, J. Fujisaki, D. Cote, D. W. Rowe, C. P. Lin & D. T. Scadden (2009). "Live-animal tracking of individual haematopoietic stem/progenitor cells in their niche." *Nature* 457(7225): 92-96

Lord, B. I., N. G. Testa & J. H. Hendry (1975). "The relative spatial distributions of CFUs and CFUc in the normal mouse femur." *Blood* 46(1): 65-72

Mackie, E. J., Y. A. Ahmed, L. Tatarczuch, K. S. Chen & M. Mirams (2008). "Endochondral ossification: how cartilage is converted into bone in the developing skeleton." *Int J Biochem Cell Biol* 40(1): 46-62

Maes, C., T. Kobayashi, M. K. Selig, S. Torrekens, S. I. Roth, S. Mackem, G. Carmeliet & H. M. Kronenberg (2010). "Osteoblast precursors, but not mature osteoblasts, move into developing and fractured bones along with invading blood vessels." *Dev Cell* 19(2): 329-344

Majumdar, M. K., M. A. Thiede, S. E. Haynesworth, S. P. Bruder & S. L. Gerson (2000). "Human marrow-derived mesenchymal stem cells (MSCs) express hematopoietic cytokines and support long-term hematopoiesis when differentiated toward stromal and osteogenic lineages." *J Hematother Stem Cell Res* 9(6): 841-848

Mangan, K. F., G. Chikkappa, L. Z. Bieler, W. B. Scharfman & D. R. Parkinson (1982). "Regulation of human blood erythroid burst-forming unit (BFU-E) proliferation by T-lymphocyte subpopulations defined by Fc receptors and monoclonal antibodies." *Blood* 59(5): 990-996

Mankani, M. H., S. A. Kuznetsov, G. W. Marshall & P. G. Robey (2008). "Creation of new bone by the percutaneous injection of human bone marrow stromal cell and HA/TCP suspensions." *Tissue Eng Part A* 14(12): 1949-1958

Mankani, M. H., S. A. Kuznetsov & P. G. Robey (2007). "Formation of hematopoietic territories and bone by transplanted human bone marrow stromal cells requires a critical cell density." *Exp Hematol* 35(6): 995-1004

Mansour, A., A. Anginot, S. J. Mancini, C. Schiff, G. F. Carle, A. Wakkach & C. Blin-Wakkach (2011). "Osteoclast activity modulates B-cell development in the bone marrow." *Cell Res* 21(7): 1102-1115

Matrosova, V. Y., I. A. Orlovskaya, N. Serobyan & S. K. Khaldoyanidi (2004). "Hyaluronic acid facilitates the recovery of hematopoiesis following 5-fluorouracil administration." *Stem Cells* 22(4): 544-555

Mayack, S. R., J. L. Shadrach, F. S. Kim & A. J. Wagers (2010). "Systemic signals regulate ageing and rejuvenation of blood stem cell niches." *Nature* 463(7280): 495-500

Mazzon, C., A. Anselmo, J. Cibella, C. Soldani, A. Destro, N. Kim, M. Roncalli, S. J. Burden, M. L. Dustin, A. Sarukhan & A. Viola (2011). "The critical role of agrin in the hematopoietic stem cell niche." *Blood* 118(10): 2733-2742

Meck, R. A., J. E. Haley & G. Brecher (1973). "Hematopoiesis versus osteogenesis in ectopic bone marrow transplants." *Blood* 42(5): 661-669

Medici, D., E. M. Shore, V. Y. Lounev, F. S. Kaplan, R. Kalluri & B. R. Olsen (2010). "Conversion of vascular endothelial cells into multipotent stem-like cells." *Nat Med* 16(12): 1400-1406

Medvinsky, A. & E. Dzierzak (1996). "Definitive hematopoiesis is autonomously initiated by the AGM region." *Cell* 86(6): 897-906

Mendez-Ferrer, S., D. Lucas, M. Battista & P. S. Frenette (2008). "Haematopoietic stem cell release is regulated by circadian oscillations." *Nature* 452(7186): 442-447

Mendez-Ferrer, S., T. V. Michurina, F. Ferraro, A. R. Mazloom, B. D. Macarthur, S. A. Lira, D. T. Scadden, A. Ma'ayan, G. N. Enikolopov & P. S. Frenette (2010). "Mesenchymal and haematopoietic stem cells form a unique bone marrow niche." *Nature* 466(7308): 829-834

Merzaban, J. S., M. M. Burdick, S. Z. Gadhoum, N. M. Dagia, J. T. Chu, R. C. Fuhlbrigge & R. Sackstein (2011). "Analysis of glycoprotein E-selectin ligands on human and mouse marrow cells enriched for hematopoietic stem/progenitor cells." *Blood* 118(7): 1774-1783

Mignini, F., V. Streccioni & F. Amenta (2003). "Autonomic innervation of immune organs and neuroimmune modulation." *Auton Autacoid Pharmacol* 23(1): 1-25

Miharada, K., T. Hiroyama, K. Sudo, I. Danjo, T. Nagasawa & Y. Nakamura (2008). "Lipocalin 2-mediated growth suppression is evident in human erythroid and monocyte/macrophage lineage cells." *J Cell Physiol* 215(2): 526-537

Moreaux, J., F. W. Cremer, T. Reme, M. Raab, K. Mahtouk, P. Kaukel, V. Pantesco, J. De Vos, E. Jourdan, A. Jauch, E. Legouffe, M. Moos, G. Fiol, H. Goldschmidt, J. F. Rossi, D. Hose & B. Klein (2005). "The level of TACI gene expression in myeloma cells is associated with a signature of microenvironment dependence versus a plasmablastic signature." *Blood* 106(3): 1021-1030

Moreaux, J., A. C. Sprynski, S. R. Dillon, K. Mahtouk, M. Jourdan, A. Ythier, P. Moine, N. Robert, E. Jourdan, J. F. Rossi & B. Klein (2009). "APRIL and TACI interact with syndecan-1 on the surface of multiple myeloma cells to form an essential survival loop." *Eur J Haematol* 83(2): 119-129

Morikawa, S., Y. Mabuchi, Y. Kubota, Y. Nagai, K. Niibe, E. Hiratsu, S. Suzuki, C. Miyauchi-Hara, N. Nagoshi, T. Sunabori, S. Shimmura, A. Miyawaki, T. Nakagawa, T. Suda, H. Okano & Y. Matsuzaki (2009). "Prospective identification, isolation, and systemic transplantation of multipotent mesenchymal stem cells in murine bone marrow." *J Exp Med* 206(11): 2483-2496

Morrison, S. J. & A. C. Spradling (2008). "Stem cells and niches: mechanisms that promote stem cell maintenance throughout life." *Cell* 132(4): 598-611

Muguruma, Y., T. Yahata, H. Miyatake, T. Sato, T. Uno, J. Itoh, S. Kato, M. Ito, T. Hotta & K. Ando (2006). "Reconstitution of the functional human hematopoietic microenvironment derived from human mesenchymal stem cells in the murine bone marrow compartment." *Blood* 107(5): 1878-1887

Murayama, E., K. Kissa, A. Zapata, E. Mordelet, V. Briolat, H. F. Lin, R. I. Handin & P. Herbomel (2006). "Tracing hematopoietic precursor migration to successive hematopoietic organs during zebrafish development." *Immunity* 25(6): 963-975

Nagasawa, T. (2006). "Microenvironmental niches in the bone marrow required for B-cell development." *Nat Rev Immunol* 6(2): 107-116

Nagasawa, T., S. Hirota, K. Tachibana, N. Takakura, S. Nishikawa, Y. Kitamura, N. Yoshida, H. Kikutani & T. Kishimoto (1996). "Defects of B-cell lymphopoiesis and bone-marrow myelopoiesis in mice lacking the CXC chemokine PBSF/SDF-1." *Nature* 382(6592): 635-638

Nagasawa, T., H. Kikutani & T. Kishimoto (1994). "Molecular cloning and structure of a pre-B-cell growth-stimulating factor." *Proc Natl Acad Sci U S A* 91(6): 2305-2309

Naiyer, A. J., D. Y. Jo, J. Ahn, R. Mohle, M. Peichev, G. Lam, R. L. Silverstein, M. A. Moore & S. Rafii (1999). "Stromal derived factor-1-induced chemokinesis of cord blood CD34(+) cells (long-term culture-initiating cells) through endothelial cells is mediated by E-selectin." *Blood* 94(12): 4011-4019

Nakamura, E., M. T. Nguyen & S. Mackem (2006). "Kinetics of tamoxifen-regulated Cre activity in mice using a cartilage-specific CreER(T) to assay temporal activity windows along the proximodistal limb skeleton." *Dev Dyn* 235(9): 2603-2612

Nathan, D. G., L. Chess, D. G. Hillman, B. Clarke, J. Breard, E. Merler & D. E. Housman (1978). "Human erythroid burst-forming unit: T-cell requirement for proliferation in vitro." *J Exp Med* 147(2): 324-339

Naveiras, O., V. Nardi, P. L. Wenzel, P. V. Hauschka, F. Fahey & G. Q. Daley (2009). "Bone-marrow adipocytes as negative regulators of the haematopoietic microenvironment." *Nature* 460(7252): 259-263

Nilsson, S. K., M. S. Dooner, C. Y. Tiarks, H. U. Weier & P. J. Quesenberry (1997). "Potential and distribution of transplanted hematopoietic stem cells in a nonablated mouse model." *Blood* 89(11): 4013-4020

Nilsson, S. K., H. M. Johnston & J. A. Coverdale (2001). "Spatial localization of transplanted hemopoietic stem cells: inferences for the localization of stem cell niches." *Blood* 97(8): 2293-2299

North, T. E., M. F. de Bruijn, T. Stacy, L. Talebian, E. Lind, C. Robin, M. Binder, E. Dzierzak & N. A. Speck (2002). "Runx1 expression marks long-term repopulating hematopoietic stem cells in the midgestation mouse embryo." *Immunity* 16(5): 661-672

O'Connor, B. P., V. S. Raman, L. D. Erickson, W. J. Cook, L. K. Weaver, C. Ahonen, L. L. Lin, G. T. Mantchev, R. J. Bram & R. J. Noelle (2004). "BCMA is essential for the survival of long-lived bone marrow plasma cells." *J Exp Med* 199(1): 91-98

Ohneda, O., C. Fennie, Z. Zheng, C. Donahue, H. La, R. Villacorta, B. Cairns & L. A. Lasky (1998). "Hematopoietic stem cell maintenance and differentiation are supported by embryonic aorta-gonad-mesonephros region-derived endothelium." *Blood* 92(3): 908-919

Ohta, M., T. Sakai, Y. Saga, S. Aizawa & M. Saito (1998). "Suppression of hematopoietic activity in tenascin-C-deficient mice." *Blood* 91(11): 4074-4083

Omatsu, Y., T. Sugiyama, H. Kohara, G. Kondoh, N. Fujii, K. Kohno & T. Nagasawa (2010). "The essential functions of adipo-osteogenic progenitors as the hematopoietic stem and progenitor cell niche." *Immunity* 33(3): 387-399

Osmond, D. G. (1990). "B cell development in the bone marrow." *Semin Immunol* 2(3): 173-180

Ottersbach, K. & E. Dzierzak (2005). "The murine placenta contains hematopoietic stem cells within the vascular labyrinth region." *Dev Cell* 8(3): 377-387

Patt, H. M., M. A. Maloney & M. L. Flannery (1982). "Hematopoietic microenvironment transfer by stromal fibroblasts derived from bone marrow varying in cellularity." *Exp Hematol* 10(9): 738-742

Peerani, R. & P. W. Zandstra (2010). "Enabling stem cell therapies through synthetic stem cell-niche engineering." *J Clin Invest* 120(1): 60-70

Peled, A., V. Grabovsky, L. Habler, J. Sandbank, F. Arenzana-Seisdedos, I. Petit, H. Ben-Hur, T. Lapidot & R. Alon (1999). "The chemokine SDF-1 stimulates integrin-mediated arrest of CD34(+) cells on vascular endothelium under shear flow." *J Clin Invest* 104(9): 1199-1211

Petit, I., M. Szyper-Kravitz, A. Nagler, M. Lahav, A. Peled, L. Habler, T. Ponomaryov, R. S. Taichman, F. Arenzana-Seisdedos, N. Fujii, J. Sandbank, D. Zipori & T. Lapidot (2002). "G-CSF induces stem cell mobilization by decreasing bone marrow SDF-1 and up-regulating CXCR4." *Nat Immunol* 3(7): 687-694

Petrini, M., S. Pacini, L. Trombi, R. Fazzi, M. Montali, S. Ikehara & N. G. Abraham (2009). "Identification and purification of mesodermal progenitor cells from human adult bone marrow." *Stem Cells Dev* 18(6): 857-866

Pfeiffer, C. A. (1948). "Development of bone from transplanted marrow in mice." *Anat Rec* 102(2): 225-243

Pilia, G., R. M. Hughes-Benzie, A. MacKenzie, P. Baybayan, E. Y. Chen, R. Huber, G. Neri, A. Cao, A. Forabosco & D. Schlessinger (1996). "Mutations in GPC3, a glypican gene, cause the Simpson-Golabi-Behmel overgrowth syndrome." *Nat Genet* 12(3): 241-247

Ponomaryov, T., A. Peled, I. Petit, R. S. Taichman, L. Habler, J. Sandbank, F. Arenzana-Seisdedos, A. Magerus, A. Caruz, N. Fujii, A. Nagler, M. Lahav, M. Szyper-Kravitz, D. Zipori & T. Lapidot (2000). "Induction of the chemokine stromal-derived factor-1 following DNA damage improves human stem cell function." *J Clin Invest* 106(11): 1331-1339

Purton, L. E., S. Dworkin, G. H. Olsen, C. R. Walkley, S. A. Fabb, S. J. Collins & P. Chambon (2006). "RARgamma is critical for maintaining a balance between hematopoietic stem cell self-renewal and differentiation." *J Exp Med* 203(5): 1283-1293

Raaijmakers, M. H., S. Mukherjee, S. Guo, S. Zhang, T. Kobayashi, J. A. Schoonmaker, B. L. Ebert, F. Al-Shahrour, R. P. Hasserjian, E. O. Scadden, Z. Aung, M. Matza, M. Merkenschlager, C. Lin, J. M. Rommens & D. T. Scadden (2010). "Bone progenitor dysfunction induces myelodysplasia and secondary leukaemia." *Nature* 464(7290): 852-857

Rafii, S., R. Mohle, F. Shapiro, B. M. Frey & M. A. Moore (1997). "Regulation of hematopoiesis by microvascular endothelium." *Leuk Lymphoma* 27(5-6): 375-386

Rafii, S., F. Shapiro, R. Pettengell, B. Ferris, R. L. Nachman, M. A. Moore & A. S. Asch (1995). "Human bone marrow microvascular endothelial cells support long-term proliferation and differentiation of myeloid and megakaryocytic progenitors." *Blood* 86(9): 3353-3363

Rafii, S., F. Shapiro, J. Rimarachin, R. L. Nachman, B. Ferris, B. Weksler, M. A. Moore & A. S. Asch (1994). "Isolation and characterization of human bone marrow microvascular endothelial cells: hematopoietic progenitor cell adhesion." *Blood* 84(1): 10-19

Roach, H. I. (1992). "Trans-differentiation of hypertrophic chondrocytes into cells capable of producing a mineralized bone matrix." *Bone Miner* 19(1): 1-20

Roach, H. I. & J. Erenpreisa (1996). "The phenotypic switch from chondrocytes to bone-forming cells involves asymmetric cell division and apoptosis." *Connect Tissue Res* 35(1-4): 85-91

Roach, H. I., J. Erenpreisa & T. Aigner (1995). "Osteogenic differentiation of hypertrophic chondrocytes involves asymmetric cell divisions and apoptosis." *J Cell Biol* 131(2): 483-494

Roberts, R., J. Gallagher, E. Spooncer, T. D. Allen, F. Bloomfield & T. M. Dexter (1988). "Heparan sulphate bound growth factors: a mechanism for stromal cell mediated haemopoiesis." *Nature* 332(6162): 376-378

Rodgers, K. D., J. D. San Antonio & O. Jacenko (2008). "Heparan sulfate proteoglycans: A GAGgle of skeletal-hematopoietic regulators." *Dev Dyn* 237(10): 2622-2642

Rosati, R., G. S. Horan, G. J. Pinero, S. Garofalo, D. R. Keene, W. A. Horton, E. Vuorio, B. de Crombrugghe & R. R. Behringer (1994). "Normal long bone growth and development in type X collagen-null mice." *Nat Genet* 8(2): 129-135

Rossi, D. J., D. Bryder, J. M. Zahn, H. Ahlenius, R. Sonu, A. J. Wagers & I. L. Weissman (2005). "Cell intrinsic alterations underlie hematopoietic stem cell aging." *Proc Natl Acad Sci U S A* 102(26): 9194-9199

Rossi, D. J., C. H. Jamieson & I. L. Weissman (2008). "Stems cells and the pathways to aging and cancer." *Cell* 132(4): 681-696

Rouleau, M. F., J. Mitchell & D. Goltzman (1990). "Characterization of the major parathyroid hormone target cell in the endosteal metaphysis of rat long bones." *J Bone Miner Res* 5(10): 1043-1053

Ryan, D. H., B. L. Nuccie, C. N. Abboud & J. M. Winslow (1991). "Vascular cell adhesion molecule-1 and the integrin VLA-4 mediate adhesion of human B cell precursors to cultured bone marrow adherent cells." *J Clin Invest* 88(3): 995-1004

Sacchetti, B., A. Funari, S. Michienzi, S. Di Cesare, S. Piersanti, I. Saggio, E. Tagliafico, S. Ferrari, P. G. Robey, M. Riminucci & P. Bianco (2007). "Self-renewing osteoprogenitors in bone marrow sinusoids can organize a hematopoietic microenvironment." *Cell* 131(2): 324-336

Sagar, B. M., S. Rentala, P. N. Gopal, S. Sharma & A. Mukhopadhyay (2006). "Fibronectin and laminin enhance engraftibility of cultured hematopoietic stem cells." *Biochem Biophys Res Commun* 350(4): 1000-1005

Sanchez, M. J., A. Holmes, C. Miles & E. Dzierzak (1996). "Characterization of the first definitive hematopoietic stem cells in the AGM and liver of the mouse embryo." *Immunity* 5(6): 513-525

Schmid, T. M. & T. F. Linsenmayer (1985). "Immunohistochemical localization of short chain cartilage collagen (type X) in avian tissues." *J Cell Biol* 100(2): 598-605

Schofield, R. (1978). "The relationship between the spleen colony-forming cell and the haemopoietic stem cell." *Blood Cells* 4(1-2): 7-25

Schwaller, J., P. Schneider, P. Mhawech-Fauceglia, T. McKee, S. Myit, T. Matthes, J. Tschopp, O. Donze, F. A. Le Gal & B. Huard (2007). "Neutrophil-derived APRIL concentrated in tumor lesions by proteoglycans correlates with human B-cell lymphoma aggressiveness." *Blood* 109(1): 331-338

Schweitzer, K. M., A. M. Drager, P. van der Valk, S. F. Thijsen, A. Zevenbergen, A. P. Theijsmeijer, C. E. van der Schoot & M. M. Langenhuijsen (1996). "Constitutive expression of E-selectin and vascular cell adhesion molecule-1 on endothelial cells of hematopoietic tissues." *Am J Pathol* 148(1): 165-175

Shackney, S. E., S. S. Ford & A. B. Wittig (1975). "Kinetic-microarchitectural correlations in the bone marrow of the mouse." *Cell Tissue Kinet* 8(6): 505-516

Siczkowski, M., D. Clarke & M. Y. Gordon (1992). "Binding of primitive hematopoietic progenitor cells to marrow stromal cells involves heparan sulfate." *Blood* 80(4): 912-919

Siebertz, B., G. Stocker, Z. Drzeniek, S. Handt, U. Just & H. D. Haubeck (1999). "Expression of glypican-4 in haematopoietic-progenitor and bone-marrow-stromal cells." *Biochem J* 344 (Pt 3): 937-943

Sipkins, D. A., X. Wei, J. W. Wu, J. M. Runnels, D. Cote, T. K. Means, A. D. Luster, D. T. Scadden & C. P. Lin (2005). "In vivo imaging of specialized bone marrow endothelial microdomains for tumour engraftment." *Nature* 435(7044): 969-973

Song, J., M. J. Kiel, Z. Wang, J. Wang, R. S. Taichman, S. J. Morrison & P. H. Krebsbach (2010). "An in vivo model to study and manipulate the hematopoietic stem cell niche." *Blood* 115(13): 2592-2600

Spiegel, A., A. Kalinkovich, S. Shivtiel, O. Kollet & T. Lapidot (2008). "Stem cell regulation via dynamic interactions of the nervous and immune systems with the microenvironment." *Cell Stem Cell* 3(5): 484-492

Spiegel, A., S. Shivtiel, A. Kalinkovich, A. Ludin, N. Netzer, P. Goichberg, Y. Azaria, I. Resnick, I. Hardan, H. Ben-Hur, A. Nagler, M. Rubinstein & T. Lapidot (2007). "Catecholaminergic neurotransmitters regulate migration and repopulation of immature human CD34+ cells through Wnt signaling." *Nat Immunol* 8(10): 1123-1131

Spiegel, A., E. Zcharia, Y. Vagima, T. Itkin, A. Kalinkovich, A. Dar, O. Kollet, N. Netzer, K. Golan, I. Shafat, N. Ilan, A. Nagler, I. Vlodavsky & T. Lapidot (2008). "Heparanase regulates retention and proliferation of primitive Sca-1+/c-Kit+/Lin- cells via modulation of the bone marrow microenvironment." *Blood* 111(10): 4934-4943

Spooncer, E., J. T. Gallagher, F. Krizsa & T. M. Dexter (1983). "Regulation of haemopoiesis in long-term bone marrow cultures. IV. Glycosaminoglycan synthesis and the stimulation of haemopoiesis by beta-D-xylosides." *J Cell Biol* 96(2): 510-514

Spranger, J., G. K. Hinkel, H. Stoss, W. Thoenes, D. Wargowski & F. Zepp (1991). "Schimke immuno-osseous dysplasia: a newly recognized multisystem disease." *J Pediatr* 119(1 (Pt 1)): 64-72

Srinivas, V. & I. M. Shapiro (2006). "Chondrocytes embedded in the epiphyseal growth plates of long bones undergo autophagy prior to the induction of osteogenesis." *Autophagy* 2(3): 215-216

Sugiyama, T., H. Kohara, M. Noda & T. Nagasawa (2006). "Maintenance of the hematopoietic stem cell pool by CXCL12-CXCR4 chemokine signaling in bone marrow stromal cell niches." *Immunity* 25(6): 977-988

Sweeney, E., M. Campbell, K. Watkins, C. A. Hunter & O. Jacenko (2008). "Altered endochondral ossification in collagen X mouse models leads to impaired immune responses." *Dev Dyn* 237(10): 2693-2704

Sweeney, E., D. Roberts, T. Corbo & O. Jacenko (2010). "Congenic mice confirm that collagen X is required for proper hematopoietic development." *PLoS One* 5(3): e9518

Taichman, R. S. & S. G. Emerson (1994). "Human osteoblasts support hematopoiesis through the production of granulocyte colony-stimulating factor." *J Exp Med* 179(5): 1677-1682

Taichman, R. S., M. J. Reilly & S. G. Emerson (1996). "Human osteoblasts support human hematopoietic progenitor cells in vitro bone marrow cultures." *Blood* 87(2): 518-524

Taichman, R. S., M. J. Reilly, R. S. Verma & S. G. Emerson (1997). "Augmented production of interleukin-6 by normal human osteoblasts in response to CD34+ hematopoietic bone marrow cells in vitro." *Blood* 89(4): 1165-1172

Tavassoli, M. (1984). "Hemopoiesis in ectopically implanted bone marrow." *Kroc Found Ser* 18: 31-54

Tavassoli, M. & W. H. Crosby (1968). "Transplantation of marrow to extramedullary sites." *Science* 161(836): 54-56

Tavassoli, M. & R. Khademi (1980). "The origin of hemopoietic cells in ectopic implants of spleen and marrow." *Experientia* 36(9): 1126-1127

Tavassoli, M., A. Maniatis & W. H. Crosby (1974). "Induction of sustained hemopoiesis in fatty marrow." *Blood* 43(1): 33-38

Tavassoli, M. & L. Weiss (1971). "The structure of developing bone marrow sinuses in extramedullary autotransplant of the marrow in rats." *Anat Rec* 171(4): 477-494

Teixido, J., M. E. Hemler, J. S. Greenberger & P. Anklesaria (1992). "Role of beta 1 and beta 2 integrins in the adhesion of human CD34hi stem cells to bone marrow stroma." *J Clin Invest* 90(2): 358-367

Tokoyoda, K., T. Egawa, T. Sugiyama, B. I. Choi & T. Nagasawa (2004). "Cellular niches controlling B lymphocyte behavior within bone marrow during development." *Immunity* 20(6): 707-718

Touw, I. & B. Lowenberg (1983). "No stimulative effect of adipocytes on hematopoiesis in long-term human bone marrow cultures." *Blood* 61(4): 770-774

Trentin, J. J. (1971). "Determination of bone marrow stem cell differentiation by stromal hemopoietic inductive microenvironments (HIM)." *Am J Pathol* 65(3): 621-628

Trinchieri, G., M. Murphy & B. Perussia (1987). "Regulation of hematopoiesis by T lymphocytes and natural killer cells." *Crit Rev Oncol Hematol* 7(3): 219-265

Verfaillie, C. M. (1993). "Soluble factor(s) produced by human bone marrow stroma increase cytokine-induced proliferation and maturation of primitive hematopoietic progenitors while preventing their terminal differentiation." *Blood* 82(7): 2045-2053

Verma, S., J. H. Rajaratnam, J. Denton, J. A. Hoyland & R. J. Byers (2002). "Adipocytic proportion of bone marrow is inversely related to bone formation in osteoporosis." *J Clin Pathol* 55(9): 693-698

Visnjic, D., I. Kalajzic, G. Gronowicz, H. L. Aguila, S. H. Clark, A. C. Lichtler & D. W. Rowe (2001). "Conditional ablation of the osteoblast lineage in Col2.3deltatk transgenic mice." *J Bone Miner Res* 16(12): 2222-2231

Visnjic, D., Z. Kalajzic, D. W. Rowe, V. Katavic, J. Lorenzo & H. L. Aguila (2004). "Hematopoiesis is severely altered in mice with an induced osteoblast deficiency." *Blood* 103(9): 3258-3264

Viviano, B. L., L. Silverstein, C. Pflederer, S. Paine-Saunders, K. Mills & S. Saunders (2005). "Altered hematopoiesis in glypican-3-deficient mice results in decreased osteoclast differentiation and a delay in endochondral ossification." *Dev Biol* 282(1): 152-162

Walkley, C. R., M. L. Fero, W. M. Chien, L. E. Purton & G. A. McArthur (2005). "Negative cell-cycle regulators cooperatively control self-renewal and differentiation of haematopoietic stem cells." *Nat Cell Biol* 7(2): 172-178

Walkley, C. R., G. H. Olsen, S. Dworkin, S. A. Fabb, J. Swann, G. A. McArthur, S. V. Westmoreland, P. Chambon, D. T. Scadden & L. E. Purton (2007). "A microenvironment-induced myeloproliferative syndrome caused by retinoic acid receptor gamma deficiency." *Cell* 129(6): 1097-1110

Walkley, C. R., J. M. Shea, N. A. Sims, L. E. Purton & S. H. Orkin (2007). "Rb regulates interactions between hematopoietic stem cells and their bone marrow microenvironment." *Cell* 129(6): 1081-1095

Wei, L., K. Kanbe, M. Lee, X. Wei, M. Pei, X. Sun, R. Terek & Q. Chen (2010). "Stimulation of chondrocyte hypertrophy by chemokine stromal cell-derived factor 1 in the chondro-osseous junction during endochondral bone formation." *Dev Biol* 341(1): 236-245

Weinstein, R., M. A. Riordan, K. Wenc, S. Kreczko, M. Zhou & N. Dainiak (1989). "Dual role of fibronectin in hematopoietic differentiation." *Blood* 73(1): 111-116

Weiss, L. (1976). "The hematopoietic microenvironment of the bone marrow: an ultrastructural study of the stroma in rats." *Anat Rec* 186(2): 161-184

Wittig, O., J. Paez-Cortez & J. Cardier (2009). "Liver Sinusoidal Endothelial Cells Promote B Lymphopoiesis from Primitive Hematopoietic Cells." *Stem Cells Dev*

Wolf, N. S. (1979). "The haemopoietic microenvironment." *Clin Haematol* 8(2): 469-500

Wolf, N. S. & J. J. Trentin (1968). "Hemopoietic colony studies. V. Effect of hemopoietic organ stroma on differentiation of pluripotent stem cells." *J Exp Med* 127(1): 205-214

Wu, J. Y., L. E. Purton, S. J. Rodda, M. Chen, L. S. Weinstein, A. P. McMahon, D. T. Scadden & H. M. Kronenberg (2008). "Osteoblastic regulation of B lymphopoiesis is mediated by Gs{alpha}-dependent signaling pathways." *Proc Natl Acad Sci U S A* 105(44): 16976-16981

Xie, Y., T. Yin, W. Wiegraebe, X. C. He, D. Miller, D. Stark, K. Perko, R. Alexander, J. Schwartz, J. C. Grindley, J. Park, J. S. Haug, J. P. Wunderlich, H. Li, S. Zhang, T.

Johnson, R. A. Feldman & L. Li (2009). "Detection of functional haematopoietic stem cell niche using real-time imaging." *Nature* 457(7225): 97-101

Yagi, K., K. Tsuji, A. Nifuji, K. Shinomiya, K. Nakashima, B. DeCrombrugghe & M. Noda (2003). "Bone morphogenetic protein-2 enhances osterix gene expression in chondrocytes." *J Cell Biochem* 88(6): 1077-1083

Yin, T. & L. Li (2006). "The stem cell niches in bone." *J Clin Invest* 116(5): 1195-1201

Yokota, T., K. Oritani, I. Takahashi, J. Ishikawa, A. Matsuyama, N. Ouchi, S. Kihara, T. Funahashi, A. J. Tenner, Y. Tomiyama & Y. Matsuzawa (2000). "Adiponectin, a new member of the family of soluble defense collagens, negatively regulates the growth of myelomonocytic progenitors and the functions of macrophages." *Blood* 96(5): 1723-1732

Yoshimoto, M., T. Shinohara, T. Heike, M. Shiota, M. Kanatsu-Shinohara & T. Nakahata (2003). "Direct visualization of transplanted hematopoietic cell reconstitution in intact mouse organs indicates the presence of a niche." *Exp Hematol* 31(8): 733-740

Youn, D. Y., D. H. Lee, M. H. Lim, J. S. Yoon, J. H. Lim, S. E. Jung, C. E. Yeum, C. W. Park, H. J. Youn, J. S. Lee, S. B. Lee, M. Ikawa, M. Okabe, Y. Tsujimoto & J. H. Lee (2008). "Bis deficiency results in early lethality with metabolic deterioration and involution of spleen and thymus." *Am J Physiol Endocrinol Metab* 295(6): E1349-1357

Zhang, C. C. & H. F. Lodish (2008). "Cytokines regulating hematopoietic stem cell function." *Curr Opin Hematol* 15(4): 307-311

Zhang, J., C. Niu, L. Ye, H. Huang, X. He, W. G. Tong, J. Ross, J. Haug, T. Johnson, J. Q. Feng, S. Harris, L. M. Wiedemann, Y. Mishina & L. Li (2003). "Identification of the haematopoietic stem cell niche and control of the niche size." *Nature* 425(6960): 836-841

Zhang, Y., A. Harada, H. Bluethmann, J. B. Wang, S. Nakao, N. Mukaida & K. Matsushima (1995). "Tumor necrosis factor (TNF) is a physiologic regulator of hematopoietic progenitor cells: increase of early hematopoietic progenitor cells in TNF receptor p55-deficient mice in vivo and potent inhibition of progenitor cell proliferation by TNF alpha in vitro." *Blood* 86(8): 2930-2937

Zhu, J., R. Garrett, Y. Jung, Y. Zhang, N. Kim, J. Wang, G. J. Joe, E. Hexner, Y. Choi, R. S. Taichman & S. G. Emerson (2007). "Osteoblasts support B-lymphocyte commitment and differentiation from hematopoietic stem cells." *Blood* 109(9): 3706-3712

Zuckerman, K. S., R. K. Rhodes, D. D. Goodrum, V. R. Patel, B. Sparks, J. Wells, M. S. Wicha & L. A. Mayo (1985). "Inhibition of collagen deposition in the extracellular matrix prevents the establishment of a stroma supportive of hematopoiesis in long-term murine bone marrow cultures." *J Clin Invest* 75(3): 970-975

Zuckerman, K. S. & M. S. Wicha (1983). "Extracellular matrix production by the adherent cells of long-term murine bone marrow cultures." *Blood* 61(3): 540-547

Zweegman, S., J. Van Den Born, A. M. Mus, F. L. Kessler, J. J. Janssen, T. Netelenbos, P. C. Huijgens & A. M. Drager (2004). "Bone marrow stromal proteoglycans regulate megakaryocytic differentiation of human progenitor cells." *Exp Cell Res* 299(2): 383-392

9

Molecular Mechanisms Underlying Bone Marrow Homing of Hematopoietic Stem Cells

Aysegul Ocal Sahin and Miranda Buitenhuis
Department of Hematology and Erasmus MC Stem Cell Institute for
Regenerative Medicine, Erasmus MC, Rotterdam,
The Netherlands

1. Introduction

The formation of blood cells, also called hematopoiesis, is a complex process that occurs in the bone marrow and depends on correct regulation of hematopoietic cell fate decisions. Aberrant regulation of hematopoiesis can result in the development of severe malignant and non-malignant hematological disorders, including leukemia. Hematopoietic stem cell transplantation is the most powerful treatment modality for a large number of those malignancies. Successful hematopoietic recovery after transplantation depends on homing of hematopoietic stem cells to the bone marrow and subsequent lodging of those cells in the bone marrow microenvironment.

Homing is a rapid, coordinated process in which circulating hematopoietic stem and progenitor cells actively enter the bone marrow within a few hours after transplantation (Figure 1). Rolling and firm adhesion of those cells to endothelial cells in small marrow sinusoids is followed by trans-endothelial migration across the endothelium/extracellular matrix barrier. Finally, in irradiated recipients, hematopoietic stem cells anchor to their specialized niches within the bone marrow compartment near osteoblasts and initiate long-term repopulation (Lo Celso et al., 2009). In absence of available niches in, for example, non-irradiated recipients, HSCs tend to be more randomly distributed throughout the bone marrow (Lo Celso et al., 2009). Since the first bone marrow transplantation decades ago, research has focused on understanding the mechanisms underlying homing of hematopoietic stem cells to the bone marrow. This chapter will focus on recent studies that have extended our understanding of the molecular mechanisms underlying adhesion, migration and bone marrow homing of hematopoietic stem cells.

2. Selectins and bone marrow homing

A first step in the process of bone marrow homing is initial tethering and rolling of hematopoietic stem and progenitor cells along the endothelial wall of blood vessels. It has been demonstrated that selectins play an important role in bone marrow homing of hematopoietic stem and progenitor cells by regulating these processes. Intravital microscopy in bone marrow sinoids and venules of mice deficient for individual selectins revealed that rolling of hematopoietic progenitor cells involves both P and E-selectin, but not L-selectin (Mazo et al.,

1998). Similarly, coating of a surface with immobilized P- or E-Selectin was sufficient to induce rolling of human CD34+ hematopoietic progenitor cells under flow conditions (Xia et al., 2004). A next step in bone marrow homing is transendothelial migration. This process requires firm adhesion of hematopoietic stem and progenitor cells to endothelial cells. Although CD34+ hematopoietic progenitor cells are capable of binding to fluid-phase P- and E-selectin (Xia et al., 2004), in vitro adhesion to bone marrow derived endothelial cells under static conditions has been shown not to depend on E-selectin (Naiyer et al., 1999). Transwell experiments performed to study the importance of E-selectin in migration of human hematopoietic progenitor cells through a confluent layer of bone marrow derived endothelial cells, precultured with IL-1B to induce E-selectin expression, yielded contradictory results. While Naiyer et al. have demonstrated with blocking antibodies that E-selectin is important for transendothelial migration (Naiyer et al., 1999), no significant inhibition in transendothelial migration could be observed by Voermans et al. who performed similar experiments (Voermans et al., 2000). Transplantation of lethally irradiated recipient mice deficient for both P-and E-selectin with wild type bone marrow cells resulted in reduced recruitment of hematopoietic progenitors to the bone marrow and enhanced levels of circulating hematopoietic progenitors, indicating that selectins indeed play an important role in bone marrow homing (Frenette et al., 1998).

Ligands for E-selectin include the PSGL-1 glycoform CLA, CD43 and the CD44 glycoform HCELL (Dimitroff et al., 2001; Merzaban et al., 2011). These ligands are all expressed on mouse Lin-Sca-1+c-Kit+ hematopoietic stem and progenitor cells and human CD34+ hematopoietic progenitor cells (Merzaban et al., 2011). Immune precipitation experiments revealed that although E-selectin can bind to CLA and CD43 in both mouse and human cells, the interaction between E-selectin and CD44 only occurs in human cells (Merzaban et al., 2011). These studies indicate that the molecular mechanism underlying bone marrow homing may be different for mouse and human hematopoietic stem cells. This hypothesis was confirmed by the observation that human CD34+ hematopoietic progenitor cells exhibit a stronger E-selectin binding capacity compared to mouse Lin-Sca-1+c-kit+ cells (Merzaban et al., 2011). In contrast to PSGL-1 which is also expressed in mature hematopoietic cells, CD44 appears to be predominantly expressed on primitive human CD34+ hematopoietic progenitor cells (Dimitroff et al., 2001). Rolling experiments performed under physiological flow conditions revealed that CD44 mediates E-selectin-dependent rolling interactions over a wider shear range in comparison to PSGL-1 and promotes rolling interactions on human bone marrow endothelial cells (Dimitroff et al., 2001). Silencing of CD44 expression in human cells with shRNAs was sufficient to decrease E-selectin binding under physiologic shear conditions, while enforced CD44 expression in Lin-Sca-1+c-kit+ cells conversely increased E-selectin adherence, resulting in improved bone marrow homing in vivo (Merzaban et al., 2011). In addition, treatment of mice with blocking antibodies against CD44 resulted in an increase in committed progenitors in the peripheral blood, suggesting that CD44 is important for lodging of hematopoietic progenitors in the bone marrow (Vermeulen et al., 1998). It has also been demonstrated that the selectin ligands must be alpha1-3 fucosylated to form glycan determinants such as sialyl Lewis x (sLe(x)). Inadequate alpha1-3 fucosylation of umbilical cord blood derived CD34+CD38-/low cells resulted in reduced interaction with both E-selectin and P-selectin, while increasing the level of cell-surface sLe(x) determinants augmented binding to fluid-phase P- and E-selectin, improved cell rolling on P- and E-selectin under flow and enhanced engraftment of human hematopoietic cells in bone marrows of irradiated NOD/SCID mice (Xia et al., 2004).

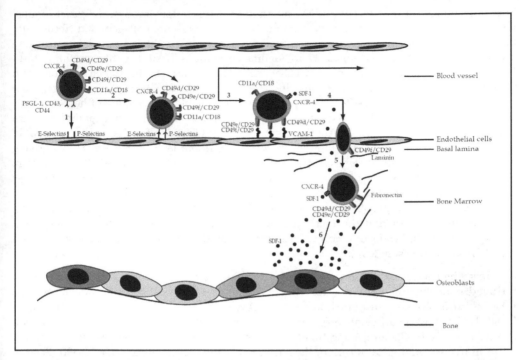

Fig. 1. Homing of hematopoietic Stem Cells to the bone marrow. 1) Initial tethering and 2) rolling are the first steps in bone marrow homing. These processes are mediated by both E- and P-selectin. 3) SDF-1 mediated integrin activation induces firm adhesion of the hematopoietic stem cells to the endothelial wall. 4) Firmly attached hematopoietic stem cells can subsequently transmigrate through the endothelial layer and 5) basal lamina, consisting of fibronectin, collagen and laminin. Integrins involved in these steps are CD49d/CD29, CD49e/CD29 and CD49f/CD29. 6) Finally, hematopoietic stem cells migrate towards the SDF-1 gradient to the osteoblasts.

3. Integrins and bone marrow homing

Integrins are, in addition to selectins, also implicated in playing an important role in regulation of bone marrow homing. Several in vitro studies with blocking antibodies have, for example, shown that both CD49d/CD29 (α4β1 or VLA-4) and CD11a/CD18 (αLβ2 or LFA-1) play an important role in adhesion of hematopoietic stem and progenitor cells to endothelial cells and subsequent transendothelial migration (Imai et al., 1999; Peled et al., 2000; Voermans et al., 2000). In addition, spontaneous migration of CD34+ hematopoietic progenitors underneath a bone marrow derived stromal cell layer, was found to be significantly inhibited by a peptide that blocks CD49d/CD29 integrin binding (Burger et al., 2003). However, adhesion of CD34+ cells to fibronectin was found to be primarily dependent on CD49e/CD29 (α5β1 or VLA-5) and not CD49d/CD29 (Peled et al., 2000). In addition, chemotaxis of peripheral blood CD34+ progenitor cells on recombinant fibronectin appears to be mediated, at least in part, by CD49e/CD29 (Carstanjen et al., 2005). The importance of both CD49d/CD29 and CD49e/CD29 in directional migration through the basal lamina, which is composed of the extracellular matrix proteins laminin, collagen, and fibronectin, has been examined utilizing a three dimensional extra cellular matrix-like gel. In contrast to the dominant role of CD49e/CD29 in facilitating static adhesion to fibronectin, SDF-1-induced directional migration of CD34+ cells was found to be dependent on both CD49d/CD29 and CD49e/CD29 integrins (Peled et al., 2000). These studies suggest that both CD49d/CD29 and CD49e/CD29 play an important role in migration of hematopoietic stem and progenitor cells in general. However, transwell migration experiments with endothelial cells from different origin showed that CD49d/CD29 is only involved in migration of hematopoietic progenitors through a confluent layer of bone marrow derived, but not human umbilical vein derived, endothelial cells (Peled et al., 2000). In addition, inhibition of CD49e/CD29 alone was not sufficient to inhibit migration through both types of endothelial cells. However, an additive effect was observed when antibodies for CD11a/CD18, CD49d/CD29 and CD49e/CD29 were mixed together (Peled et al., 2000). These results suggest that the mechanisms underlying hematopoietic stem cell migration through endothelial walls of blood vessels depends on the origin of the endothelial cells and the VCAM-1 expression level.

As described above, deletion of both P- and E-selectin in recipient mice significantly reduced bone marrow homing after transplantation of wild type HPCs. Treatment of these mice with a blocking antibody against VCAM-1, thereby prohibiting interaction with CD49d/CD29, was sufficient to further reduce bone marrow homing after transplantation (Frenette et al., 1998), suggesting that both selectins and integrins are important for optimal bone marrow homing. In addition, the capacity of cells either deficient for CD49d (Scott et al., 2003) or pretreated with CD49d antibodies (Vermeulen et al., 1998; Papayannopoulou et al., 2001; Qian et al., 2006; Carstanjen et al., 2005) to migrate to bone marrow has been shown to be impaired resulting in delayed short-term engraftment (Scott et al., 2003). Furthermore, treatment of mice with blocking antibodies against CD49d resulted in an increase in the number of committed progenitors in the peripheral blood, suggesting that CD49d is also important for lodging of hemaopoietic progenitors in the bone marrow (Vermeulen et al., 1998). Since antibodies directed against mouse CD49d can bind to both CD49d/CD29 and CD49d/ITGB7 ($\alpha 4\beta 7$), and CD49d/ITGB7 is also expressed on mouse Lin-Sca-1+c-Kit+ cells, it was hypothesized that in addition to CD49d/CD29, CD49d/ITGB7 could also be involved in bone marrow homing. Indeed, inhibition of CD49d/ITGB7or its substrate MadCam-1 significantly reduced, but not completely abrogated, bone marrow homing after transplantation (Katayama et al., 2004). In contrast, other integrins, including CD11a, appear not be involved in bone marrow homing (Vermeulen et al., 1998). Transplantation studies with hematopoietic stem cells deficient for CD18 indicated that also CD18 is not essential for bone marrow homing. However, since inhibition of CD49d/CD29 in CD18 deficient hematopoietic stem cells resulted in more dramatic reduction in bone marrow homing in comparison to inhibition of CD49d/CD29 in wild type mice, it was suggested that CD18 can contribute to bone marrow homing when the function of CD49d/CD29 is compromised (Papayannopoulou et al., 2001). In addition to CD49d, CD49e/CD29 has also been implicated in playing a role in regulation of bone marrow homing. Treatment of hematopoietic progenitors with an antibody directed against CD49e/CD29 was sufficient to partially reduce homing of those cells to the bone marrow but not to the spleen (Wierenga et al., 2006; Carstanjen et al., 2005). Another integrin implicated in regulation of bone marrow homing is CD49f (α6). In contrast to CD49d that appears to primarily be involved in bone marrow homing of short-term repopulating hematopoietic stem cells, CD49f is thought to be important for homing of both short-term and long-term stem cells (Qian et al., 2006). In contrast, similar experiments with fetal liver cells revealed that, in contrast to CD49d which appeared to be important for homing of both hematopoietic stem and progenitor cells, CD49f is only important for homing of hematopoietic progenitors but not stem cells (Qian et al., 2007). These studies indicate that CD49d and Cd49f play differential roles during homing of cord blood and fetal liver derived hematopoietic stem and progenitor cells (Qian et al., 2007). In contrast, bone marrow homing was not affected in a more recent study in which also mouse bone marrow derived hematopoietic stem and progenitor cells pretreated with blocking antibodies directed against CD49f were transplanted in recipient mice (Bonig et al., 2009). In addition, blocking CD49f in human and primate bone marrow derived hematopoietic stem and progenitor cells, but not mobilized peripheral blood or cord blood derived cells that express little or no CD49f, resulted in enhanced bone marrow homing in a xenogeneic transplant model and significantly improved engraftment levels (Bonig et al., 2009). Finally, intravenous injection of anti-CD49f antibodies, in contrast to antibodies against CD49d integrin, did not mobilize progenitors or enhance cytokine-induced mobilization by G-CSF, suggesting that CD49f is not essential for lodging of hematopoietic stem and progenitor cells in the bone marrow (Qian et al., 2006). Additional research is required to investigate whether or not CD49f regulates bone marrow homing.

4. Chemoattractants involved in migration of hematopoietic stem cells

Chemoattractants play an important role in directing migration of hematopoietic stem and progenitor cells to the bone marrow. Several studies have demonstrated that Stromal cell Derived Factor 1 (SDF-1), also known as CXC chemokine ligand 12 (CXCL12) (Tashiro et al., 1993) acts as a chemoattractant for hematopoietic stem and progenitor cells and is important for their transendothelial migration (Aiuti et al., 1997; Naiyer et al., 1999; Mohle et al., 1998; Kim & Broxmeyer, 1998; Glass et al., 2011). Further investigation, utilizing a large panel of CC and CXC chemokines, suggested that the only chemokine capable of inducing migration of murine hematopoietic stem and progenitor cells appears to be SDF-1 (Liesveld et al., 2001; Wright et al., 2002). Although the chemokine receptors CCR3 and CCR9 were also expressed at mRNA level, their ligands could not induce migration (Wright et al., 2002). Similarly, examination of a panel of chemokines and cytokines in transendothelial migration assays revealed that SDF-1 is also important for migration of human hematopoietic progenitors through a confluent layer of endothelial cells (Liesveld et al., 2001). However, to a lesser extent, also other chemokines and cytokines, including CCL2 (MCP-1), CCL5 (RANTES), CXCL10 (IP-10), IL-8 and SCF could also induce transendothelial migration (Liesveld et al., 2001). In addition, LTD4, a ligand for CysLT(1), a G protein-coupled receptor recognizing inflammatory mediator of the cysteinyl leukotriene family, which is highly expressed in hematopoietic progenitors, has been demonstrated to up-regulate CD49d/CD29 and CD49e/CD29 dependent adhesion of hematopoietic progenitors (Boehmler et al., 2009) and to induce chemotaxis and in vitro transendothelial migration (Bautz et al., 2001). Recently, a role for the proteolysis-resistant bioactive lipids sphingosine-1-phosphate and ceramide-1-phosphate in regulation of bone marrow homing has been suggested. Conditioning of mice for transplantation resulted in enhanced levels of these lipids in the bone marrow. In addition, both lipids appear to be chemoattractants for hematopoietic stem and progenitor cells (Kim et al., 2011).

The role of SDF-1 in migration of hematopoietic stem and progenitor cells will be discussed below in more detail.

4.1 SDF-1 and bone marrow homing

SDF-1 is produced by several types of bone marrow cells (Maekawa & Ishii, 2000). In the adult human bone marrow, SDF-1 was found to be expressed by endothelial cells and along the endosteum region (Peled et al., 2000; Ponomaryov et al., 2000). SDF-1 plays an important role in many processes, including immune surveillance, proliferation, differentiation and survival of many cell types (Aiuti et al., 1997; Bleul et al., 1996; Bleul et al., 1998; Cashman & Eaves, 2000; Lataillade et al., 2000). In addition, SDF-1 is considered to be essential for migration of hematopoietic stem cells to the bone marrow (Imai et al., 1999; Peled et al., 1999a; Wright et al., 2002). To date, two receptors for SDF-1 have been identified, of which CXCR4 (LESTR/fusin), a seven-transmembrane domain G-protein coupled receptor, appears to be the most prominent (Heesen et al., 1997; Loetscher et al., 1994). CXCR4 is expressed by a variety of cell types, including hematopoietic stem and progenitor cells, T lymphocytes, endothelial, stromal and neuronal cells (Nagasawa et al., 1996; Ma et al., 1998; Mohle et al., 1998; Loetscher et al., 1994). Recently, CXCR7, another SDF-1 receptor, has been identified (Tarnowski et al., 2010). However, CXCR7 is expressed at low levels in normal human CD34+ hematopoietic stem and progenitor cells and does not appear to be important for migration of those cells. In contrast, CXCR7 is highly expressed in several human myeloid leukemic cell lines and is thought to play a role in adhesion and, to a lesser extent, also in migration of those cells (Tarnowski et al., 2010).

Mouse transplantation studies have been performed to investigate the importance of SDF-1 in migration of hematopoietic stem cells to the bone marrow. Pre-treatment of human CD34+CD38-/low cells with a blocking antibody against CXCR4 has, for example, been demonstrated to be sufficient to impair their capacity to home to the bone marrow of immune deficient NOD/SCID mice or β2m deficient NOD/SCID mice (Peled et al., 1999b; Kollet et al., 2001; Kollet et al., 2002; Oberlin et al., 1996). In addition, up-regulation of CXCR4 expression by incubation with hematopoietic cytokines (SCF and IL-6) (Peled et al., 1999b) or over-expression of CXCR4 by viral transduction (Brenner et al., 2004; Kahn et al., 2004) resulted in enhanced bone marrow homing of human CD34+ and CD34+CD38- cells in NOD/SCID mice, which correlated with enhanced engraftment levels 6 weeks after transplantation (Peled et al., 1999b; Kollet et al., 2001; Kollet et al., 2002). Similarly, fetal liver hematopoietic stem and progenitor cells deficient for CXCR4 displayed a reduced bone marrow homing capacity compared to wild type cells (Ma et al., 1998). In addition to bone marrow homing, SDF-1 also appears to play a critical role in retention of hematopoietic stem cells in the hematopoietic stem cell niche. Enhancing the level of SDF-1 in plasma, but not bone marrow, utilizing adenoviral vectors (Hattori et al., 2001) or sulfated glycans (Sweeney et al., 2000; Frenette & Weiss, 2000; Sweeney et al., 2002) resulted in mobilization of CXCR4 expressing hematopoietic stem and progenitor cells (Hattori et al., 2001; Sweeney et al., 2002). Similarly, treatment of C3H/HeJ mice or healthy human volunteers with AMD3100, a selective CXCR4 antagonist, enhanced the number of HSCs and neutrophils in peripheral blood, again suggesting a role for CXCR4 and SDF-1 in HSC retention in BM (Broxmeyer et al., 2005).

4.2 Regulation of SDF-1 activity

Several proteolytic enzymes have been implicated in negatively regulating migration of hematopoietic stem cells by cleaving and inactivating SDF-1, including matrix metalloproteinases (MMP) 2/9 (Heissig et al., 2002; Sweeney et al., 2002; McQuibban et al., 2001), CD26 (Christopherson et al., 2002), carboxypeptidase M (Marquez-Curtis et al., 2008), carboxypeptidase N (Davis et al., 2005), neutrophil elastase (Petit et al., 2002; Levesque et al., 2002), cathepsin G (Petit et al., 2002; Levesque et al., 2002) and cathepsin K (Kollet et al., 2006). Cleavage of SDF-1 by several individual MMPs at Ser^4-Leu^5 bond of SDF-1 N-terminal domain has, for example, been demonstrated to result in reduced binding capacity of SDF-1 for CXCR-4 and reduced chemoattractant activity for hematopoietic stem and progenitor cells (McQuibban et al., 2001; Cho et al., 2010). Another protein involved in regulation of the activity of SDF-1 is the membrane-bound extracellular peptidase CD26 (DPPIV). It has been shown that a small number of umbilical cord blood derived CD34+CXCR4+ cells express CD26 and can therefore cleave the N-terminal part of SDF-1 at 2-proline (Christopherson et al., 2002). Functional studies showed that truncated SDF-1 lacks the ability to induce migration of CD34+ cells. In addition, inhibition of endogenous CD26 activity appears to be sufficient to enhance the migratory capacity of CD34+ cells towards SDF-1, indicating that CD26 abrogates SDF-1 induced migration of hematopoietic progenitors (Christopherson et al., 2002; Christopherson et al., 2003; Christopherson et al., 2006).

A third class of SDF-1 inhibitors includes the carboxypeptidases M and N (Marquez-Curtis et al., 2008; Davis et al., 2005). Carboxypeptidase N, which is present in human serum and plasma (Davis et al., 2005), can efficiently and specifically cleave SDF-1 at the carboxy-terminal lysine (K68) resulting in reduced SDF-1 activity and inhibition of SDF-1 mediated induction of migration of hematopoietic progenitors (Davis et al., 2005). In contrast, carboxypeptidase M is a membrane bound zinc-dependent peptidase that cleaves carboxy-terminal basic residues. This particular carboxypeptidase is expressed by stromal cells and CD34+ cells from both bone marrow and mobilized peripheral blood (Skidgel & Erdos, 1998; Marquez-Curtis et al., 2008). Carboxypeptidase M mediated cleavage of SDF-1 results in reduced chemotactic activity of hematopoietic stem and progenitor cells, which can be rescued by addition of the carboxypeptidase inhibitor DL-2-mercaptomethyl-3-guanidino-ethylthiopropanoic acid (Marquez-Curtis et al., 2008).

Whereas high SDF-1 expression in the bone marrow is essential for normal bone marrow homing of hematopoietic stem and progenitor cells and lodging of those cells in the hematopoietic stem cell niche, during mobilization SDF-1 levels should conversely be decreased. Upon administration of G-CSF, which is used to mobilize HSPCs, an accumulation of various proteolytic enzymes including MMP-9, neutrophil elastase and cathepsin G or K (Petit et al., 2002; Levesque et al., 2002) has been observed in mouse bone marrow which correlated with a gradual decrease in SDF-1 in the bone marrow, but not circulation (Petit et al., 2002). In addition, also an enhanced SDF-1 plasma level was shown to result in up-regulation of MPP-9 in bone marrow cells and mobilization of hematopoietic stem and progenitor cells (Heissig et al., 2002). The importance of MPP-9 for mobilization of hematopoietic stem cells was demonstrated utilizing MMP-9 deficient mice. A high SDF-1 level in plasma was not sufficient to induce mobilization of hematopoietic progenitors in these mice (Heissig et al., 2002). In addition, in primary myelofibrosis, which is a chronic myeloproliferative neoplasm characterized by constitutive mobilization of hematopoietic stem and progenitor cells into the peripheral blood (Migliaccio et al., 2008), both a high level of truncated SDF-1 and enhanced levels of proteases, including dipeptidyl peptidase-IV (CD26), neutrophil elastase, matrix metalloproteinase-2 (MMP-2), MMP-9, and cathepsin G have been observed (Cho et al., 2010). Taken together, these studies demonstrated that SDF-1 plays an important role in integrin-mediated firm arrest of human HSPCs, facilitate their transendothelial migration, and regulate bone marrow homing and retention of HSPCs in the hematopoietic stem cell niche.

4.3 Molecular mechanisms underlying SDF-1 mediated regulation of migration

To understand the molecular mechanism underlying migration of hematopoietic stem and progenitor cells, research has focused on identifying the downstream effectors of SDF-1 and CXCR4. SDF-1 has been demonstrated to induce the activity of the integrins CD11a/CD18 (Peled et al., 2000) and CD49/CD29 (Hidalgo et al., 2001; Peled et al., 2000) on CD34+ cells which allows interaction with their substrates ICAM-1 and VCAM-1, respectively.

Small guanosine triphosphatases (GTPases) that belong to the Ras superfamily of GTPases , including Rho, Rac and Cdc42, have been demonstrated to be involved in SDF-1 mediated homing and migration of hematopoietic stem and progenitor cells (Fuhler et al., 2008; del Pozo et al., 1999). The activity of Rho GTPases can be induced by tyrosine kinase receptors (Taylor & Metcalfe, 2000; Timokhina et al., 1998), integrin receptors (del Pozo et al., 2004) and chemokine receptors including SDF-1 (Cancelas et al., 2005; del Pozo et al., 1999; Fuhler et al., 2008; Shirvaikar et al., 2011). It has been demonstrated in *in vitro* assays that SDF-1 induced chemo-attraction is mediated, at least in part, by Rac (del Pozo et al., 1999; Shirvaikar et al., 2011; Wysoczynski et al., 2005). In addition, analysis of Rac2 deficient mice revealed that Rac2 is essential for lodging of HSPCs in the bone marrow. Deletion of Rac2 resulted, for example, in reduced adhesion and enhanced mobilization of hematopoietic stem cells to the circulation. Furthermore, Rac2 deficiency resulted in enhanced SDF-1 induced migration of hematopoietic stem and progenitor cells (Yang et al., 2001). An enhanced activation of Cdc42 and Rac1 was observed in these cells, suggesting a compensatory role of Cdc42 and Rac1 with regard to migration, but not adhesion (Yang et al., 2001). In addition, it was shown that SDF-1 mediated Rac activation is impaired in CD34+ cells from MDS patients. CD34+ cell from patients with myelodysplastic syndrome exhibit reduced F-actin polymerization and migration towards SDF-1 compared to normal CD34+ cells (Fuhler et al., 2008). While pharmacological inhibition of Rac1 activity in a human myeloblastic cell line (HL-60) with NSC23766 was sufficient to abrogate SDF-1 induced actin assembly and migration, over-expression of active Rac in HL-60 cells conversely restored both F-actin polymerization and migration, suggesting that Rac is essential for SDF-1–induced migration in these cells (Fuhler et al., 2008). Although over-expression of active Rac in CD34+ cells from patients with myelodysplastic syndrome resulted in increased F-actin polymerization and enhanced motility, directional migration toward SDF-1 was not improved (Fuhler et al., 2008). These studies suggest that SDF-1 mediated induction of Rac activity is important for migration of both normal and malignant hematopoietic progenitors (Fuhler et al., 2008). The role of the hematopoietic-specific guanine nucleotide exchange factor Vav1, which is an upstream regulator of Rac activity, in localization and engraftment of hematopoietic stem and progenitor cells has also been investigated. Deletion of Vav1 in hematopoietic stem cells has been demonstrated to result in impaired responses to SDF1α, dysregulated Rac/Cdc42 activation and a reduction of in vitro migration. In addition, intravital microscopy assays revealed that transplantation of Vav1 deficient hematopoietic stem and progenitor cells results in impaired early localization near nestin(+) perivascular mesenchymal stem cells after transplantation (Sanchez-Aguilera et al., 2011). Recently, another upstream regulator of Rac activity has been identified. In contrast to Rac, the activity of R-Ras, a member of the Ras family, is inhibited upon SDF-1 stimulation. Deletion of R-Ras resulted in enhanced levels of Rac1/2 activity, while expression of a constitutively active R-Ras mutant resulted in down-regulation of Rac1-activity. Deletion of R-Ras in hematopoietic stem and progenitor cells resulted in increased directional migration. This phenotype could be reversed by inhibition of Rac. Furthermore, R-Ras deficient mice showed enhanced responsiveness to G-CSF for progenitor cell mobilization and exhibited decreased bone marrow homing (Sanchez-Aguilera et al., 2011).

Another important mediator of hematopoietic progenitor cell migration is the GTPase Rho (Bug et al., 2002; Ghiaur et al., 2006; Gottig et al., 2006). It has been demonstrated that SDF-1 mediated release of intracellular Ca^{2+} stores requires activation of Rho GTPases, but not Rac or Cdc42 (Henschler et al., 2003). Depletion of intracellular Ca^{2+} resulted in reduced SDF-1 induced migration and bone marrow homing of hematopoietic progenitors (Henschler et al., 2003). In addition, over-expresssion of dominant negative RhoA by retroviral transduction in mouse cells (C57BL/6J mice) resulted in decreased migration of hematopoietic progenitor cells towards SDF-1 and reduced integrin-mediated adhesion (Henschler et al., 2003). Furthermore, over-expression of RhoH, a GTPase deficient type of Rho (Sahai & Marshall, 2002), in hematopoietic stem and progenitor cells resulted in impaired activation of Rac GTPases, defective actin polymerization and impaired chemotaxis. In contrast, inhibition of RhoH expression in these cells conversely stimulated SDF-1–induced migration in vitro (Gu et al., 2005). In addition, it has been demonstrated that Epac1, a nucleotide exchange protein for the GTPase Rap1, which is directly activated by cAMP, can also improve the adhesive and migratory capacity CD34+ hematopoietic progenitor cells (Carmona et al., 2008), suggesting that Rap1 may also play a role in bone marrow homing.

Endolyn (CD164), a type I integral transmembrane silomucin (Chan et al., 2001; Zannettino et al., 1998), which is recruited to CXCR4 upon SDF-1 slimulation (Forde et al., 2007) was shown to play an important role in SDF-1 mediated migration of human CD133+ hematopoietic stem and progenitor cells (Forde et al., 2007). Inhibition of CD164 in CD133+ cells with 103B2, a specific mAb, resulted in a reduction of migration towards SDF-1, but not CCL1, CCL5, CCL17, CCL19, CCL20, CCL21, CCL22 and CXCL3. A similar inhibition in SDF-1 mediated migration of CD133+ cells was observed after siRNA mediated knock-down of CD164 (Forde et al., 2007). Knock-down of CD164 resulted in a significant reduction in SDF-1 mediated activation of PI3K and PKCζ (Forde et al., 2007). Both PI3K and PKCζ have been implicated in playing an important role in SDF-1 mediated migration of CD34$^+$ cells. Inhibition of PKCζ, for example, reduced SDF-1 induced migration of CD34+ cells and reduced engraftment levels after transplantation (Petit et al., 2005). Furthermore, injection of inhibitory PKCζ pseudosubstrate peptides resulted in mobilization of murine progenitors to the circulation, suggesting an important role for PKCζin SDF-1-dependent regulation of hematopoietic stem and progenitor cell motility and localization (Petit et al., 2005) The role of PI3K in regulation of bone marrow homing will be discussed in the next section.

In addition to regulating the activity of downstream effectors, SDF-1 has also been demonstrated to regulate the expression of specific target genes. Stimulation of peripheral blood mononuclear, Jurkat or HeLa cells has, for example, been demonstrated to result in a rapid increase in expression of the ubiquitin-specific protease 17 (USP17) (de la Vega et al., 2011). A role for this protease in regulation of migration of hematopoietic progenitor cells has been examined in vitro. Inhibition of USP17 in these cells showed decreased chemotaxis towards SDF-1, whereas over-expression of USP17 conversely resulted in increased chemotaxis. Interestingly, CXCR4 levels were not affected by inhibition or over-expression of USP17, suggesting that USP17 modulates the down-stream signaling of the CXCR4 receptor. shRNA mediated inhibition of USP17 expression resulted in decreased polymerization of actin and tubulin and reduced membrane ruffling. In addition, upon SDF-1 stimulation, the GTPases, RAC1, Cdc42 and RhoA were not transported to the plasma membrane, thereby prohibiting their activiation (de la Vega et al., 2011). In addition, CD9, a member of the tetraspanin superfamily (Boucheix et al., 1991) that is widely expressed in hematopoietic and non-hematopoietic cells, has been shown to be a SDF-1 responsive gene. Microarray analysis with human umbilical cord blood derived CD34+ cells revealed that short-term exposure to SDF-1 resulted in up-regulation of CD9 mRNA expression both in CD34$^+$ CD38$^+$ and CD34$^+$ CD38$^{-/low}$ cells (Leung et al., 2011). A role for CD9 in migration and adhesion of human cord blood derived hematopoietic stem and progenitor cells was investigated utilizing a neutralizing CD9 antibody (Leung et al., 2011). Although actin polymerization was not affected, the calcium influx and transendothelial migration towards a SDF-1 gradient was reduced by this antibody (Leung et al., 2011). In contrast, adhesion of progenitor cells to fibronectin and human umbilical vein endothelial cells was enhanced (Leung et al., 2011). Transplantation experiments revealed that in NOD/SCID mice, pre-treatment of human CD34+ cells with a neutralizing CD9 antibody resulted in inhibition of homing to bone marrow and spleen. However, enhanced CD9 expression in CD34+ cells with ingenol 3,20-dibenzoate (IDB), a protein kinase C agonist which was shown to induce CD9 expression in CD34+ cells, did not result in enhanced bone marrow homing (Desmond et al., 2011).

5. The PI3K/PKB signalling module and bone marrow homing

Correct regulation of the Phosphatidylinositol-3-Kinase (PI3K) / Protein Kinase B (PKB/c-Akt) signaling module is essential for multiple processes during hematopoiesis. Phosphatidylinositol 4,5 bisphosphate (PI(4,5)P$_2$, the most important substrate for PI3K, can be phosphorylated upon extracellular stimulation, resulting in the formation of phosphatidylinositol 3,4,5 trisphosphate (PI(3,4,5)P$_3$) (Hawkins et al., 2006). PI(3,4,5)P$_3$ subsequently serves as an anchor for pleckstrin homology (PH) domain-containing proteins, such as Protein Kinase B (PKB/ c-akt) (Burgering & Coffer, 1995). Activation of PI3K and its downstream effector Protein Kinase B (PKB/c-Akt) has been observed in leukemic cell lines stimulated with SDF-1 (Ganju et al., 1998). A positive role for PI3K/PKB in regulation of SDF-1 induced migration of hematopoietic stem cells was therefore suggested. However, it has been shown that Protein Phosphatase 2A plays an important role in positively regulating SDF-1 mediated migration of human hematopoietic progenitors by inhibition of PKB activity (Basu et al., 2007). Similarly, inhibition of PKB activity in CD34$^+$ cells for over 24 hours appears to be sufficient to reduce their adhesion to bone marrow derived stromal cells and to induce their basal migratory capacity (Buitenhuis et al., 2010). Transwell migration experiments through a confluent layer of human umbilical vein endothelial cells revealed that the observed reduction in firm adhesion does not ameliorate the induced migratory capacity of CD34+ cells pre-treated with a PKB inhibitor (Buitenhuis et al., 2010). In addition, ectopic expression of constitutively active PKB in CD34+ cells conversely induced firm adhesion and reduced the basal level of migration. Although it cannot be excluded that transient activation of PI3K/PKB activity by SDF-1 is important for induction of migration, these studies suggest that prolonged activation of PKB activity is detrimental for migration of CD34+ cells. The role of PI3K in regulation of bone marrow homing was initially examined utilizing mice deficient for SHIP (SH2-containing inositol-5'-phosphatase), a negative regulator of PI3K (Damen et al., 1996). Transplantation of lethally irradiated recipients with HSCs from SHIP deficient mice resulted in diminished repopulation, suggesting that constitutive activation of PI3K impairs the ability of HSCs to home to and to be retained in the hematopoietic stem cell niche in the bone marrow. Assessment of bone marrow homing revealed that SHIP-/- hematopoietic stem and progenitor cells indeed traffic to the bone marrow and spleen with significantly reduced efficiency compared to wild type cells. Although it is evident that constitutive activation of PI3K plays a critical role in regulation of hematopoiesis per se (Buitenhuis et al., 2008), these results indicate that the inability of SHIP deficient hematopoietic stem cells to engraft and sustain long-term hematopoiesis can be, at least partially, explained by their impaired ability to home to the bone marrow (Desponts et al., 2006). Deletion of Phosphate and tensin homologue (PTEN), another critical negative regulator of PI3K signaling that dephosphorylates $PI(3,4,5)P_3$ resulting in the formation of $PI(4,5)P_2$ (Maehama & Dixon, 1998) only decreased bone marrow homing when PTEN deficient HSCs were transplanted into non-irradiated recipients. These results suggest that, although PTEN deficient hematopoietic stem cells are capable of migrating to the bone marrow, their performance is reduced compared to competeting wild-type hematopoietic stem cells when vacant niches are limited (Zhang et al., 2006). Although both PTEN and SHIP act on the main product of PI3K activity, $PI(3,4,5)P_3$, the products generated are distinct, which could explain the differences between SHIP and PTEN deficient hematopoietic stem cells in terms of bone marrow homing (Dowler et al., 2000; Golub & Caroni, 2005). Recent findings demonstrated that, similar to deletion of SHIP, constitutive activation of PKB in human hematopoietic progenitors cells is sufficient to significantly inhibit homing of these cells to the bone marrow and spleen of β2 microglobulin -/- NOD/SCID mice (Buitenhuis et al., 2010). In contrast, although transplantation of C57 BL/6 mice with bone marrow cells from 5-fluorouracil treated mice that ectopically expressed constitutively active PKB resulted in reduced engraftment levels, bone marrow homing was only modestly impaired 18 hours after transplantation (Kharas et al., 2010). To investigate whether inhibition of PKB activity would be sufficient to conversely improve bone marrow homing, human hematopoietic progenitor cells, pre-treated with a PKB inhibitor for 24 or 48 hours, were injected into recipient mice. Flow cytometric analysis, 22 hours after transplantation, revealed that transient inhibition of PKB activity prior to transplantation is sufficient to improve bone marrow homing (Buitenhuis et al., 2010). In addition, while constitutive activation of PKB appears to be detrimental for bone marrow homing, engraftment levels and hematopoietic recovery, inhibition of PKB activity prior to transplantation, resulting in an induction of bone marrow homing, conversely enhanced engraftment levels in recipient mice. Together, these studies demonstrated that correct regulation of PI3K/PKB is essential for migration of hematopoietic stem and progenitor cells to the bone marrow after transplantation, which is essential for optimal engraftment and hematopoietic recovery (Buitenhuis et al., 2010; Desponts et al., 2006; Kharas et al., 2010).

The molecular mechanisms underlying PKB mediated regulation of migration and bone marrow homing are, thus far, incompletely understood. Although PKB mediated inhibition of migration has been demonstrated to involve RAC1 (Farooqui et al., 2006), NFAT (Yiu & Toker, 2006; Yoeli-Lerner et al., 2005) and p27Kip1 (Baldassarre et al., 2005; Viglietto et al., 2002; Wu et al., 2006) in non-hematopoietic cell lines, their importance for migration of hematopoietic stem and progenitor cells remains to be investigated. As described above, adhesion and migration of HSCs depend on correct integrin and selectin expression and regulation of integrin activity. PKB and its downstream effector GSK-3 have initially been shown to play an important role in recycling of the CD49e/CD29 and CD51/CD61 ($\alpha v \beta 3$) integrins to the membrane in NIH 3T3 fibroblasts, resulting in enhanced cell spreading and adhesion (Roberts et al., 2004). Ectopic expression of PKB in human hematopoietic stem and progenitor cells has been demonstrated to enhance the level of CD49d, while inhibition of PKB activity conversely reduces expression of both CD49d and CD18 (Buitenhuis et al., 2010), providing a potential mechanism by which PKB induces adhesion and inhibits migration. Although it is evident that integrins play an important role in adhesion and migration of cells, the importance of these molecules in PKB mediated inhibition of migration remains to be investigated. In addition, CXCR4 expression has been demonstrated to be reduced in SHIP deficient hematopoietic stem cells, suggesting that activation of PI3K also impairs their response to SDF-1(Zhang et al., 2006).

6. Conclusion

Allogeneic HSC transplantation is the preferred treatment modality for a number of hematological malignancies. To allow normal long-term hematopoiesis to occur after transplantation, correct regulation of homing of hematopoietic stem and progenitor cells to the bone marrow and subsequent lodging of those cells into the hematopoietic stem cell niche is essential. As described above, this is a coordinated multistep process that is regulated by chemokines, integrins and selectins. Initial tethering and rolling of hematopoietic stem and progenitor cells along the endothelial wall of blood vessels are the first steps in this process. It has been demonstrated that both P and E-selectin play an important role in rolling of HSCs. In addition to selectins, integrins are also implicated in playing an important role in regulation of bone marrow homing. Both studies with blocking antibodies and knockout mice have revealed that CD49d/CD29, CD49e/CD29, CD49f, and CD49d/ITGB7 play an important role in adhesion of hematopoietic stem and progenitor cells to endothelial cells and subsequent transendothelial migration. In addition, both CD49d/CD29 and CD49e/CD29 integrins appear to be involved in mediation of SDF-1–induced directional migration of CD34+ cells through the basal lamina. In addition, although, under normal circumstances, CD18 appears not to be essential for bone marrow homing of hematopoietic stem cells, CD18 can contribute to bone marrow homing when the function of CD49d/CD29 is compromised. Although multiple chemokines are capable of inducing transendothelial migration of hematopoietic stem cells, the chemokine SDF-1 appears to be the most prominent chemokine involved in bone marrow homing. In addition, SDF-1 also appears to play a critical role in retention of hematopoietic stem cells in the hematopoietic stem cell niche. Regulation of SDF-1 activity by a variety of proteolytic enzymes has been demonstrated to play an important role in migration of hematopoietic stem cells to and from the bone marrow. The molecular mechanism underlying SDF-1 mediated regulation of HSC migration has been investigated extensively. Thus far, multiple downstream effectors have been identified, including CD164, the GTPases Rac, Rho, and Cdc42, and the signalling molecules PI3K and PKCζ. In addition, the SDF-1 responsive genes CD9, USP17, both implicated in regulation of hematopoietic stem cell migration, have been indentified. Finally, SDF-1 has been demonstrated to induce the activity of integrins which allows interaction with their substrates. Although activation of PI3K and its downstream effector Protein Kinase B (PKB/c-Akt) has been observed in leukemic cell lines stimulated with SDF-1, suggesting a positive role for PI3K/PKB in regulation of SDF-1 induced migration of hematopoietic stem cells, the above described studies clearly implicate the PI3K/PKB signalling module in playing a critical role in negatively regulating migration of HSCs and bone marrow homing.

7. References

Aiuti A, Webb IJ, et al. (1997). The chemokine SDF-1 is a chemoattractant for human CD34+ hematopoietic progenitor cells and provides a new mechanism to explain the mobilization of CD34+ progenitors to peripheral blood *Journal of Experimental Medicine*, Vol. 185, No. 1, pp. 111-20, 0022-1007

Baldassarre G, Belletti B, et al. (2005). p27(Kip1)-stathmin interaction influences sarcoma cell migration and invasion *Cancer Cell*, Vol. 7, No. 1, pp. 51-63, ISSN 1535-6108.

Basu S, Ray NT, et al. (2007). Protein phosphatase 2A plays an important role in stromal cell-derived factor-1/CXC chemokine ligand 12-mediated migration and adhesion of CD34+ cells *Journal of Immunology*, Vol. 179, No. 5, pp. 3075-85, ISSN 0022-1767.

Bautz F, Denzlinger C, et al. (2001). Chemotaxis and transendothelial migration of CD34(+) hematopoietic progenitor cells induced by the inflammatory mediator leukotriene D4 are mediated by the 7-transmembrane receptor CysLT1 *Blood*, Vol. 97, No. 11, pp. 3433-40, ISSN 0006-4971.

Bleul CC, Fuhlbrigge RC, et al. (1996). A highly efficacious lymphocyte chemoattractant, stromal cell-derived factor 1 (SDF-1) *Journal of Experimental Medicine*, Vol. 184, No. 3, pp. 1101-9, ISSN 0022-1007.

Bleul CC, Schultze JL, et al. (1998). B lymphocyte chemotaxis regulated in association with microanatomic localization, differentiation state, and B cell receptor engagement *Journal of Experimental Medicine*, Vol. 187, No. 5, pp. 753-62, ISSN 0022-1007.

Boehmler AM, Drost A, et al. (2009). The CysLT1 ligand leukotriene D4 supports alpha4beta1- and alpha5beta1-mediated adhesion and proliferation of CD34+ hematopoietic progenitor cells *Journal of Immunology*, Vol. 182,No. 11, pp. 6789-98, ISSN 1550-6606.

Bonig H, Priestley GV, et al. (2009). Blockade of alpha6-integrin reveals diversity in homing patterns among human, baboon, and murine cells *Stem Cells Develoment*, Vol. 18, No. 6, pp. 839-44, ISSN 1557-8534.

Boucheix C, Benoit P, et al. (1991). Molecular cloning of the CD9 antigen. A new family of cell surface proteins *Journal of Biological Chemistry*, Vol. 266, No. 1, pp. 117-22, ISSN 0021-9258.

Brenner S, Whiting-Theobald N, et al. (2004). CXCR4-transgene expression significantly improves marrow engraftment of cultured hematopoietic stem cells *Stem Cells*, Vol. 22, No. 7, pp. 1128-33, ISSN 1066-5099.

Broxmeyer HE, Orschell CM, et al. (2005). Rapid mobilization of murine and human hematopoietic stem and progenitor cells with AMD3100, a CXCR4 antagonist *Journal of Experimental Medicine*, Vol. 201, No. 8, pp. 1307-18, ISSN 0022-1007.

Bug G, Rossmanith T, et al. (2002). Rho family small GTPases control migration of hematopoietic progenitor cells into multicellular spheroids of bone marrow stroma cells *Journal of Leukocyte Biology*, Vol. 72, No. 4, pp. 837-45, ISSN 0741-5400.

Buitenhuis M, van der Linden E, et al. (2010). Protein kinase B (PKB/c-akt) regulates homing of hematopoietic progenitors through modulation of their adhesive and migratory properties *Blood*, Vol. 116, No. 13, pp. 2373-84, ISSN 1528-0020.

Buitenhuis M, Verhagen LP, et al. (2008). Protein kinase B (c-akt) regulates hematopoietic lineage choice decisions during myelopoiesis *Blood*, Vol. 111, No. 1, pp. 112-21, ISSN 0006-4971.

Burger JA, Spoo A, et al. (2003). CXCR4 chemokine receptors (CD184) and alpha4beta1 integrins mediate spontaneous migration of human CD34+ progenitors and acute myeloid leukaemia cells beneath marrow stromal cells (pseudoemperipolesis) *British Journal of Haematology*, Vol. 122, No. 4, pp. 579-89, ISSN 0007-1048.

Burgering BM and Coffer PJ. (1995). Protein kinase B (c-Akt) in phosphatidylinositol-3-OH kinase signal transduction *Nature*, Vol. 376, No. 6541, pp. 599-602, ISSN 0028-0836.

Cancelas JA, Lee AW, et al. (2005). Rac GTPases differentially integrate signals regulating hematopoietic stem cell localization *Nature Medicine*, Vol. 11, No. 8, pp. 886-91, ISSN 1078-8956.

Carmona G, Chavakis E, et al. (2008). Activation of Epac stimulates integrin-dependent homing of progenitor cells *Blood*, Vol. 111, No. 5, pp. 2640-6, ISSN 0006-4971.

Carstanjen D, Gross A, et al. (2005). The alpha4beta1 and alpha5beta1 integrins mediate engraftment of granulocyte-colony-stimulating factor-mobilized human hematopoietic progenitor cells *Transfusion*, Vol. 45, No. 7, pp. 1192-200, ISSN 0041-1132.

Cashman JD and Eaves CJ. (2000). High marrow seeding efficiency of human lymphomyeloid repopulating cells in irradiated NOD/SCID mice *Blood*, Vol. 96, No. 12, pp. 3979-81, ISSN 0006-4971.

Chan JY, Lee-Prudhoe JE, et al. (2001). Relationship between novel isoforms, functionally important domains, and subcellular distribution of CD164/endolyn *Journal of Biological Chemistry*, Vol. 276, No. 3, pp. 2139-52, ISSN 0021-9258.

Cho SY, Xu M, et al. (2010). The effect of CXCL12 processing on CD34+ cell migration in myeloproliferative neoplasms *Cancer Research*, Vol. 70, No. 8, pp. 3402-10, ISSN 1538-7445.

Christopherson KW, 2nd, Cooper S, et al. (2003). Cell surface peptidase CD26/DPPIV mediates G-CSF mobilization of mouse progenitor cells *Blood*, Vol. 101, No. 12, pp. 4680-6, ISSN 0006-4971.

Christopherson KW, 2nd, Hangoc G, et al. (2002). Cell surface peptidase CD26/dipeptidylpeptidase IV regulates CXCL12/stromal cell-derived factor-1 alpha-mediated chemotaxis of human cord blood CD34+ progenitor cells *Journal of Immunology*, Vol. 169, No. 12, pp. 7000-8, ISSN 0022-1767.

Christopherson KW, 2nd, Uralil SE, et al. (2006). G-CSF- and GM-CSF-induced upregulation of CD26 peptidase downregulates the functional chemotactic response of

CD34+CD38- human cord blood hematopoietic cells *Experimental Hematology*, Vol. 34, No. 8, pp. 1060-8, ISSN 0301-472X.

Damen JE, Liu L, et al. (1996). The 145-kDa protein induced to associate with Shc by multiple cytokines is an inositol tetraphosphate and phosphatidylinositol 3,4,5-triphosphate 5-phosphatase *Procedures National Academy Sciencies U S A*, Vol. 93, No. 4, pp. 1689-93, ISSN 0027-8424.

Davis DA, Singer KE, et al. (2005). Identification of carboxypeptidase N as an enzyme responsible for C-terminal cleavage of stromal cell-derived factor-1alpha in the circulation *Blood*, Vol. 105, No. 12, pp. 4561-8, ISSN 0006-4971.

de la Vega M, Kelvin AA, et al. (2011). The deubiquitinating enzyme USP17 is essential for GTPase subcellular localization and cell motility *Nature Communications*, Vol. 2, pp. 259, ISSN 2041-1723.

del Pozo MA, Alderson NB, et al. (2004). Integrins regulate Rac targeting by internalization of membrane domains *Science*, Vol. 303, No. 5659, pp. 839-42, ISSN 1095-9203.

del Pozo MA, Vicente-Manzanares M, et al. (1999). Rho GTPases control migration and polarization of adhesion molecules and cytoskeletal ERM components in T lymphocytes *European Journal of Immunology*, Vol. 29, No. 11, pp. 3609-20, ISSN 0014-2980.

Desmond R, Dunfee A, et al. (2011). CD9 up-regulation on CD34+ cells with ingenol 3,20-dibenzoate does not improve homing in NSG mice *Blood*, Vol. 117, No. 21, pp. 5774-6, ISSN 1528-0020.

Desponts C, Hazen AL, et al. (2006). SHIP deficiency enhances HSC proliferation and survival but compromises homing and repopulation *Blood*, Vol. 107, No. 11, pp. 4338-45, ISSN 0006-4971.

Dimitroff CJ, Lee JY, et al. (2001). CD44 is a major E-selectin ligand on human hematopoietic progenitor cells *Journal of Cell Biology*, Vol. 153, No. 6, pp. 1277-86, ISSN 0021-9525.

Dowler S, Currie RA, et al. (2000). Identification of pleckstrin-homology-domain-containing proteins with novel phosphoinositide-binding specificities *Biochemical Journal*, Vol. 351, No. Pt 1, pp. 19-31, ISSN 0264-6021.

Farooqui R, Zhu S, et al. (2006). Glycogen synthase kinase-3 acts upstream of ADP-ribosylation factor 6 and Rac1 to regulate epithelial cell migration *Experimental Cell Research*, Vol. 312, No. 9, pp. 1514-25, ISSN 0014-4827.

Forde S, Tye BJ, et al. (2007). Endolyn (CD164) modulates the CXCL12-mediated migration of umbilical cord blood CD133+ cells *Blood*, Vol. 109, No. 5, pp. 1825-33, ISSN 0006-4971.

Frenette PS, Subbarao S, et al. (1998). Endothelial selectins and vascular cell adhesion molecule-1 promote hematopoietic progenitor homing to bone marrow *Procedures National Academy Sciences U S A*, Vol. 95, No. 24, pp. 14423-8, ISSN 0027-8424.

Frenette PS and Weiss L. (2000). Sulfated glycans induce rapid hematopoietic progenitor cell mobilization: evidence for selectin-dependent and independent mechanisms *Blood*, Vol. 96, No. 7, pp. 2460-8, ISSN 0006-4971.

Fuhler GM, Drayer AL, et al. (2008). Reduced activation of protein kinase B, Rac, and F-actin polymerization contributes to an impairment of stromal cell derived factor-1 induced migration of CD34+ cells from patients with myelodysplasia *Blood*, Vol. 111, No. 1, pp. 359-68, ISSN 0006-4971.

Ganju RK, Brubaker SA, et al. (1998). The alpha-chemokine, stromal cell-derived factor-1alpha, binds to the transmembrane G-protein-coupled CXCR-4 receptor and activates multiple signal transduction pathways *Journal of Biological Chemistry*, Vol. 273, No. 36, pp. 23169-75, ISSN 0021-9258.

Ghiaur G, Lee A, et al. (2006). Inhibition of RhoA GTPase activity enhances hematopoietic stem and progenitor cell proliferation and engraftment *Blood*, Vol. 108, No. 6, pp. 2087-94, ISSN 0006-4971.

Glass TJ, Lund TC, et al. (2011). Stromal cell-derived factor-1 and hematopoietic cell homing in an adult zebrafish model of hematopoietic cell transplantation *Blood*, Vol. 118, No. 3, pp. 766-74, ISSN 1528-0020.

Golub T and Caroni P. (2005). PI(4,5)P2-dependent microdomain assemblies capture microtubules to promote and control leading edge motility *Journal of Cell Biology*, Vol. 169, No. 1, pp. 151-65, ISSN 0021-9525.

Gottig S, Mobest D, et al. (2006). Role of the monomeric GTPase Rho in hematopoietic progenitor cell migration and transplantation *European Journal of Immunology*, Vol. 36, No. 1, pp. 180-9, ISSN 0014-2980.

Gu Y, Jasti AC, et al. (2005). RhoH, a hematopoietic-specific Rho GTPase, regulates proliferation, survival, migration, and engraftment of hematopoietic progenitor cells *Blood*, Vol. 105, No. 4, pp. 1467-75, ISSN 0006-4971.

Hattori K, Heissig B, et al. (2001). Plasma elevation of stromal cell-derived factor-1 induces mobilization of mature and immature hematopoietic progenitor and stem cells *Blood*, Vol. 97, No. 11, pp. 3354-60, ISSN 0006-4971.

Hawkins PT, Anderson KE, et al. (2006). Signalling through Class I PI3Ks in mammalian cells *Biochemical Society Transactions*, Vol. 34, No. Pt 5, pp. 647-62, ISSN 0300-5127.

Heesen M, Berman MA, et al. (1997). Alternate splicing of mouse fusin/CXC chemokine receptor-4: stromal cell-derived factor-1alpha is a ligand for both CXC chemokine receptor-4 isoforms *Journal of Immunology*, Vol. 158, No. 8, pp. 3561-4, ISSN 0022-1767.

Heissig B, Hattori K, et al. (2002). Recruitment of stem and progenitor cells from the bone marrow niche requires MMP-9 mediated release of kit-ligand *Cell*, Vol. 109, No. 5, pp. 625-37, ISSN 0092-8674.

Henschler R, Piiper A, et al. (2003). SDF-1alpha-induced intracellular calcium transient involves Rho GTPase signalling and is required for migration of hematopoietic progenitor cells *Biochemical Biophysical Research Communnications*, Vol. 311, No. 4, pp. 1067-71, ISSN 0006-291X.

Hidalgo A, Sanz-Rodriguez F, et al. (2001). Chemokine stromal cell-derived factor-1alpha modulates VLA-4 integrin-dependent adhesion to fibronectin and VCAM-1 on bone marrow hematopoietic progenitor cells *Experimental Hematology*, Vol. 29, No. 3, pp. 345-55, ISSN 0301-472X.

Imai K, Kobayashi M, et al. (1999). Selective transendothelial migration of hematopoietic progenitor cells: a role in homing of progenitor cells *Blood*, Vol. 93, No. 1, pp. 149-56, ISSN 0006-4971.

Kahn J, Byk T, et al. (2004). Overexpression of CXCR4 on human CD34+ progenitors increases their proliferation, migration, and NOD/SCID repopulation *Blood*, Vol. 103, No. 8, pp. 2942-9, ISSN 0006-4971.

Katayama Y, Hidalgo A, et al. (2004). Integrin alpha4beta7 and its counterreceptor MAdCAM-1 contribute to hematopoietic progenitor recruitment into bone marrow following transplantation *Blood*, Vol. 104, No. 7, pp. 2020-6, ISSN 0006-4971.

Kharas MG, Okabe R, et al. (2010). Constitutively active AKT depletes hematopoietic stem cells and induces leukemia in mice *Blood*, Vol. 115, No. 7, pp. 1406-15, ISSN 1528-0020.

Kim CH and Broxmeyer HE. (1998). In vitro behavior of hematopoietic progenitor cells under the influence of chemoattractants: stromal cell-derived factor-1, steel factor, and the bone marrow environment *Blood*, Vol. 91, No. 1, pp. 100-10, ISSN 0006-4971.

Kim CH, Wu W, et al. (2011). Conditioning for hematopoietic transplantation activates the complement cascade and induces a proteolytic environment in bone marrow: a novel role for bioactive lipids and soluble C5b-C9 as homing factors *Leukemia*, ISSN 1476-5551.

Kollet O, Dar A, et al. (2006). Osteoclasts degrade endosteal components and promote mobilization of hematopoietic progenitor cells *Nature Medicine*, Vol. 12, No. 6, pp. 657-64, ISSN 1078-8956.

Kollet O, Petit I, et al. (2002). Human CD34(+)CXCR4(-) sorted cells harbor intracellular CXCR4, which can be functionally expressed and provide NOD/SCID repopulation *Blood*, Vol. 100, No. 8, pp. 2778-86, ISSN 0006-4971.

Kollet O, Spiegel A, et al. (2001). Rapid and efficient homing of human CD34(+)CD38(-/low)CXCR4(+) stem and progenitor cells to the bone marrow and spleen of NOD/SCID and NOD/SCID/B2m(null) mice *Blood*, Vol. 97, No. 10, pp. 3283-91, ISSN 0006-4971.

Lataillade JJ, Clay D, et al. (2000). Chemokine SDF-1 enhances circulating CD34(+) cell proliferation in synergy with cytokines: possible role in progenitor survival *Blood*, Vol. 95, No. 3, pp. 756-68, ISSN 0006-4971.

Leung KT, Chan KY, et al. (2011). The tetraspanin CD9 regulates migration, adhesion, and homing of human cord blood CD34+ hematopoietic stem and progenitor cells *Blood*, Vol. 117, No. 6, pp. 1840-50, ISSN 1528-0020.

Levesque JP, Hendy J, et al. (2002). Mobilization by either cyclophosphamide or granulocyte colony-stimulating factor transforms the bone marrow into a highly proteolytic environment *Experimental Hematology*, Vol. 30, No. 5, pp. 440-9, ISSN 0301-472X.

Liesveld JL, Rosell K, et al. (2001). Response of human CD34+ cells to CXC, CC, and CX3C chemokines: implications for cell migration and activation *Journal of Hematotherapy and Stem Cell Research*, Vol. 10, No. 5, pp. 643-55, ISSN 1525-8165.

Lo Celso C, Fleming HE, et al. (2009). Live-animal tracking of individual haematopoietic stem/progenitor cells in their niche *Nature*, Vol. 457, No. 7225, pp. 92-6, ISSN 1476-4687.

Loetscher M, Geiser T, et al. (1994). Cloning of a human seven-transmembrane domain receptor, LESTR, that is highly expressed in leukocytes *Journal of Biological Chemistry*, Vol. 269, No. 1, pp. 232-7, ISSN 0021-9258.

Ma Q, Jones D, et al. (1998). Impaired B-lymphopoiesis, myelopoiesis, and derailed cerebellar neuron migration in CXCR4- and SDF-1-deficient mice *Procedures National Academy Sciences U S A*, Vol. 95, No. 16, pp. 9448-53, ISSN 0027-8424.

Maehama T and Dixon JE. (1998). The tumor suppressor, PTEN/MMAC1, dephosphorylates the lipid second messenger, phosphatidylinositol 3,4,5-trisphosphate *Journal of Biological Chemistry*, Vol. 273, No. 22, pp. 13375-8, ISSN 0021-9258.

Maekawa T and Ishii T. (2000). Chemokine/receptor dynamics in the regulation of hematopoiesis *Internal Medicine*, Vol. 39, No. 2, pp. 90-100, ISSN 0918-2918.

Marquez-Curtis L, Jalili A, et al. (2008). Carboxypeptidase M expressed by human bone marrow cells cleaves the C-terminal lysine of stromal cell-derived factor-1alpha: another player in hematopoietic stem/progenitor cell mobilization? *Stem Cells*, Vol. 26, No. 5, pp. 1211-20, ISSN 1549-4918.

Mazo IB, Gutierrez-Ramos JC, et al. (1998). Hematopoietic progenitor cell rolling in bone marrow microvessels: parallel contributions by endothelial selectins and vascular cell adhesion molecule 1 *Journal of Experimental Medicine*, Vol. 188, No. 3, pp. 465-74, ISSN 0022-1007.

McQuibban GA, Butler GS, et al. (2001). Matrix metalloproteinase activity inactivates the CXC chemokine stromal cell-derived factor-1 *Journal of Biological Chemistry*, Vol. 276, No. 47, pp. 43503-8, ISSN 0021-9258.

Merzaban JS, Burdick MM, et al. (2011). Analysis of glycoprotein E-selectin ligands on human and mouse marrow cells enriched for hematopoietic stem/progenitor cells *Blood*, ISSN 1528-0020.

Migliaccio AR, Martelli F, et al. (2008). Altered SDF-1/CXCR4 axis in patients with primary myelofibrosis and in the Gata1 low mouse model of the disease *Experimental Hematology*, Vol. 36, No. 2, pp. 158-71, ISSN 0301-472X.

Mohle R, Bautz F, et al. (1998). The chemokine receptor CXCR-4 is expressed on CD34+ hematopoietic progenitors and leukemic cells and mediates transendothelial migration induced by stromal cell-derived factor-1 *Blood*, Vol. 91, No. 12, pp. 4523-30, ISSN 0006-4971.

Nagasawa T, Hirota S, et al. (1996). Defects of B-cell lymphopoiesis and bone-marrow myelopoiesis in mice lacking the CXC chemokine PBSF/SDF-1 *Nature*, Vol. 382, No. 6592, pp. 635-8, ISSN 0028-0836.

Naiyer AJ, Jo DY, et al. (1999). Stromal derived factor-1-induced chemokinesis of cord blood CD34(+) cells (long-term culture-initiating cells) through endothelial cells is mediated by E-selectin *Blood*, Vol. 94, No. 12, pp. 4011-9, ISSN 0006-4971.

Oberlin E, Amara A, et al. (1996). The CXC chemokine SDF-1 is the ligand for LESTR/fusin and prevents infection by T-cell-line-adapted HIV-1 *Nature*, Vol. 382, No. 6594, pp. 833-5, ISSN 0028-0836.

Papayannopoulou T, Priestley GV, et al. (2001). Molecular pathways in bone marrow homing: dominant role of alpha(4)beta(1) over beta(2)-integrins and selectins *Blood*, Vol. 98, No. 8, pp. 2403-11, ISSN 0006-4971.

Peled A, Grabovsky V, et al. (1999a). The chemokine SDF-1 stimulates integrin-mediated arrest of CD34(+) cells on vascular endothelium under shear flow *Journal of Clinical Investigation*, Vol. 104, No. 9, pp. 1199-211, ISSN 0021-9738.

Peled A, Kollet O, et al. (2000). The chemokine SDF-1 activates the integrins LFA-1, VLA-4, and VLA-5 on immature human CD34(+) cells: role in transendothelial/stromal migration and engraftment of NOD/SCID mice *Blood*, Vol. 95, No. 11, pp. 3289-96, ISSN 0006-4971.

Peled A, Petit I, et al. (1999b). Dependence of human stem cell engraftment and repopulation of NOD/SCID mice on CXCR4 *Science*,Vol. 283,No. 5403,pp. 845-8, ISSN 0036-8075.

Petit I, Goichberg P, et al. (2005). Atypical PKC-zeta regulates SDF-1-mediated migration and development of human CD34+ progenitor cells *Journal of Clinical Investigation*, Vol. 115, No. 1, pp. 168-76, ISSN 0021-9738.

Petit I, Szyper-Kravitz M, et al. (2002). G-CSF induces stem cell mobilization by decreasing bone marrow SDF-1 and up-regulating CXCR4 *Nature Immunology*, Vol. 3, No. 7, pp. 687-94, ISSN 1529-2908.

Ponomaryov T, Peled A, et al. (2000). Induction of the chemokine stromal-derived factor-1 following DNA damage improves human stem cell function *Journal of Clinical Investigation*, Vol. 106, No. 11, pp. 1331-9, ISSN 0021-9738.

Qian H, Georges-Labouesse E, et al. (2007). Distinct roles of integrins alpha6 and alpha4 in homing of fetal liver hematopoietic stem and progenitor cells *Blood*, Vol. 110, No. 7, pp. 2399-407, ISSN 0006-4971.

Qian H, Tryggvason K, et al. (2006). Contribution of alpha6 integrins to hematopoietic stem and progenitor cell homing to bone marrow and collaboration with alpha4 integrins *Blood*, Vol. 107, No. 9, pp. 3503-10, ISSN 0006-4971.

Roberts MS, Woods AJ, et al. (2004). Protein kinase B/Akt acts via glycogen synthase kinase 3 to regulate recycling of alpha v beta 3 and alpha 5 beta 1 integrins *Molecular Cell Biology*, Vol. 24, No. 4, pp. 1505-15, ISSN 0270-7306.

Sahai E and Marshall CJ. (2002). RHO-GTPases and cancer *Nature Reviews Cancer*, Vol. 2, No. 2, pp. 133-42, ISSN 1474-175X.

Sanchez-Aguilera A, Lee YJ, et al. (2011). Guanine nucleotide exchange factor Vav1 regulates perivascular homing and bone marrow retention of hematopoietic stem and progenitor cells *Procedures Nationall Academy Sciences U S A*, Vol. 108, No. 23, pp. 9607-12, ISSN 1091-6490.

Sauer G, Windisch J, et al. (2003). Progression of cervical carcinomas is associated with down-regulation of CD9 but strong local re-expression at sites of transendothelial invasion *Clinical Cancer Research*, Vol. 9, No. 17, pp. 6426-31, ISSN 1078-0432.

Scott LM, Priestley GV, et al. (2003). Deletion of alpha4 integrins from adult hematopoietic cells reveals roles in homeostasis, regeneration, and homing *Molecular Cell Biology*, Vol. 23, No. 24, pp. 9349-60, ISSN 0270-7306.

Skidgel RA and Erdos EG. (1998). Cellular carboxypeptidases *Immunology Reviews*, Vol. 161, pp. 129-41, ISSN 0105-2896.

Sweeney EA, Lortat-Jacob H, et al. (2002). Sulfated polysaccharides increase plasma levels of SDF-1 in monkeys and mice: involvement in mobilization of stem/progenitor cells *Blood*, Vol. 99, No. 1, pp. 44-51, ISSN 0006-4971.

Sweeney EA, Priestley GV, et al. (2000). Mobilization of stem/progenitor cells by sulfated polysaccharides does not require selectin presence *Procedures National Academy Sciences U S A*, Vol. 97, No. 12, pp. 6544-9, ISSN 0027-8424.

Tarnowski M, Liu R, et al. (2010). CXCR7: a new SDF-1-binding receptor in contrast to normal CD34(+) progenitors is functional and is expressed at higher level in human malignant hematopoietic cells *European Journal of Haematology*, Vol. 85, No. 6, pp. 472-83, ISSN 1600-0609.

Tashiro K, Tada H, et al. (1993). Signal sequence trap: a cloning strategy for secreted proteins and type I membrane proteins *Science*, Vol. 261, No. 5121, pp. 600-3, ISSN 0036-8075.

Taylor ML and Metcalfe DD. (2000). Kit signal transduction *Hematology/Oncology Clinics North America*, Vol. 14, No. 3, pp. 517-35, ISSN 0889-8588.

Timokhina I, Kissel H, et al. (1998). Kit signaling through PI 3-kinase and Src kinase pathways: an essential role for Rac1 and JNK activation in mast cell proliferation *EMBO Journal*, Vol. 17, No. 21, pp. 6250-62, ISSN 0261-4189.

Vermeulen M, Le Pesteur F, et al. (1998). Role of adhesion molecules in the homing and mobilization of murine hematopoietic stem and progenitor cells *Blood*, Vol. 92, No. 3, pp. 894-900, ISSN 0006-4971.

Viglietto G, Motti ML, et al. (2002). Cytoplasmic relocalization and inhibition of the cyclin-dependent kinase inhibitor p27(Kip1) by PKB/Akt-mediated phosphorylation in breast cancer *Nature Medicine*, Vol. 8, No. 10, pp. 1136-44, ISSN 1078-8956.

Voermans C, Rood PM, et al. (2000). Adhesion molecules involved in transendothelial migration of human hematopoietic progenitor cells *Stem Cells*, Vol. 18, No. 6, pp. 435-43, ISSN 1066-5099.

Wierenga PK, Weersing E, et al. (2006). Differential role for very late antigen-5 in mobilization and homing of hematopoietic stem cells *Bone Marrow Transplantation*, Vol. 38, No. 12, pp. 789-97, ISSN 0268-3369.

Wright DE, Bowman EP, et al. (2002). Hematopoietic stem cells are uniquely selective in their migratory response to chemokines *Journal of Experimental Medicine*, Vol. 195, No. 9, pp. 1145-54, ISSN 0022-1007.

Wu FY, Wang SE, et al. (2006). Reduction of cytosolic p27(Kip1) inhibits cancer cell motility, survival, and tumorigenicity *Cancer Research*, Vol. 66, No. 4, pp. 2162-72, ISSN 0008-5472.

Wysoczynski M, Reca R, et al. (2005). Incorporation of CXCR4 into membrane lipid rafts primes homing-related responses of hematopoietic stem/progenitor cells to an SDF-1 gradient *Blood*, Vol. 105, No. 1, pp. 40-8, ISSN 0006-4971.

Xia L, McDaniel JM, et al. (2004). Surface fucosylation of human cord blood cells augments binding to P-selectin and E-selectin and enhances engraftment in bone marrow *Blood*, Vol. 104, No. 10, pp. 3091-6, ISSN 0006-4971.

Yang FC, Atkinson SJ, et al. (2001). Rac and Cdc42 GTPases control hematopoietic stem cell shape, adhesion, migration, and mobilization *Procedures National Academy Sciences U S A*, Vol. 98, No. 10, pp. 5614-8, ISSN 0027-8424.

Yiu GK and Toker A. (2006). NFAT induces breast cancer cell invasion by promoting the induction of cyclooxygenase-2 *Journal of Biological Chemistry*, Vol. 281, No. 18, pp. 12210-7, ISSN 0021-9258.

Yoeli-Lerner M, Yiu GK, et al. (2005). Akt blocks breast cancer cell motility and invasion through the transcription factor NFAT *Molecular Cell*, Vol. 20, No. 4, pp. 539-50, ISSN 1097-2765.

Zannettino AC, Buhring HJ, et al. (1998). The sialomucin CD164 (MGC-24v) is an adhesive glycoprotein expressed by human hematopoietic progenitors and bone marrow stromal cells that serves as a potent negative regulator of hematopoiesis *Blood*, Vol. 92, No. 8, pp. 2613-28, ISSN 0006-4971.

Zhang J, Grindley JC, et al. (2006). PTEN maintains haematopoietic stem cells and acts in lineage choice and leukaemia prevention *Nature*, Vol. 441, No. 7092, pp. 518-22, ISSN 1476-4687.

10

Searching for the Key to Expand Hematopoietic Stem Cells

Jeanne Grosselin[1,2], Karine Sii-Felice[1,2],
Philippe Leboulch[1,2,3] and Diana Tronik-Le Roux[1,2]
[1]*CEA, Institute of Emerging Diseases and
Innovative Therapies (iMETI), Fontenay-aux-Roses,*
[2]*Inserm U962 and University Paris 11, CEA-iMETI, Fontenay-aux-Roses,*
[3]*Harvard Medical School and Genetics Division, Brigham & Women's Hospital, Boston,*
[1,2]*France*
[3]*USA*

1. Introduction

Stem cells are characterized by their capacity to self renew and differentiate into progressively restricted cells that ultimately become limited to a specific cell fate. The two broad types of mammalian stem cells are: embryonic stem cells and adult stem cells.

Embryonic stem cells (ESC) are mostly derived from the undifferentiated inner mass cells of a blastocyst. These cells give rise during development of the embryo to all derivatives of the three primary germ layers: ectoderm, endoderm and mesoderm. They do not contribute to the extra-embryonic membranes or the placenta. Ex-vivo, they can be cultured for extended periods of time and under the appropriate conditions, they can be also directed to differentiate into many specialized types of cells. These particular features are being exploited to use ESC as starting material for treatment of degenerative diseases and replacement of damaged organs. Although their potential is great, the promise of ESC-derived therapies will be unfulfilled unless several challenges are overcome. For example, the quite small production of ESC-derived cells obtained or the active immune rejection of the ESC-derived graft.

Unlike embryonic stem cells, the adult stem cells are already partially specialized. They have been found in most self-renewing tissues, including the skin, the brain, the intestinal epithelium and the hematopoietic system and have the primary role of maintaining and repairing the tissue in which they are found. They are located deep within organs in specialized areas known as the "stem cell niche" (Scadden, 2006). This microenvironment allows for their survival, self renewal, regulated proliferation and maintenance of their quiescence for long periods of time until the moment in which they are activated. *Ex vivo*, however, the capacity of stem cells to self-renew is limited, they exhibit poor survival and consequently their numbers sharply declines during experimental manipulation.

One of the more intriguing but highly debated areas of stem cell biology was the phenomenon described as plasticity or transdifferentiation. Numerous reports expressed opposing views about this ability of stem cells to cross organ/tissue boundaries. These discrepancies have now been mostly passed over by current research showing that cell populations of one lineage might produce cells from other lineages by changing gene expression in response to micro-environmental cues (Jang and Sharkis, 2005; Theise, 2010).

Owing to their unique characteristic of plasticity, self-renewal capacity and potential to generate functional cell types, stem cells are particularly attractive for developing therapeutic settings that range from drug discovery protocols to cell transplantation and regenerative therapies. Nevertheless, several challenges including the need to identify the signals that influence the stem cell fate decisions and the application of this information towards the design of stem cell bioprocesses have to be overcome to accomplish the transition from fundamental science to functional technologies.

1.1 Hematopoietic stem cells

Hematopoietic stem cells (HSC) are probably the best characterized adult stem cell and often serve as a paradigm for other stem cells. Even though no morphological criteria to unequivocally identify such cells exist, HSC have been proven to be invaluable in the clinic. They are the only stem cells used routinely in cell based therapies, to treat numerous hematologic and non-hematologic malignancies as well as a range of both inherited and acquired diseases. This is typically due i) to the availability of a straight forward purification protocols using cell surface antigen selection and ii) to the possibility to perform reconstitution assays that rely on their clonal ability to reconstitute the entire hematopoietic system following transplantation into myeloablated recipients (Fig. 1). The same cell surface antigens, however, do not always conform to the same stem cell functional phenotype (Simonnet et al., 2009) and therefore the transplantation procedure constitutes undoubtedly the "gold standard" method for proving that a cell is indeed an HSC.

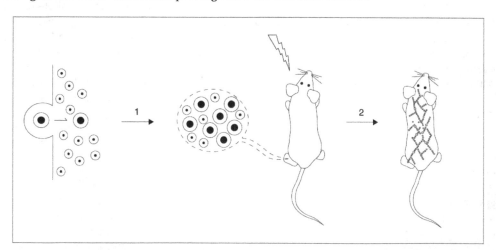

Fig. 1. A diagrammatic representation of a stem cell in its micro-environment and one stem cell induced to move out of the niche where it will undergo development. Following BM removal and cell surface antigen selection (1), cells are cultured *in vitro* and infused in a myeloablated mouse. Several weeks after (2), blood cells are regenerated in the transplanted mouse.

To maintain the steady-state of the stem cell compartment and to allow the regeneration of hematopoietic cells after transplantation or after hematopoietic injury, HSC divide asymmetrically or symmetrically. In an asymmetric self-renewing division, the two daughter cells adopt different fates, resulting in only one cell maintaining stem-cell properties. The symmetric self-renewing division refers to the process whereby both daughter cells retain stem cell properties. This type of cell division expands the stem-cell pool and is therefore critical for sustaining the HSC compartment and thus is a requirement for lifelong hematopoiesis.

The HSC fate decisions are dependent on concomitantly intrinsic HSC fate determinants and extrinsic signals delivered by the bone marrow (BM) niches were HSC resides. These niches are small cavities formed by heterogeneous types of cells, named stroma, that are positioned close to the BM longitudinal axis of the femur with more differentiated cells disposed in a graduated manner as the central longitudinal axis of the bone is approached. The attachment of HSC to the stroma via a network of adhesion molecules provide an environment that optimally balances signals that control self-renewal, proliferation and differentiation. Under normal physiological conditions, HSC are kept in a relatively low proliferative, quiescent state, protecting them from stress and preventing their depletion due to excessive proliferation (Jang and Sharkis, 2007). Recent data imply that these areas where HSC reside are hypoxic (Parmar et al., 2007).

To take advantage of the HSC plasticity capacities for therapeutic use, HSC may be withdrawn from their original niches, and placed on a novel non-hematopoietic environment. Once located in this novel medium, the reprogramming of the cell genome occurs and directs and/or contributes to their conversion into unrelated cell types (Fig. 2). The unexpected flexibility of HSC to produce non-hematopoietic cells was described for several cells/tissues (Quesenberry et al., 2010) including liver cells (Almeida-Porada et al., 2010; Jang et al., 2004), neurones (Mezey et al., 2000), lung epithelial (Abe et al., 2003) or connective tissues (Ogawa et al., 2010).

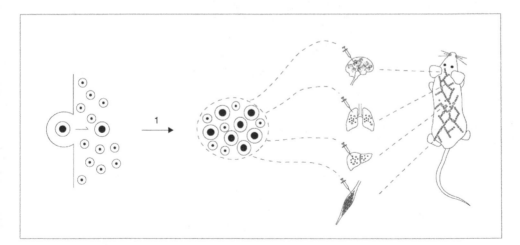

Fig. 2. A schematic representation of HSC plasticity. Hematopoietic cell are removed from the femoral bone (1) and the HSC-enriched population is cultured *in vitro*. Following an optional genetic modification, cells may be used to generate *in vivo* non-hematopoietic cell types.

The development of HSC-based therapies however, is to some extent prevented by the scarce representation of HSC in the BM and their finite lifespan *ex vivo*. Increasing their utilisation needs enhancement of hematopoietic stem cells availability or *de novo* generation of HSC. This presumes i) the development of robust methods to efficiently control HSC regulatory processes; ii) the therapeutic *in vivo* or *in vitro* expansion of HSC number and iii) the utilisation of optimized protocols to generate available HSC from ESC or IPSC.

2. Physiological pathways involved in the regulation of stem cells

HSC fate decisions are supported by the orchestration of several pathways such as Wnt, Notch and Hedgehog pathways that critically balance cell cycling and quiescence, leading to proliferation and apoptosis, self-renewal or differentiation (Fig. 3). The ultimate decision is dependent on hundreds of inputs including concentrations of different growth factors, cytokines, hormones, oxygen levels that must be integrated to subsequently activate these different signal transduction cascades. Understanding their regulation might led to the effective and more spread out utilization of HSC in clinical settings. The most relevant aspects of these pathways are briefly resumed below.

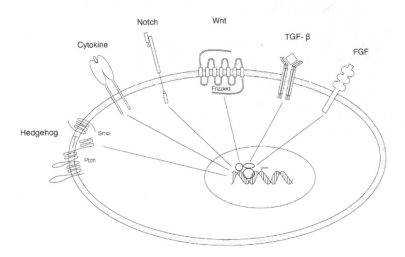

Fig. 3. A schematic representation of signaling pathways collectively influencing stem cell fate.

2.1 The hedgehog (Hh) signaling

In adult tissues, Hh signaling is involved in the maintenance of stem cells, regeneration and tissue repair where it governs processes like cell proliferation, cell renewal and differentiation. The three Hh ligand homologues: Sonic Hh, Indian Hh, and Desert Hh bind interchangeably the two related twelve-pass membrane Patched (Ptc) receptors. They relieve the inhibition of smoothened (SMO), a serpentine receptor resembling G protein–coupled receptors allowing activation of a family of zinc-finger transcription factors called GLI and the modification of the expression Hh target genes (Kasper et al., 2009).

The role of Hh signaling in HSC is controversial. Bhardwaj et al provided evidence for a role of Hh signaling in HSC (Bhardwaj et al., 2001). In this study, suppression of Hh signaling inhibited proliferation of HSC and addition of soluble SHh induced expansion of hematopoietic repopulating cells (Bhardwaj et al., 2001). More recent reports confirmed that suppression of the Hh pathway leads to a severe defect in HSC functions (Merchant et al., 2010; Trowbridge et al., 2006) whereas others reported that this pathway can be dispensable for HSC biology (Gao et al., 2009; Hofmann et al., 2009). In $Ptc1+/-$ mice, which have increased Hh activity, activation of the Hh signaling pathway induces expansion of primitive blood cells under homeostatic conditions. However, when HSC are challenged to regenerate the blood system, persistent Hh activation leads to HSC exhaustion (Trowbridge et al., 2006). Furthermore, Indian Hh gene transfer can confer enhanced hematopoietic support ability to BM stromal cells, suggesting that it is involved in the interaction between HSC and the stromal cells. This leads to an increase in proliferation and repopulating capacity of primitive hematopoietic cells (Kobune et al., 2004). These results suggest a role for Hh signaling in balancing homeostasis and regeneration *in vivo*. In contrast, other reports show that Hh signaling is dispensable for adult HSC functions (Gao et al., 2009; Hofmann et al., 2009). In these studies conditional deletion of SMO, the only non redundant component of the Hh cascade, or pharmacologic inhibition of Hh signaling have no apparent effect on adult hematopoietic, including peripheral blood count, number or cell cycle status of stem or progenitor cells, hematopoietic colony-forming potential or long-term repopulating activity in *in vivo* assays. In agreement with this notion, genome-wide transcriptome analysis revealed that silencing the Hh signaling does not significantly alter the HSC-specific gene expression "signature." Taken together, these conflicting data suggest that Hh signaling may influence HSC through more complex networks such as cell-niche interactions.

2.2 Fibroblast growth factor (FGF) signaling

FGF belongs to a family of heparin-binding polypeptides that shows multiple functions, including effects on cell proliferation, differentiation and survival (Baird, 1994). Twenty-four members of the FGF family have been identified in human and mice. FGFs bind and activate their cognate FGFRs that are encoded by four genes (FGFR1– 4). This results in receptor dimerization, tyrosine kinase autophosphorylation, and recruitment of signaling complexes. The FGF signal transduction proceeds by one, or a combination, of three main pathways: Ras/mitogen-activated protein kinase (MAPK) signaling; planar cell polarity/calcium; phosphoinotitide-3-kinase (PI3K)/Akt (extensively reviewed by Bottcher and Niehrs, 2005). Both FGF-1 and FGF-2 support HSC expansion when unfractionated mouse BM cells are cultured in serum-free medium (de Haan et al., 2003; Yeoh et al., 2006). Crcareva et al. confirmed that FGF-1 stimulates ex-vivo expansion of HSC (Crcareva et al., 2005). Conditional derivatives of FGFR-1 have also been used to support short-term HSC expansion and long-term HSC survival (Weinreich et al., 2006). This factor seems to also support *ex vivo* expansion of murine and human HSC in combination with other cytokines, i.e stem cell factor [SCF], thrombopoietin [TPO], insulin-like growth factor-2 [IGF-2], and fibroblast growth factor-1 [FGF-1] (Zhang and Lodish, 2005). Moreover, a recent study showed that addition of SCF, TPO, and FGF-1 to a mesenchymal stem cells (MSC) culture stimulates proliferation, maintenance of primitive immunophenotype, and expansion of CFU-initiating cells. This supports the notion that expansion of HSC requires complex stimulation of different signal cascades activated by soluble growth factors as well as adhesion proteins (Walenda et al., 2011).

2.3 Notch signaling

The Notch pathway is also an evolutionarily conserved mechanism that plays a fundamental role in regulating cell-fate decisions (Bolos et al., 2007). Four types of Notch receptors (Notch 1-4) and five Notch ligands (Jagged 1 and 2, Delta 1, 3 and 4) have been identified in vertebrates. Notch ligands are single-pass transmembrane proteins consisting of multiple EGF-like repeats and a characteristic DSL (Delta, Serrate, and LAG-2) domain (see for review Ohishi et al., 2003; Shimizu et al., 2000). One characteristic of this signaling pathway is the dual role of Notch as both a transmembrane receptor and a transcription factor in a system where no second messengers are used (Matsuno et al., 1995). Notch can have opposite functions in different self-renewing organs indicating that the outcome of Notch activation depends to a great extent on the cell context and the specific growth factors present in the microenvironment. For example, activation of Notch1 by Delta ligands 1 and 4 is required for inducing T-cell and inhibiting B-cell differentiation whereas Notch2 activation by Jagged1, and possibly Delta1, acts on HSC (Han et al., 2002; Radtke et al., 1999; Varnum-Finney et al., 2011).

A role for Notch in hematopoietic was initially suggested by detection of the human Notch1 gene in CD34$^+$ or lineage (Lin)$^-$CD34$^+$ hematopoietic cells (Milner et al., 1994). Transduction of murine HSC with a retrovirus expressing a constitutively active form of Notch1 induced the emergence of an immortalized pluripotent cytokine-dependent cell line capable of both myeloid and lymphoid repopulation *in vivo*, thereby demonstrating a role for Notch in HSC self-renewal (Varnum-Finney et al., 2000). Similar results were obtained using an immobilized form of the Notch ligand Delta-1 since incubation of murine HSC with immobilized Delta-1 and cytokines led to a several-log expansion of cells capable of short-term *in vivo* reconstitution (Varnum-Finney et al., 2003).

In contrast to the murine studies, only a modest or no increase in the progenitor numbers was achieved by expressing activated Notch-1 in human CD34$^+$ cord blood cells (Carlesso et al., 1999; Chadwick et al., 2007) or by incubation with Delta-1 (Jaleco et al., 2001), Delta-4 (Lauret et al., 2004) or Jagged-1 (Karanu et al., 2000; Karanu et al., 2001; Walker et al., 1999). This contrast with other reports showing that incubation of human cord blood cells with the immobilized Delta-1 combined with fibronectin fragments and cytokines induce a 100-fold increase in the number of CD34$^+$ cells compare to controls (Ohishi et al., 2002) and a 16-fold increase in SCID Repopulating Cells (SRC) number compared to uncultured cells. *In vivo* transplanted cells persisted 9 weeks post-transplantation and in secondary recipients, suggesting the presence of both long-term and short-term repopulating cells following culture of human cord blood cells on Delta-1 ligand (Delaney et al., 2010). The SRC enhancement by relatively low density of immobilized ligand and the preference to promote differentiation toward the T-cell lineage at higher ligand density revealed important ligand dose-dependent effects of Notch signaling (Delaney et al., 2005).

The engineered Notch ligand approach for *ex vivo* expansion of human cord blood cells is now under clinical investigation (http://clinicaltrials.gov/ct2/show/record/NCT00343798). In this phase 1 clinical trial, patients undergoing a myeloablative double cord blood transplantation are receiving one non-manipulated cord blood unit along with a second cord blood unit that has undergone Notch-mediated *ex vivo* expansion. These cells were safely infused and led to a significant reduction in the time needed for neutrophil recovery (16 days in patients receiving the expanded unit, compared to 26 days in patients of the concurrent cohort). Similarly, preliminary evaluation of time needed for platelet recovery compared favourably in those patient receiving the expanded cell product compared with those receiving non-manipulated cells (Dahlberg et al., 2011). In addition, comparable overall survival and graft-versus-host disease risk of patient receiving non-manipulated cells was observed within the average follow-up of 354 days. The expanded cell population may also have retained long-term repopulating capacities as two patients display *in vivo* persistence of cultured donor cells. The lack of *in vivo* persistence in the remaining patients may either be due to loss of stem cell self-renewal capacity during *ex vivo* culture or to immune mediated rejection. Indeed, it has been well documented that in most of the patients who received two non-manipulated cord blood units for transplantation, only one contributes to persistent long-term engraftment. The mechanism responsible for this single donor dominance remains yet to be defined. Larger phase II/III studies are required to evaluate whether co-infusion of this expanded cell product decreases the occurrence of serious infection, improves survival, or affects duration of hospital stay (Delaney et al., 2010).

2.4 The transforming growth factor beta (TGFβ) superfamily

The TGFβ superfamily consist of a large collection of secreted proteins that regulate cell growth, differentiation, apoptosis, cellular homeostasis, and other functions in both the adult organism and the developing embryo. The more than 30 TGFβ family ligands are organized into three subgroups (reviewed in (Lyssiotis et al., 2011)). The TGFβ (which comprises SMAD and Activin/Nodal ligands), bone morphogenetic protein (BMP), and the growth differentiation factors (GDF). The TGFβ signaling leads to the phosphorylation of Smads by activated receptors resulting in their partnering with the common signaling transducer Smad4, and translocation to the nucleus. Once activated, Smads regulate diverse biological effects by partnering with transcription factors resulting in cell-state specific modulation of transcription (Kaivo-Oja et al., 2003).

A significant number of studies have demonstrated that TGFβ inhibits proliferation of both murine and human HSC *in vitro*. It was suggest that TGFβ induces quiescence in HSC since its neutralization was showed to release early hematopoietic progenitors cells from quiescence (Hatzfeld et al., 1991; Yamazaki et al., 2009). In agreement with studies performed *in vitro*, injection of TGFβ1 into the femoral artery of mice effectively inhibits proliferation of multipotent hematopoietic progenitors in the BM, establishing an inhibitory role of TGFβ1 also *in vivo* (Goey et al., 1989). Despite a key role *in vitro*, TGFβ did not seem to provide the necessary signals that maintain quiescence and the stem cell pool *in vivo* (Larsson et al., 2005).

To block the entire Smad signaling pathway, the Smad7 was overexpressed in murine HSC using a retroviral gene transfer approach. Forced expression of Smad7 significantly increased the self-renewal capacity of HSC *in vivo* (Blank et al., 2006). In a similar approach using human hematopoietic cells, overexpression of Smad7 resulted in a shift from lymphoid-dominant engraftment toward the myeloid lineage, and an increase of the myeloid-committed clonogenic progenitor frequency in NOD-SCID mice (Chadwick et al., 2005). Instead, Smad4-deficient HSC displayed a significantly reduced repopulative capacity of primary and secondary recipients (Karlsson et al., 2007). Because overexpression of Smad7 versus deletion of Smad4 would be anticipated to yield similar hematopoietic phenotypes, it is conceivable that Smad4 functions as a positive regulator of self-renewal independently of its role as a central mediator of the canonical Smad pathway. In the context of adult hematopoiesis, a high concentration of BMP-4 was shown to promote maintenance of human cord blood cells *in vitro*, while lower concentration of BMP4, BMP2 and BMP7 induced proliferation and differentiation of HSC (Bhatia et al., 1999).

2.5 Wingless-type (Wnt) pathway

Wnt proteins are secreted morphogens necessary for basic developmental processes, such as cell-fate specification, progenitor-cell proliferation and the control of asymmetric cell division, in many different species and organs (Bejsovec, 2005; Moon et al., 2004). Wnt proteins bind to cell surface receptors of the Frizzled family which can translocate the signals to the nucleus and function as transcriptional activators through intracellular β-catenin. Different Wnt pathways are known but their clear separation and their independence remain controversial. There is one canonical pathway that acts on the stability of β-catenin and interacts with T cell transcription factors in the nucleus. There are many non-canonical pathways like the PCP and Wnt/Calcium pathways. The most distinctive differences between the canonical and non-canonical pathways include the specific ligands activating each pathway, ß-Catenin, LRP5/6 co-receptor, and Dsh-DEP domain independence, respectively, and the ability of the non-canonical pathways to inhibit the canonical pathway. Ligands that activate the non-canonical pathways are Wnt4, Wnt5a, and Wnt11.

Recent evidence based on genetic models suggests that canonical Wnt signaling, regulates HSC self-renewal. Active β-catenin promotes HSC proliferation and inhibits differentiation (Kirstetter et al., 2006; Scheller et al., 2006) whereas deficiency in β-catenin inhibits HSC self-renewal (Cobas et al., 2004; Luis et al., 2009; Zhao et al., 2007). Moreover, purified Wnt3a treatment of adult HSC increases self-renewal of murine HSC, as determined by *in vivo* reconstituting assays (Willert et al., 2003) and of human Lin⁻CD34⁺ cells as measured by immunophenotype and colony assays (Van Den Berg et al., 1998).

The role of the non-canonical pathways is not well defined, but surprisingly, their activation and consequently inhibition of the canonical pathway, appears also to be able to expand HSC. Murdoch et al. demonstrated that injecting mice with Wnt5a conditioned media prior to transplant of human umbilical cord blood cells increased engraftment more than 3-fold (Murdoch et al., 2003). Furthermore, culturing Lin⁻Sca-1⁺c-Kit⁺ (LSK) cells with recombinant murine Wnt5a resulted in an enhancement of hematopoietic reconstitution in a BM transplant assay. Wnt5a seems to activate the non-canonical signaling pathways leading to a 3.5- fold more HSC in G0 phase (Nemeth et al., 2007).

Overexpression of Wnt4 led to a modest increase in HSC frequency as measured by phenotype and limiting dilution transplant assays and Wnt4-/- mice showed decreased frequencies of HSC in BM. Similar to the results obtained using Wnt5a, overexpression of Wnt4 led to an increase in the percentage of HSC in G0 (Louis et al., 2008). Whether Wnt4 and Wnt5a inhibit the canonical pathway in a similar fashion remains to be elucidated. These results show the importance of a balanced regulation of these two overlapping Wnt signaling pathways.

2.6 Cross-talk between these pathways

The individual contribution of these pathways to the hematopoietic development of HSC have been extensively addressed (Cerdan and Bhatia, 2010). However, there are many potential intersections along them and therefore the impact of their collective contribution towards influencing the fate of HSC should be carefully considered. Some of these intersection points are resumed below.

Ducan et al. provide a model for how HSC may integrate multiple signals to maintain the stem cell state. They showed that although the proliferation and survival of HSC exposed to Wnt proteins seem unaffected when Notch signaling is impaired, their ability to remain undifferentiated is substantially altered (Duncan et al., 2005). These results demonstrated that the Notch pathway is imperative in maintaining HSC in an undifferentiated state. These findings do not preclude the possibility that a stronger Wnt signal, such as activated β-catenin, may be able to overcome the consequences of loss of Notch signaling. Moreover, Wnt3a regulates the expression of established Notch target genes (Duncan et al., 2005) and the inhibition of GSK-3, a downstream target of Wnt signaling that affects HSC fate through mechanisms involving both Wnt and Notch target genes (Trowbridge et al., 2006). These findings suggest that these pathways could play a role in HSC self renewal using a common network of regulatory circuits with Wnt enhancing proliferation and survival, and Notch preventing differentiation (Blank et al., 2008).

Furthermore, there is substantial evidence for the cross-talk between the Wnt signaling pathway and FGFs and TGF-b by means of the association between Smad4 and Hox proteins. *Homeobox (hox)* genes encode transcription factors that function as regulators of hematopoiesis and are frequently dysregulated in human leukemia, particularly acute myeloid leukemia (Kroon et al., 1998). Recently, Wang et al described a mechanism whereby TGF-β/BMP inhibited the BM transformation capacity of HoxA9 and HoxA9-Nup98 fusion protein through a Smad4-dependent mechanism. Accordingly, Smad4 was shown to interact directly with HoxA9 and Nup98-HoxA9 fusion protein, thus precluding their DNA binding capacity and subsequent transcriptional activity (Wang et al., 2006). Smad4 also seems to participate in other signaling cascades such as Wnt or Notch (Itoh et al., 2004; Labbe et al., 2000).

These studies show the high interdependence between the different pathways, and the impact of their collective contribution on HSC self-renewal. This should be carefully considered when trying to expand HSC for clinical purposes.

2.7 Epigenetic control and HSC self-renewal

Epigenetic modifications, in addition to the intracellular pathways described in the previous section also play an essential role in regulating self-renewal, differentiation and tissue development. They induce gene expression regulation and can be grouped into three main categories: i) DNA methylation, ii) Histone modifications and iii) Nucleosome positioning. Recent studies suggest that epigenetic mechanisms contribute to establish the HSC unique characteristics. The following is a description of some of these examples.

2.7.1 Methylation of DNA

The most widely studied epigenetic modification in humans is cytosine methylation. DNA methylation occurs almost exclusively in the context of CpG dinucleotides that tend to cluster in regions called CpG islands. A group of enzymes, the DNA methyltransferases (DNMTs) tightly regulate both the initiation and maintenance of these methyl marks. DNA methylation can inhibit gene expression by various mechanisms. Methylated DNA can promote the recruitment of methyl-CpG-binding domain proteins which in turn recruit histone-modifying and chromatin-remodeling complexes to methylated sites. DNA methylation can also directly inhibit transcription by precluding the recruitment of DNA binding proteins from their target sites. In contrast, unmethylated CpG islands generate a chromatin structure favorable for gene expression (Portela and Esteller, 2010).

Methylation is controlled by at least 3 DNMTs: DNMT3a and DNMT3b for *de novo* methylation and DNMT1 for methylation maintenance. Conditionally disruption of *Dnmt3a*, *Dnmt3b*, or both *Dnmt3a* and *Dnmt3b* (*Dnmt3a/Dnmt3b*) showed that Dnmt3a and Dnmt3b function as *de novo* DNA methyltransferases during differentiation of hematopoietic cells. Unexpectedly, *in vitro* colony assays showed that both myeloid and lymphoid lineage differentiation potentials were maintained in Dnmt3a-, Dnmt3b-, and Dnmt3a/Dnmt3b-deficient HSC. However, Dnmt3a/Dnmt3b-deficient HSC, but not Dnmt3a- or Dnmt3b-deficient HSC, were incapable of long-term reconstitution in transplantation assays, suggesting a role for DNA methylation by Dnmt3a and Dnmt3b in HSC self-renewal (Tadokoro et al., 2007).

Conditional disruption of Dnmt1 in the mouse hematopoietic system revealed defects in self-renewal, niche retention, and in the ability of cells to give rise to multilineage hematopoiesis. Loss of Dnmt1 had specific impact on myeloid progenitor cells, causing enhanced cell cycling and inappropriate expression of mature lineage genes (Trowbridge et al., 2009). Consistent with these results, Broske et *al.* showed that Dnmt1 is essential for HSC self-renewal but dispensable for homing, cell cycle control and suppression of apoptosis but also implicated Dnmt1 in lymphoid differentiation (Broske et al., 2009).

2.7.2 Histone modifications and nucleosome positioning

A nucleosome is a histone octamer composed by a histone H3-H4 tetramer and two H2A-H2B dimers, around which DNA, 147 base pairs in length, is wrapped in 1.75 superhelical turns. Nucleosomes are connected by the so-called linker DNA and the histone H1. Histones post-transcriptional modifications, including acetylation, methylation, phosphorylation, ubiquitination, SUMOylation and ADP-ribosylation, occur predominantly in histone tails. They have important roles in transcriptional regulation as they can provide either an ON or OFF signature which result in the tight regulation of gene expression but display also important roles in DNA repair, DNA replication, alternative splicing and chromosome condensation. Nucleosomes act as barriers to transcription. They block access of activators and transcription factors to their sites on DNA and inhibit the elongation of the transcripts. The packaging of DNA into nucleosomes appears to affect all stages of transcription, thereby regulating gene expression. Nucleosome positioning plays also an important role in shaping the methylation landscape (Portela and Esteller, 2010).

Polycomb group (PcG) and Trithorax group (TrxG) proteins have emerged as key players in gene regulation and are thought to function coordinately to orchestrate DNA accessibility. These epigenetic regulators act antagonistically to either promote (TrxG) or repress (PcG) transcription through regulation of specific amino acid modifications in histones. It is not known how the PcG and TrxG proteins switch and balance between transcriptionally silenced heterochromatin (for example, enriched in histone H3 lysine 27 trimethylation, H3K27me3) and transcriptionally competent euchromatin (for example, enriched in histone H3 lysine 4 trimethylation, H3K4me3), respectively, during development.

In vertebrates, polycomb group proteins participate mainly in two complexes, Polycomb Repressive Complex (PRC) 1 and PRC2. Probably the best example of a chromatin-associated factor involved in self-renewal is BMI1, which is a component of PRC1. BMI1 is expressed in HSC and its expression decreases upon differentiation towards myeloid or erythroid cells, but is retained within the lymphoid compartments. Upon deletion of BMI1, no changes in the number of HSC in the fetal liver were observed, but in postnatal BMI1$^{-/-}$ mice, the number of HSC was markedly reduced. Targeted deletion of BMI1 in murine HSC impaired their competitive repopulation capacity (Park et al., 2003). *In vitro*, BMI1$^{-/-}$ HSC proliferated poorly and displayed an accelerated loss of multilineage differentiation potential and overexpression of BMI1 enhanced the self-renewal of HSC and enhanced their engraftment potential (Iwama et al., 2004).

Overexpression of BMI1 in cord blood CD34$^+$ cells resulted in stem cell maintenance. After an *in vitro* culture period of 10 days, BMI1-overexpressing cells display a much better engraftment in NOD-SCID mice. Although the mechanisms involved remain to be elucidated, it was observed in single-cell assays that the percentage of CD34$^+$/CD38$^-$ HSC undergoing apoptosis was reduced, whereas the percentage of quiescent HSC not undergoing cell cycle progression was increased upon BMI1 overexpression (Rizo et al., 2008). Lentiviral downmodulation of BMI1 in human cord blood CD34$^+$ cells impaired long-term expansion, progenitor-forming capacity and stem cell frequencies, both in cytokine-driven liquid cultures and in BM stromal cocultures. This was associated with higher expression of p14ARF and p16INK4A and enhanced apoptosis, which coincided with increased levels of intracellular reactive oxygen species (ROS) and reduced FOXO3A expression (Rizo et al., 2008).

Another example of a chromatin-associated factor involved in self-renewal is the mixed lineage leukemia (MLL) protein, which encodes a trithorax-group chromatin regulator. Using *Mll*-deficient ESC to generate chimeras, Ernst et al. showed a cell-intrinsic requirement for MLL in the generation of lymphoid and myeloid populations in adult animals (Ernst et al., 2004). Moreover, MLL is often fused to the AF9 protein in leukemia and have been reported to impart leukaemia stem cell properties on committed hematopoietic progenitors. The leukemia stem cells generated can maintain the global identity of the progenitor from which they arose while activating a limited stem-cell- or self-renewal-associated programme (Krivtsov et al., 2006). Moreover, this MLL-AF9 fusion drives high-level expression of multiple *Hox* genes and can overcome Bmi1-deficiency to establish leukemic stem cells (Smith et al., 2011).

The studies described in this section establish that epigenetic alterations can modulate the self-renewal process. Epigenetic state in stem cells can be stably heritable or can be erased (partly or completely) by cell division. These changes might facilitate the transition of a progenitor cell to a self-renewing stem cell, or might prompt a stem cell to differentiate, divide or lose its ability to self-renew.

3. Compounds modifying HSC capacities

As described in the previous section, the strategy for stem-cell expansion involves activation of regulators that encourage HSC self-renewal and/or inhibition of pathways that mediate, differentiation or apoptosis by using primarily genetic modification approaches. An alternative strategy might imply pharmacological intervention by using a variety of small molecules. The term "small molecule" refers to a molecular entity that interacts with one or more molecular targets and effects a change in biological state while having minimal side effects. These small molecules, defined by a known structure, may be chemicals, proteins, small interfering RNAs or antibodies. Some of the most effective compounds for *ex vivo* maintaining or expanding HSC are reviewed below.

3.1 Regulation by cytokines

Cytokines are secreted proteins that regulate many aspects of hematopoiesis, such as, immune responses and inflammation. Numerous attempts have been made to use classic hematopoietic cytokines for the purpose of expanding HSC *in vitro*. Many interleukins, including interleukin (IL)-3, IL-6, and IL-11, Flt-3 ligand, TPO and SCF have extensively been investigated. In most cases, efforts to expand HSC have failed because of differentiation of HSC and subsequent loss of their reconstitution capacity. The combination of these molecules has however allowed maintaining HSC in culture for several days allowing their use in protocols for gene or cell therapies. Here we describe some examples of cytokines that were used to maintain HSC levels in culture.

3.1.1 Thrombopoietin (TPO)

TPO, acting through its receptor c-MPL, is the chief cytokine that regulates megakaryocyte production. However, several studies suggest that TPO can act to increase the *ex-vivo* expansion of HSC (Sitnicka et al., 1996). This effect was far more effective when used in combination with other cytokines including SCF, fms-like tyrosine kinase 3 ligand (FLT3-L), IL-3 or IL-6. Human cord blood cells expanded with this cytokine cocktail were shown to provide good short- and long-term platelet recovery and lymphomyeloid reconstitution in NOD-SCID mice (Ohmizono et al., 1997; Pineault et al., 2010). Further, a non peptidyl molecule agonist of c-MPL, NR-101, was found to be more efficient than TPO in expanding HSC. Indeed, 7 days culture of human cord blood CD34+ or CD34+CD38-, treated with NR-101 induced a 2-fold increase in their number compare to TPO and a 2.9-fold or 2.3-fold increase in SRC numbers compared to freshly isolated CD34+ cells or TPO-expanded cells respectively. As it was not more efficient than TPO in inducing megakaryocyte expansion, its effect seemed to be HSC specific. NR-101 treatment appeared to persistently activate STAT5 and to induce a long-term accumulation of HIF-1α (Nishino et al., 2009).

3.1.2 Angiopoietin-like 5 (ANGPLT5) and insulin-like growth factor binding protein 2 (IGFBP2)

Soluble growth factors, such as ANGPLT5 and IGFBP2, produced by the endothelium may enhance HSC expansion *ex vivo* when used with conventional cytokines. Although the addition of ANGPLT5 and/or IGFBP2 to a 10 days-human CD133+ cord blood cells culture has no effect upon the total nucleated cells number *in vitro*, it significantly enhances *in vivo* repopulation of NOD-SCID mice 2 months post-transplantation as well as secondary transplantation (Zhang et al., 2008a). These results were confirmed recently using human cord blood CD34$^+$CD133$^+$ cells cultured for 10 days in the presence of IGFBP2 and ANGPLT5. Expanded cells were shown to be capable of long-term multi-lineage and multi-site hematopoiesis in serial reconstitution in NSG mice (Drake et al., 2011).

3.1.3 Pleiotropin (Ptn)

Pleiotropin, which have mitogenic and angiogenic activities, has been found to be essential for maintenance of murine HSC. Mice transplanted with LSK CD34$^-$ cells treated with Ptn and a standard cocktail of cytokines showed 6-fold increase in HSC frequency compared to cells treated with cytokines alone. *In vivo*, systemic administration of Ptn was found to increase the number of BM LSK cells both in irradiated and nonirradiated mice, suggesting a role for this factor in the *in vivo* regeneration of HSC. Treatment of human cord blood Lin$^-$ CD34$^+$CD38$^-$ cells with Ptn for 7 days induced a 4-fold increase in CFC content and a 3- or 7-fold improved engraftment at 4 or 7 weeks respectively in NOD-SCID mice compared with controls. This factor may activate the PI3-Kinase/AKT and Notch pathways by alleviating activation of its receptor, RPTP-β/ξ (Himburg et al., 2010).

3.2 Transcription factors: The HOX- family

3.2.1 HOXB4

The homeobox gene family member HoxB4 is the most investigated transcription factor for its potential to increase the self-renewal potential of HSC. HOXB4 belongs to a large family of transcription factors that share a highly conserved DNA-binding domain, the homeodomain. In mammals, there are 39 *Hox* genes grouped in four clusters referred to as A, B, C and D. In the hematopoietic system, 16 different *Hox* genes are transcribed during normal hematopoiesis. Primitive subpopulations express primarily genes of the A and B cluster (Giampaolo et al., 1995; Pineault et al., 2002; Sauvageau et al., 1994). Mice transplanted with marrow overexpressing HOXB4 resulted in a 47-fold increase of the competitive repopulating unit (CRU) numbers and did not develop leukemic transformation (Sauvageau et al., 1995). *HOXB4* overexpression in mouse HSC cultured for 14 days induced a primitive cell-specific growth advantage contrary to a progressive depletion of HSC usually observed under these conditions. Total cell growth (mostly mature cells) was enhanced by 2-fold, progenitors by 3-fold and HSC by 1000-fold in cells overexpressing HOXB4 (Antonchuk et al., 2002).

In humans, transient overexpression of HOXB4 in hematopoietic cord blood cells, did not increase proliferation of primitive progenitors, frequency of CFC, and LTC-ICs but induced an iincrease in myeloid differentiation (Brun et al., 2003). Other studies showed that enforced high level of HOXB4 expression in human hematopoietic cord blood cells cultured for 24 hours induced a 5-10-fold increase in LTC-IC and a 4-fold increase in SRC (Buske et al., 2002). However, this HOXB4 overexpression markedly impaired the lymphoid and myeloerythroid differentiation (Schiedlmeier et al., 2003). Altogether these studies demonstrated that high levels of HOXB4 perturbed the myeloid differentiation program both *in vivo* and *in vitro* and are consistent with a dose dependant activity of HOXB4 to control the differentiation or self-renewal of HSC (Klump et al., 2005).

To increase the effect of HOXB4, a *NUP98-HOXB4* fusion gene was engeeniered since the fusion of *Hox* genes with the nucleoporine gene *NUP98* is often reported in leukemia. Ohta et *al.* observed, in a murine transplantation model, a 300-fold increase in CRUs among NUP98-HOXB4-overexpressing cells compared to only 80-fold increase with HOXB4 alone. An even higher increase (2000-fold) was observed using the *NUP98-HOXA10* fusion gene that, in contrast to HOXB4, blocks terminal differentiation and leads to a sustained output of cells with a "primitive" phenotype (Pineault et al., 2005; Pineault et al., 2004). The authors did not observe any long-term hematological defect in recipients repopulated with NUP98-HOXA10 expanded HSC (Ohta et al., 2007). However, these results contrast with those obtained by Watts et al. in a nonhuman primate stem cell transplantation model. Transplantation of comparable doses of HOXB4- and NUP98-NUP98-HOXA10-overexpressing cells revealed that HOXB4 contributed more to early hematopoiesis whereas NUP98-HOXA10 contributed more to later hematopoeisis. The emergence of a deleterious effect, such as leukaemia, could not be monitored due to the short survey period of the study (Watts et al., 2011).

In 2006, Zhang et al. investigate the ability of HOXB4 to expand HSC in a clinically relevant nonhuman primate competitive repopulation model. They found an initial 56-fold advantage for the *HOXB4*-transduced cells which decline significantly over time (Zhang et al., 2006). In addition, the first appearence of myeloid leukemia linked to HOXB4 expression were observed two years later, both in the original group of monkeys (1 out of 2) and in dogs (2 out of 2) that received cells transduced with a HOXB4 expressing vector (Zhang et al., 2008b). None of the 40 dogs and monkeys that received cells transduced with control vectors developed leukemia. Besides, a profound growth inhibition and a rapid cell differentiation was induced by siRNA knocking down HOXB4 using a cell line derived from the leukemic cells of one animal. The direct implication of HOXB4 in the development of leukemia can not be certify since analysis of the vector insertion sites in the genome of all tumors revealed insertion of the transgene near or within protooncogenes, such as *c-myb* and *PRDM16* (Zhang et al., 2008b).

To avoid the use of retroviral vectors, Amsellem et al. generate an MS-5 stromal cell line secreting HOXB4 to expand human cord blood hematopoietic cells. Using a 5-week long term culture system, they show a 4-fold increase in LTC-IC and 2.5-fold increase in SRC in NOD-SCID mice. This expansion did not appear to interfere with myeloid or lymphoid differentiation. However, the coculture system might not be suitable for clinical applications (Amsellem et al., 2003). To avoid this issue, Krosl et al. used a soluble recombinant HOXB4 protein fused to a small peptide derived from the HIV TAT protein. TAT-HOXB4 treatment of murine HSC for 4 days expanded approximately 4- to 6-fold and were 8-20 times more numerous than non treated HSC. This TAT-HOXB4 expanded population retained its normal *in vivo* potential for differentiation and long-term repopulation (Krosl et al., 2003).

The capacity of soluble HOXB4 to expand human HSC was verified using several recombinant human HOXB4 proteins. The N-terminal-tat and C-terminal histidine-tagged version of HOXB4 (T-HOXB4-H) had the highest activity in expanding CFC (10-fold) and LTC-IC (15-fold), and a 1.5- to 2.7-fold increase in SRC (Tang et al., 2009).

3.2.2 Other HOX family proteins

Surveys of *Hox* gene expression in HSC enriched populations showed dominancy of the *Hox*A cluster. In d14.5 fetal liver populations enriched for HSC, the expression of HOXA4 is a log higher than that of HOXB4. The fact that during this phase of development HSC undergo their major expansion, combined with the high homology and functional redundancy found within *Hox* paralog groups, suggests a putative role of HOXA4 to expand HSC with negligible or null oncogenic potential. HOXA4 overexpressing HSC expanded 6.6-fold after a week of culture. Although HOXA4 expressing HSC produced mature myeloid and lymphoid progeny in irradiated recipient mice, B-cell progenitors were preferentially expanded compared to myeloid progenitors (Fournier et al., 2011).

HOXC4, another member of the *Hox* family, is also expressed in proliferating hematopoietic cells suggesting a role in the control of normal proliferation. Using retroviral gene transfer in human CD34+ cells, Daga et *al.* showed that HOXC4 induced an *in vitro* expansion of committed cells and early hematopoietic progenitors, with the most striking effect on LTC-IC (13-fold expansion) (Daga et al., 2000). These results are consistent with those of Amsellem and Fichelson who showed a more efficient expansion of human CD34+/CD38low cells on MS-5 cell line secreting HOXC4 compared to those secreting HOXB4. The simultaneous presence of HOXB4 and HOXC4 seems synergize to improve expansion (Amsellem and Fichelson, 2006). However, the *in vivo* effect of HOXC4 still remains to be established.

All these observations clearly implicated Hox family proteins in HSC self renewal but further studies are required to determine if the use of these compounds could be suitable for clinical applications.

3.3 Chemical compounds

The low efficiency obtained with purified proteins and the safety concerns when attempting to expand HSC with viral vector-mediated gene transfer (Baum et al., 2003) lead to searching for alternative and safer approaches. One of these promising strategies involved the use of chemical compounds.

Chemical molecules constitute a particularly useful tool for modifying biological signaling pathways since they can be arrayed in chemical libraries for high-throughput analysis, and they can be withdrawn from the biological system once the desired effect is obtained. The use of a small molecule allows the study of the kinetics of a response in a more subtle and graduated way that is not possible with gene disruption techniques. These molecules may be further transposed into drugs for therapeutic use. Their use is rapid and cost-effective.

What are the sources of molecules available?

Historically, the pharmaceutical companies gathered the collections of molecules accumulated during the year in-house companies. These molecules can come from two different sources, one from natural origin and the other from chemically-synthesized compounds. Several companies have pooled their collections through partnerships to increase the size and diversity. At present, a large collection of oriented chemical libraries is available. In the milieu of academia, access to these collections is almost impossible unless a very restrictive partnership is framed. The number of screenable drug candidates have dramatically increased in the last years, and might account for 10 000 to 1 000 000 compounds. The difficulty to use these large collections resides in the ability to order millions of natural products, many of which are available in only limited amounts and are not yet completely characterized or even purified. Further, to identify a molecule producing the desired biological effect, different concentrations covering several orders of magnitude should be initially screened. This is why their widespread use has not yet been generalized and most discoveries to date are mainly available through the pharmaceutical industry. During the past ten years, various companies have specialized in the provision of all-purpose or targeted libraries. ChemBridge, ChemDiv, Asinex, Prestwick, Maybridge, enamine, Interbioscreen, TimTec can be mentioned as examples of commercially available collections. These libraries are relatively diverse and oriented "drug-like" (Kugawa et al., 2007). Small-molecule compounds approved for use as drugs may also be "repurposed" for new indications and studied to determine the mechanisms of their beneficial and adverse effects. A comprehensive collection of all small-molecule drugs approved for human use would be invaluable for systematic repurposing across human diseases, particularly for rare and neglected diseases, for which the cost and time required for development of a new chemical entity are often prohibitive. Major efforts are now underway to produce comprehensive collections of these small molecules amenable to high-throughput screening (Huang et al., 2011).

During the last ten years, cell-based phenotypic and pathway-specific screens using synthetic small molecules have provided new insights into stem cell biology and help to identify a number of small molecules that can be used to selectively (a) control self-renewal of embryonic and adult stem cells; (b) expand therapeutically desirable mature cell types; (c) control lineage commitment; and (d) enhance the reversion of lineage-restricted cells back to the multipotent or pluripotent state. All four practices are beginning to find application in therapeutic settings.

In this section we will focus on chemical compounds that were used to expand HSC. However, the most important question to keep in mind is whether the *in vitro* expanded cells preserve their capacities to regenerate hematopoiesis *in vivo* (Fig. 4).

3.3.1 Chromatin-modifying agents

Valproic acid (VPA) and chlamydocin are histone deacetylase (HDAC) inhibitors that exert their activity by interacting with the catalytic site of HDACs.

VPA was first studied by De Felice et al. on human CD34$^+$ cells isolated from cord blood, mobilized peripheral blood and BM. They showed that VPA preserves the CD34+ population after 1 week (40-89%) or 3 weeks (21-52%) of culture with cytokines and VPA increases H4 acetylation levels at specific sites on *HOXB4* and AC133 (De Felice et al., 2005).

In 2008, using a two step culture system, Seet et al. showed that VPA induced a 2-fold expansion of human cord blood CD34+CD45+ cells. Higher numbers of treated cells resided in the S phase compare to controls. VPA-treated cells reconstituted hematopoiesis in NOD-SCID mouse with a 6-fold higher efficiency compare to control cells. The advantage of using VPA resides on the fact that this molecule is clinically well-known since it has been used for more than 25 years to treat neurologic disorders (Seet et al., 2009). Chlamydocin, was showed to enhance Thy-1 expression on human CD34+ cells and to display a 4-fold increase in SRC in NOD-SCID (Young et al., 2004).

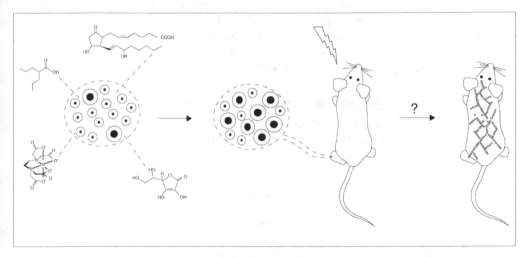

Fig. 4. A diagrammatic representation of an experimental design typology to test the effect of molecules on HSC expansion. Each molecule is added individually to the *in vitro* culture of HSC and the expansion capacities are then measured. However, infusion of the treated cells in myeloablated mice is essential to answer the question (?) on whether the HSC treated with the selected molecule have still the capacity to regenerate blood cells in transplanted animals.

Another HDAC inhibitor, trichostatin A (TSA), and 5-aza-2'-deoxycytidine (5azaD), a DNA methyl transferase inhibitor where shown to act in synergy to yield a 12.5-fold increase of human CD34+CD90+ cells after 9 days of culture in comparison to the input cell numbers, a 9.8-fold increase in the numbers of CFU and a 9.6-fold increase in SRC. Several genes implicated in HSC self-renewal including *HOXB4*, *BMI1*, *GATA2*, *P21*, and *P27* were up-regulated in the 5azaD/TSA-treated cells (Araki et al., 2006; Araki et al., 2007).

3.3.2 Copper chelator tetraethylenepentamine (TEPA)

Several clinical observations have suggested that copper plays a role in regulating HSC development. Peled et al. reported that modulation of cellular copper content might shift the balance between self-renewal and differentiation (Peled et al., 2005; Peled et al., 2002). This group cultured human CD34+ cord blood cells with the copper chelator TEPA during extended periods of time and showed a higher percentage of early progenitors (CD34+CD38-, CD34+CD38-Lin-) in the TEPA-treated cultures compared with controls and a 1- to 3-log-fold expansion of CD34+ cells compare with that of controls. They cultured human CD133+ cord blood cells during 3 weeks, in order to use a clinically suitable protocol, and found that the median output value of CD34+ cells increased by 89-fold, CD34+CD38- by 30-fold and CFU by 172-fold over the input values. Moreover, the CD34+ cells expanded with TEPA appeared to show improved NOD-SCID engraftment compare to control cells (Peled et al., 2004a; Peled et al., 2004b). Based on these data, a phase 1 trial was initiated. In this study, a portion of a single cord blood unit was cultured with TEPA and cytokines for 21 days and co-infused with the remainder of the untreated cell fraction. Although this methodology showed a 219-fold expansion of total nucleated cells *in vitro*, it did not improve the time to neutrophil or platelet recovery (de Lima et al., 2008). A phase 2/3 study is under way in more than 28 centers in the United States, Europe, and Israel, to evaluate the safety and efficacy of this approach ("StemEx") in 100 patients with advanced hematologic malignancies (http://clinicaltrials.gov/ct2/show/NCT00469729).

3.3.3 Oxygen, reactive oxygen species and antioxidants

Low oxygen levels were also described to play a beneficial role on HSC expansion *in vitro*. This is consistent with the observation that protection of HSC *in vivo* is achieved by a predominantly low-oxygen environment of the stem-cell niche (Cipolleschi et al., 1993; Eliasson and Jonsson, 2010).

The positive effect of hypoxia on the survival and/or self-renewal of the HSC population *in vitro* was demonstrated quantitatively on human marrow cells with Lin-CD34+CD38- phenotype which are enriched in SRC. A significant increase in SRC after 4 days was found in cultures under 1.5% O_2 compared to normoxic conditions. The positive effect of hypoxia on SRCs is short-lived but their engraftment into immmunocompromised mice was to some extent improved (Danet et al., 2003).

Similar studies have been performed with cord blood cells (Hermitte et al., 2006). The authors reported preferential survival of primitive HSC among cord blood CD34+ cells in cultures under 0.1% O_2. After 72 hours, cells were 1.5 and 2.5 times more in quiescence (G0) at 3% and 0.1% O2. At 0.1% O2, 46.5%+/-19.1% of divided cells returned to G0 compared with 7.9%+/-0.3% at 20%. This shows a return of the cycling CD34+ cells into G0, a quiescent state that characterizes steady-state HSC.

During the process of HSC purification or mobilization from the BM to the peripheral blood, the cells go across different levels of oxygenation until reach maxima in culture assays. Furthermore, cell factors added to these cultures can lead to an abnormal increase in reactive oxygen species (ROS) in the HSC and to a ROS stress that might change their properties and functions (Hao et al., 2011; Ito et al., 2006; Pervaiz et al., 2009). These ROS are unstable reactive molecular species possessing an unpaired electron that are produced continuously in cells as a byproduct of metabolism. They participate in vital signal transduction pathways but they can also oxidize DNA, proteins, and lipids leading to cell differentiation, senescence, and apoptosis. Notably, the mouse long-term repopulating HSC capacities were found in a Ros[low] population (Jang and Sharkis, 2007). This cell population has a higher self-renewal activity than a Ros[high] population both *in vitro* and *in vivo*. Moreover, distinct metabolic profiles of HSC reflect their location in the hypoxic niche (Simsek et al., 2010; Takubo et al., 2010).

The continual production of ROS in the *in vitro* culture (Iiyama et al., 2006) might be overcome by the addition of antioxidants. These molecules will maintain the ROS at a low level, thereby regulating the proliferation, growth, signal transduction, and gene expression of the cells (Chen et al., 2008).

Antioxidants are classified into enzyme and non-enzyme antioxidants. Enzyme antioxidants include superoxide dismutase, catalase, and glutathione peroxidase. Non-enzyme antioxidant includes vitamin C.

The application of enzyme antioxidants is limited because of the poor stability and ease of inactivation (Wojcik et al., 2010). However, when culturing mouse HSC in the presence of catalase, the number of short-term or long-term HSC with LSK immune markers was significantly increased and the stem cells begin to degenerate as the catalase is removed (Gupta et al., 2006).

Ascorbic acid (vitamin C) is a natural water-soluble antioxidant but under some conditions such as the air, heat, light, alkaline substances, enzymes and trace amount of copper oxide and iron, oxidation of vitamin C could be accelerated and the oxidative products lead to the damage of cellular DNA. The ascorbic acid 2-phosphate (AA2P), one derivative of vitamin C, is stable at 37°C in cell culture media and has no cytotoxic effect; therefore it might constitute an advantageous antioxidant (Duarte et al., 2009). Reducing oxidative stress by N-acetyl-L-cysteine (NAC) may enhance the viability and engraftment of HSC as treatment of gene corrected BM mononuclear cells or purified CD34(+) cells from FANCA patients with the reducing agent NAC showed increased CFC (Becker et al., 2010).

Although the current amplification under normal oxygen can expand a certain number of HSC, the application of glutathione for stem cell mobilization and re-infusion as well as the application of AA2P in the *in vitro* amplification culture of cells may become effective methods for protecting the hematopoietic reconstitution capacity of HSC (Hao et al., 2011). Moreover, *in vitro* culturing HSC-enriched samples under O2 concentrations that more closely resemble the BM environment (low O2 concentrations, 1–3%) might also improve their expansion and preserve proper stem cell functions for engraftment.

3.3.4 PGE2

Prostaglandin E2 (PGE2) was first identified as capable of enhancing HSC formation in zebrafish, following a high-toughput chemical screen. This effect was also tested using murine transplantation assays. When murine BM cells where briefly treated *ex vivo* by PGE2, a 3-fold increase in the CFU number and a 3.3-fold increase of SRC 6 weeks post transplantation were observed (North et al., 2007). Hoggatt et al. confirmed enhanced murine HSC engraftment following PGE2 exposure as they observed a 4-fold increase in HSC 20 weeks after transplantation. The increase in chimerism was still present in primary recipient 32 weeks post-transplant and in secondary recipients without additional PGE2 treatment. Several studies were performed to determine whether the action of PGE2 on HSC could be the result of an increase in HSC numbers, homing capability, proliferation, survival, or a combination thereof. Hoggatt et al. observed a significant increase in homing of PGE2-treated LSK cells. This was partially attributed to an increase in CXCR4 expression, a SDF1α specific receptor. This effect also occurs in human HSC, since PGE2-treated cord blood cells transplanted into NOD-SCID mice displayed an enhanced homing to marrow. In addition, PGE2 treatment increased survivin expression, reduced intracellular active caspase-3 that lead to enhanced HSC survival and increased the percentage of cycling cells (Hoggatt et al., 2009). Frish et al. treated mice *in vivo* with PGE2 by intraperitoneal injection twice a day for 16 days. They observed a significant increase of the LSK population without inhibiting their differentiation. The treatment expands preferentially the short-term-HSC/MPP subpopulation since this advantage was lost 6 weeks post-transplant in primary recipients and in secondary transplants. The disparities between these studies may be the result of the extended exposure of mice to PGE2 compared with a short term pulse used hitherto (Frisch et al., 2009).

Goessling et al. briefly treated human cord blood CD34+ cells *in vitro* with dimethyl-PGE2 (dmPGE2). They showed that dmPGE2 treatment decreased apoptosis, increased 1.4-fold the CFU number and enhanced engraftment of unfractionated and CD34+ cord blood cells after xenotransplantation in NOD-SCID mice. Using a non-human primate transplantation model, they found no significant enhancement of CD34+-treated cells engraftment but showed that dmPGE2 treatment had no negative impact on HSC function, including multilineage repopulation, even 1 year post-transplantation. They suggested that these results reflect suboptimal compound dosing and anticipate the use of 50μM rather than 10μM of dmPGE2 in future transplantation assays (Goessling et al., 2011). Based on these data, this brief *ex vivo* incubation with dmPGE2 is currently being tested in a phase 1 clinical trial in which adults with hematologic malignancies receive a non-myeloablative conditioning treatment followed by double-unit cord blood transplantation in which 1 of the 2 cord blood units has been incubated with dmPGE2 before infusion (http://clinicaltrials.gov/ct2/show/ NCT00890500).

3.3.5 Aryl Hydrocarbon receptor (AhR) antagonists

Using a high-throughput screen based on CD34/CD133 expression, Boitano et al identified a purine derivative (StemRegenin1 or SR1) capable of *in vitro* enhancing the levels of a CD34+ cell population derived from blood of mobilized donors. SR1 added to human CD34+ cells cultured for 5 weeks led to a 10-fold increase in total nucleated cells, a 47-fold increase in CD34+ cells and a 65-fold increase in CFU. CD34+ cord blood cells cultured in the presence of SR1 for 3 weeks revealed a 17-fold increase in SRC content in NOD-SCID Gamma (NSG) primary recipient and a 12-fold increase in the number of secondary SRC compared to input (Boitano et al., 2010). Additional screens followed by a quantitative structure-activity relationship identified three novel compounds (i.e SR2, SR3 and SR4), structurally distinct from SR1, that expand the number of human CD34+ cells. Experiments that aimed to determine the ability of cord blood derived human HSC expanded with these molecules to engraft NSG mice are still undergoing (Bouchez et al., 2011). SR1, SR2, SR3 and SR4 were showed to act as antagonists of AhR signaling. Indeed, this receptor has been implicated in HSC biology and hematopoietic disease through numerous factors including c-MYC, HES-1, PU.1, C/EBP, β-catenin, CXCR4, and STAT-5 (Singh et al., 2009). However, the precise mechanism whereby an AhR inhibitor might induce HSC self-renewal remains unknown.

3.3.6 SALL4

The transcription factor SALL4 was reported to play a role in maintaining ES cell pluripotency through interaction with Oct4 and Nanog (Wu et al., 2006; Yang et al., 2010). It was recently showed that overexpression of SALL4 can expand *ex vivo* human mobilized HSC from peripheral blood (Aguila et al., 2011). SALL4-transduced cells seemed capable of *ex vivo* expansion of both, CD34+CD38- and CD34+CD38+ cells and showed enhanced stem cell engraftment and long term repopulation capacity in NOD-SCID mice. Moreover, human CD34+ cells cultured 3 to 4 days with a soluble SALL4 fusion protein (TAT-SALL4B) showed a 10-fold increase in total mononuclear cells, a 8-fold increase in CD34+ cells and a 10-fold increase in the CFU number compare to controls (Aguila et al., 2011). However, *in vivo* studies with this fusion protein still have to be conducted to validate that these expanded cells are still able to reconstitute hematopoiesis in transplanted recipients.

4. *De novo* generation of HSC

Considering the interest in HSC expansion for treatment of both malignant and non-malignant diseases as well as their use in gene therapy and the difficulty to obtain *ex vivo* expansion of HSC without loss of their regeneration capacities, relevant methods to produce *de novo* HSC have emerged.

4.1 Obtaining HSC from ESC

One of these methods was initiated 20 years ago when ESC could be cultivated *in vitro* and directed to generate hematopoietic cells (Wiles and Keller, 1991). Since then, culture conditions were constantly optimized and allowed the differentiation into specific hematopoietic lineages such as erythroid and myeloid lineages, T and B lymphocytes and megakaryocytes (for review see Sakamoto et al., 2010). These protocols were then adapted to human (h) ESC. These cells like their murine counterparts, are karyotypically stable, capable of prolonged self-renewal, and might differentiate into most cell types. These properties might be exploited for therapeutic benefits to cure many human degenerative diseases and resulted in intense biomedical studies.

Different methods were established to generate hematopoietic progenitors and specific lineages from mouse ESC including embryoid bodies formation, coculture with stromal cells, and direct differentiation in coated plates using a mixture of cytokines and growth factors without stromal cells (Tian and Kaufman, 2008). These protocols were then optimized for efficient differentiation of hESC into early mesodermal cells (Bernardo et al., 2011) and for obtaining defined hematopoietic precursors from ES cells (Chiang and Wong, 2011; Salvagiotto et al., 2011).

The ultimate goal of these strategies is to produce HSC capable of robust, long-term, multilineage engraftment to alleviate blood cells diseases; however the numbers and the capacities of the *de novo* cells generated are not quite sufficient to fulfill the clinical challenge. At present, multipotent hematopoietic progenitors (short-term HSC) with limited engrafting ability in transplanted mice were obtained (Woods et al., 2011). Other groups reported efficient generation of cells that mostly produce the myeloid lineage following long term engraftment or produce CD34+ hematopoietic precursors that have phenotype similar to adult HSC but might best correspond to the embryonic stage of yolk-sac, aortogonadal-mesonephros (AGM), and/or fetal liver stage of hematopoiesis (Melichar et al., 2011; Narayan et al., 2006 and for review : Tian and Kaufman, 2008). More recently, the polycomb group protein Bmi1 was shown to promote more than 100-fold increase of hematopoietic cell development from ESC (Ding et al., 2011).

Since short-term HSC could be generated from ESC, an attractive option to increase the number of clinically competent HSC would be to find a molecule that dedifferentiate from short-term or mature hematopoietic cells to the long-term HSC population. Such a strategy might be valuable, since de-differentiation of somatic cells mediated by a chemical has been achieved in other systems. This is the case for reversine or 2-(4-morpholinoanilino)-6-cyclo-hexylaminopurine. This chemical compound was reported to induce reversal of mouse myoblast cell line, C2C12, to become multipotent progenitor cells, which can re-differentiate into osteoblasts and adipocytes (Chen et al., 2004). The de-differentiation activity of reversine however is not conserved across all cell lineages, since in certain cell types, it acts as a potent differentiation-inducing molecule (D'Alise et al., 2008).

To support the generation of long-term repopulating HSC from mouse ESC, other groups tested intrinsic regulators of adult HSC (Schuringa et al., 2004; Wang et al., 2005b). However, the use of many of these compounds, such as HoxB4, did not improve the expected engraftment efficiency *in vivo* (Wang et al., 2005a).

An unfavorable complication for the use of ESC in producing HSC is that lifelong use of drugs is required to prevent rejection of the transplanted cells. In order to make ESC practical for therapeutic use, it would be necessary to create a new stem cell line for each patient that needs treatment. Serious technical and ethical problems are associated with this issue.

4.2 Obtaining HSC from induced pluripotent stem cells

An alternative to the utilization of ES cells to produce *de novo* HSC arise from one of the most transformative accomplishments performed in the last years: the discovery that transient overexpression of a small number of defined transcription factors can reprogram the differentiated cells and become pluripotent populations. These cells are commonly referred to as Induced Pluripotent Stem Cells (iPSC) and have definitively broken the dogma commonly accepted that differentiated cell types generally lack the ability to revert back to a less specialized state.

4.2.1 Reprogramming somatic cells to pluripotency

The direct reprogramming of somatic cells to pluripotency was demonstrated in 2006, when Takahashi and Yamanaka converted adult mouse fibroblasts to iPSC by overexpressing four transcription factors: octamer-binding transcription factor 4 (OCT4), sex determining region Y-box 2 (SOX2), Kruppel-like factor 4 (KLF4), and cytoplasmic Myc (c-MYC) in mouse embryonic fibroblasts using retroviruses (Takahashi and Yamanaka, 2006). The transcription factors originally used for reprogramming differentiated cells are not stringently necessary to achieve this process as some of them can be replaced by other factors. Yu et al. were able to reprogram human fibroblasts with a distinct set of transcription factors comprising OCT4,

SOX2, NANOG, and LIN28 (Yu et al., 2007). Krüppel-like transcription factors (Klf2 and Klf5) and the orphan nuclear receptor, Esrrb, can replace Klf4 (Nakagawa et al., 2008 and for review see Feng et al., 2009).

The derived iPSC exhibited typical ESC morphology and were similar to ESC in their regenerative potential (Takahashi and Yamanaka, 2006) and their capacity to differentiate into cells of all three germ layers, the ectoderm, mesoderm, and endoderm. Because iPSC are generated without the need to destroy an embryo, their discovery has further energized the field of regenerative medicine and stem cell biology. Patient-specific therapeutic cells derived from induced pluripotent stem iPSC may bypass the ethical issues associated with ESC and avoid potential immunological reactions associated with allogenic transplantation. These human disease–specific iPSC provide a unique and previously unavailable resource for studying the pathophysiology of various important human diseases.

The therapeutical hope of iPSC is based on three issues: 1) The ability to generate iPSC from any tissue of the organism, and further differentiate them according to the patient needs, particularly into a wide range of primary human cell types, many of which are unavailable for routine use; 2) The ability to generate iPSC from patients with any disease; 3) The possibility of using patient-derived iPSC for drug development.

The therapeutic potential of such iPSC (schematized in Fig. 5) was demonstrated in a proof-of-principle study using a humanized sickle cell anemia mouse model (Hanna et al., 2007). In this study, mice could be rescued after transplantation with hematopoietic progenitors obtained *in vitro* from autologous iPSC. This was achieved after correction of the human sickle hemoglobin allele by gene-specific targeting.

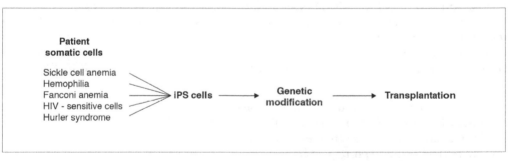

Fig. 5. Studies performed to validate the therapeutic potential of iPSC.

Also in mice, Xu et al. cured hemophilia by transplantation of cells that were generated from murine wild-type iPSC. These murine experiments suggest that human iPSC can be utilized for regenerative and therapeutic applications (Xu et al., 2009). Most recently, patient-specific iPSC have been established. Raya et al. reprogrammed dermal fibroblasts and/or epidermal keratinocytes of Fanconi anemia patients to generate iPSC, which were genetically corrected with lentiviral vectors encoding FANCA or FANCD2, to obtain hematopoietic progenitors of the myeloid and erythroid lineages that are phenotypically normal, that is, disease-free (Raya et al., 2009). Similar strategies were performed to correct the Hurler syndrome (Tolar et al., 2011) and for the production of macrophages from iPSCs which were resistant to HIV infection (Kambal et al., 2011).

The enthusiasm surrounding the clinical potential of iPSC is tempered by key issues regarding their safety, efficacy, and long-term benefits. Fully realizing the biomedical potential of iPSC in a clinical setting will require addressing certain limitations inherent to the process. First, need to find alternative strategies to remove non-viral or non-integrative vectors to overcome their potential deleterious effects. Although expression of the exogenous reprogramming factors is eventually silenced during iPSC cell generation, there is a significant risk of tumorigenesis if these exogenous genes are inadvertently reactivated. Second, it will be essential to increase the number of cells with specific phenotype. Third, it will be necessary to improve the efficiency of reprogramming (0.001–3% of cells are reprogrammed) since this is a slow and inefficient process (Jaenisch and Young, 2008; Nakagawa et al., 2008; Wernig et al., 2008).

4.2.2 Improving reprogramming somatic cells to pluripotency

To overcome the potential deleterious effects of viral vectors or oncogenes, and to improve the efficiency of the process toward a potential clinical application, a powerful alternative is offered by using small molecules. Several small molecules were reported to improve the reprogramming process by lowering the epigenetic barrier to initiate pluripotency (for reviews see Feng et al., 2009; Lyssiotis et al., 2011). Consistent with this notion, small molecules that affect reorganization of chromatin architecture, a rate limiting step during the reprogramming of a somatic genome, have been identified (Blelloch et al., 2006; Hochedlinger and Jaenisch, 2006; Huangfu et al., 2008a). In particular, the HDAC inhibitor VPA was shown to strongly increase reprogramming efficiency in the absence of c-Myc in both mouse and human cells and to allow 2-factor reprogramming (Oct4 and Sox2) of human fibroblasts in the absence of Klf4 and c-Myc (Huangfu et al., 2008b). Other epigenetic regulators such as BIX01294, a G9a histone methyltransferase inhibitor; BayK8644, an L-type calcium channel agonist and the two DNA methyltransferase inhibitors, AzaC and RG108 (summarized in Fig. 6), substantially increased reprogramming efficiency (Lukaszewicz et al., 2010; Shi et al., 2008).

The low efficiency of reprogramming (Hong et al., 2009) might also result from the accumulation of ROS (Parrinello et al., 2003). Consistent with this, Esteban et al. found that vitamin C strongly increases the reprogramming efficiency (Esteban et al., 2010). This is in line with the study reporting that hypoxic conditions improve the efficiency of iPSC production generated from mouse or human somatic cells (Yoshida et al., 2009). Co-treatment with VPA synergizes this effect. Other molecules including the MEK inhibitor PD0325901, the GSK3 inhibitor CHIR99021 combined with tranylcypromine, kenpaullone, SB-431542, and the TGF-β signaling inhibitor called RepSox (Ichida et al., 2009) were reported to enhance reprogramming or to replace viral vectors or oncogenes (Li and Ding, 2009; Pan and Thomson, 2007).

With the continued use of high-throughput screening to identify more chemicals that could assist in reprogramming, we may be closer to the goal of using a chemical-only cocktail to reprogram somatic cells to iPSC. These pluripotency gene activators may be then used in combination with specific differentiation modulators to achieve the production of the desired cell type.

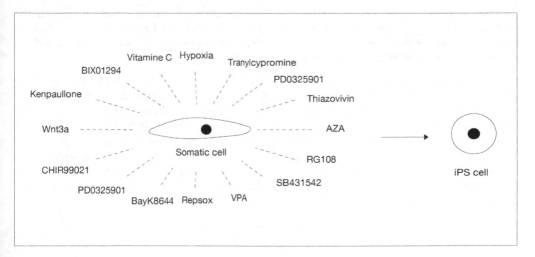

Fig. 6. Chemicals used to enhance reprogramming or to replace core reprogramming factors.

4.2.3 Obtaining HSC from induced pluripotent stem cells

Differentiation of iPSC into hematopoietic lineage have been achieved using a combination of specific cytokines and growth factors (Sakamoto et al., 2010) and have already demonstrated from both mouse and human iPSC (Lengerke et al., 2009; Niwa et al., 2009; Woods et al., 2011). However, the number of cells obtained in view of therapeutic use is still insufficient and small molecules that might expand the production of hematopoietic cells have yet to be found. Studies in this direction are beginning to emerge. For example, Wnt signaling, in particular WNT3a, mediates the stimulation of hemoangiogenic cell development and increase hematopoietic differentiation from ESC and iPSC (Wang and Nakayama, 2009; Wang et al., 2010). However, the conditions to generate human HSC capable of robust, long-term, multilineage engraftment from iPSC are still hoped for.

5. Conclusion

The ex-vivo expansion of HSC represents a promising approach to obtain large enough quantities for therapeutic intervention in cell and gene therapy protocols. Derivatives of hESCs and iPS cells are also expected to be employed as *de novo* HSC source for therapeutic settings. However, as described in the previous section, practical and ethical issues must be settled before clinical practice can begin. In both cases, the chemical biology approach using small molecules as tools or drugs holds unquestionably greater promise in the outcome of the final goal.

Even though a few molecules are being tested in clinical assays, the ideal soluble factor that enables to increase the number of rare HSC during the *ex vivo* growth culture without limiting their regeneration capacities has yet to be found. Most attempts have been unsuccessful because i) suitable expansion *in vitro* has been mostly correlated with loss of the regenerative capacities of HSC *in vivo*; ii) no straight forward method allows the association of *in vitro* observations with the *in vivo* outcome; iii) testing the *in vivo* effect of each molecule independently would be costly, time-consuming and would need an imposing number of mice which is ethically inconceivable.

In an attempt to develop new tools that might overcome some of these limitations, we have developed an innovative screening strategy to identify molecules for their potential to improve the *in vitro* HSC self-renewal and proliferation while preserving the HSC regenerative capacities *in vivo* (Sii Felice K, Grosselin J, Leboulch P, Tronik-Le Roux D, manuscript in preparation). Our approach is based on stem cells labeling with specific barcodes before exposure to the molecules (Fig. 7). Then, prior to their infusion in myeloablated mice, all the treated cells are pooled. Several weeks after transplantation, the identification of barcodes present in the blood and the BM of transplanted mice will enable the precise retrospective quantification of the initial effect of the molecule.

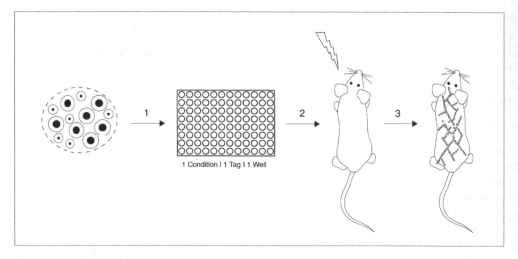

1 Condition I 1 Tag I 1 Well

Fig. 7. Schematic representation of the strategy developed to simultaneously test dozens of molecules. Each well contains barcoded-HSC (1) treated by a particular molecule. After several days of *in vitro* culture (2), all the cells are pooled, infused in myeloablated mice. The identification of barcodes in blood and BM of transplanted mice will enable the precise retrospective quantification of the initial effect of the molecule.

This strategy might facilitate the development of high-throughput screening for fast and effective identification of small molecules that can be used to burst the production of HSC. This will undoubtedly accelerate the promise of regenerative medicine as a routine therapeutic modality for many blood diseases as well as for gene and cell therapy.

6. Acknowledgments

We are grateful to Eliane Le Roux for graphic illustrations and Matthew Uselman for critical reading of the manuscript. We sincerely apologize to our colleagues whose relevant work was omitted in this review because of space limitations.

7. References

Abe, S., Lauby, G., Boyer, C., Rennard, S. I. & Sharp, J. G. (2003). *Transplanted BM and BM side population cells contribute progeny to the lung and liver in irradiated mice.* Cytotherapy 5, 523-533.

Aguila, J. R., Liao, W., Yang, J., Avila, C., Hagag, N., Senzel, L. & Ma, Y. (2011). *SALL4 is a robust stimulator for the expansion of hematopoietic stem cells.* Blood 118, 576-585.

Almeida-Porada, G., Zanjani, E. D. & Porada, C. D. (2010). *Bone marrow stem cells and liver regeneration.* Exp Hematol 38, 574-580.

Amsellem, S. & Fichelson, S. (2006). *Ex vivo expansion of human hematopoietic stem cells by passive transduction of the HOXB4 homeoprotein.* J Soc Biol 200, 235-241.

Amsellem, S., Pflumio, F., Bardinet, D., Izac, B., Charneau, P., Romeo, P. H., Dubart-Kupperschmitt, A. & Fichelson, S. (2003). *Ex vivo expansion of human hematopoietic stem cells by direct delivery of the HOXB4 homeoprotein.* Nat Med 9, 1423-1427.

Antonchuk, J., Sauvageau, G. & Humphries, R. K. (2002). *HOXB4-induced expansion of adult hematopoietic stem cells ex vivo.* Cell 109, 39-45.

Araki, H., Mahmud, N., Milhem, M., Nunez, R., Xu, M., Beam, C. A. & Hoffman, R. (2006). *Expansion of human umbilical cord blood SCID-repopulating cells using chromatin-modifying agents.* Exp Hematol 34, 140-149.

Araki, H., Yoshinaga, K., Boccuni, P., Zhao, Y., Hoffman, R. & Mahmud, N. (2007). *Chromatin-modifying agents permit human hematopoietic stem cells to undergo multiple cell divisions while retaining their repopulating potential.* Blood 109, 3570-3578.

Baird, A. (1994). *Fibroblast growth factors: activities and significance of non-neurotrophin neurotrophic growth factors.* Curr Opin Neurobiol 4, 78-86.

Baum, C., Dullmann, J., Li, Z., Fehse, B., Meyer, J., Williams, D. A. & von Kalle, C. (2003). *Side effects of retroviral gene transfer into hematopoietic stem cells.* Blood 101, 2099-2114.

Becker, P. S., Taylor, J. A., Trobridge, G. D., Zhao, X., Beard, B. C., Chien, S., Adair, J., Kohn, D. B., Wagner, J. E., Shimamura, A. & Kiem, H. P. (2010). *Preclinical correction of human Fanconi anemia complementation group A bone marrow cells using a safety-modified lentiviral vector.* Gene Ther 17, 1244-1252.

Bejsovec, A. (2005). *Wnt pathway activation: new relations and locations.* Cell 120, 11-14.

Bernardo, A. S., Faial, T., Gardner, L., Niakan, K. K., Ortmann, D., Senner, C. E., Callery, E. M., Trotter, M. W., Hemberger, M., Smith, J. C., et al. (2011). *BRACHYURY and CDX2 Mediate BMP-Induced Differentiation of Human and Mouse Pluripotent Stem Cells into Embryonic and Extraembryonic Lineages.* Cell Stem Cell 9, 144-155.

Bhardwaj, G., Murdoch, B., Wu, D., Baker, D. P., Williams, K. P., Chadwick, K., Ling, L. E., Karanu, F. N. & Bhatia, M. (2001). *Sonic hedgehog induces the proliferation of primitive human hematopoietic cells via BMP regulation.* Nat Immunol 2, 172-180.

Bhatia, M., Bonnet, D., Wu, D., Murdoch, B., Wrana, J., Gallacher, L. & Dick, J. E. (1999). *Bone morphogenetic proteins regulate the developmental program of human hematopoietic stem cells.* J Exp Med 189, 1139-1148.

Blank, U., Karlsson, G. & Karlsson, S. (2008). *Signaling pathways governing stem-cell fate.* Blood 111, 492-503.

Blank, U., Karlsson, G., Moody, J. L., Utsugisawa, T., Magnusson, M., Singbrant, S., Larsson, J. & Karlsson, S. (2006). *Smad7 promotes self-renewal of hematopoietic stem cells.* Blood *108*, 4246-4254.

Blelloch, R., Wang, Z., Meissner, A., Pollard, S., Smith, A. & Jaenisch, R. (2006). *Reprogramming efficiency following somatic cell nuclear transfer is influenced by the differentiation and methylation state of the donor nucleus.* Stem Cells 24, 2007-2013.

Boitano, A. E., Wang, J., Romeo, R., Bouchez, L. C., Parker, A. E., Sutton, S. E., Walker, J. R., Flaveny, C. A., Perdew, G. H., Denison, M. S., et al. (2010). *Aryl hydrocarbon receptor antagonists promote the expansion of human hematopoietic stem cells.* Science *329*, 1345-1348.

Bolos, V., Grego-Bessa, J. & de la Pompa, J. L. (2007). *Notch signaling in development and cancer.* Endocr Rev *28*, 339-363.

Bottcher, R. T. & Niehrs, C. (2005). *Fibroblast growth factor signaling during early vertebrate development.* Endocr Rev *26*, 63-77.

Bouchez, L. C., Boitano, A. E., de Lichtervelde, L., Romeo, R., Cooke, M. P. & Schultz, P. G. (2011). *Small-molecule regulators of human stem cell self-renewal.* Chembiochem *12*, 854-857.

Broske, A. M., Vockentanz, L., Kharazi, S., Huska, M. R., Mancini, E., Scheller, M., Kuhl, C., Enns, A., Prinz, M., Jaenisch, R., et al. (2009). *DNA methylation protects hematopoietic stem cell multipotency from myeloerythroid restriction.* Nat Genet *41*, 1207-1215.

Brun, A. C., Fan, X., Bjornsson, J. M., Humphries, R. K. & Karlsson, S. (2003). *Enforced adenoviral vector-mediated expression of HOXB4 in human umbilical cord blood CD34+ cells promotes myeloid differentiation but not proliferation.* Mol Ther *8*, 618-628.

Buske, C., Feuring-Buske, M., Abramovich, C., Spiekermann, K., Eaves, C. J., Coulombel, L., Sauvageau, G., Hogge, D. E. & Humphries, R. K. (2002). *Deregulated expression of HOXB4 enhances the primitive growth activity of human hematopoietic cells.* Blood *100*, 862-868.

Carlesso, N., Aster, J. C., Sklar, J. & Scadden, D. T. (1999). *Notch1-induced delay of human hematopoietic progenitor cell differentiation is associated with altered cell cycle kinetics.* Blood *93*, 838-848.

Cerdan, C. & Bhatia, M. (2010). *Novel roles for Notch, Wnt and Hedgehog in hematopoesis derived from human pluripotent stem cells.* Int J Dev Biol *54*, 955-963.

Chadwick, K., Shojaei, F., Gallacher, L. & Bhatia, M. (2005). *Smad7 alters cell fate decisions of human hematopoietic repopulating cells.* Blood *105*, 1905-1915.

Chadwick, N., Nostro, M. C., Baron, M., Mottram, R., Brady, G. & Buckle, A. M. (2007). *Notch signaling induces apoptosis in primary human CD34+ hematopoietic progenitor cells.* Stem Cells *25*, 203-210.

Chen, C., Liu, Y., Liu, R., Ikenoue, T., Guan, K. L., Liu, Y. & Zheng, P. (2008). *TSC-mTOR maintains quiescence and function of hematopoietic stem cells by repressing mitochondrial biogenesis and reactive oxygen species.* J Exp Med *205*, 2397-2408.

Chen, S., Zhang, Q., Wu, X., Schultz, P. G. & Ding, S. (2004). *Dedifferentiation of lineage-committed cells by a small molecule.* J Am Chem Soc *126*, 410-411.

Chiang, P. M. & Wong, P. C. (2011). *Differentiation of an embryonic stem cell to hemogenic endothelium by defined factors: essential role of bone morphogenetic protein 4.* Development *138*, 2833-2843.

Cipolleschi, M. G., Dello Sbarba, P. & Olivotto, M. (1993). *The role of hypoxia in the maintenance of hematopoietic stem cells.* Blood 82, 2031-2037.

Cobas, M., Wilson, A., Ernst, B., Mancini, S. J., MacDonald, H. R., Kemler, R. & Radtke, F. (2004). *Beta-catenin is dispensable for hematopoiesis and lymphopoiesis.* J Exp Med 199, 221-229.

Crcareva, A., Saito, T., Kunisato, A., Kumano, K., Suzuki, T., Sakata-Yanagimoto, M., Kawazu, M., Stojanovic, A., Kurokawa, M., Ogawa, S., et al. (2005). *Hematopoietic stem cells expanded by fibroblast growth factor-1 are excellent targets for retrovirus-mediated gene delivery.* Exp Hematol 33, 1459-1469.

D'Alise, A. M., Amabile, G., Iovino, M., Di Giorgio, F. P., Bartiromo, M., Sessa, F., Villa, F., Musacchio, A. & Cortese, R. (2008). *Reversine, a novel Aurora kinases inhibitor, inhibits colony formation of human acute myeloid leukemia cells.* Mol Cancer Ther 7, 1140-1149.

Daga, A., Podesta, M., Capra, M. C., Piaggio, G., Frassoni, F. & Corte, G. (2000). *The retroviral transduction of HOXC4 into human CD34(+) cells induces an in vitro expansion of clonogenic and early progenitors.* Exp Hematol 28, 569-574.

Dahlberg, A., Delaney, C. & Bernstein, I. D. (2011). *Ex vivo expansion of human hematopoietic stem and progenitor cells.* Blood 117, 6083-6090.

Danet, G. H., Pan, Y., Luongo, J. L., Bonnet, D. A. & Simon, M. C. (2003). *Expansion of human SCID-repopulating cells under hypoxic conditions.* J Clin Invest 112, 126-135.

De Felice, L., Tatarelli, C., Mascolo, M. G., Gregorj, C., Agostini, F., Fiorini, R., Gelmetti, V., Pascale, S., Padula, F., Petrucci, M. T., et al. (2005). *Histone deacetylase inhibitor valproic acid enhances the cytokine-induced expansion of human hematopoietic stem cells.* Cancer Res 65, 1505-1513.

de Haan, G., Weersing, E., Dontje, B., van Os, R., Bystrykh, L. V., Vellenga, E. & Miller, G. (2003). *In vitro generation of long-term repopulating hematopoietic stem cells by fibroblast growth factor-1.* Dev Cell 4, 241-251.

de Lima, M., McMannis, J., Gee, A., Komanduri, K., Couriel, D., Andersson, B. S., Hosing, C., Khouri, I., Jones, R., Champlin, R., et al. (2008). *Transplantation of ex vivo expanded cord blood cells using the copper chelator tetraethylenepentamine: a phase I/II clinical trial.* Bone Marrow Transplant 41, 771-778.

Delaney, C., Heimfeld, S., Brashem-Stein, C., Voorhies, H., Manger, R. L. & Bernstein, I. D. (2010). *Notch-mediated expansion of human cord blood progenitor cells capable of rapid myeloid reconstitution.* Nat Med 16, 232-236.

Delaney, C., Varnum-Finney, B., Aoyama, K., Brashem-Stein, C. & Bernstein, I. D. (2005). *Dose-dependent effects of the Notch ligand Delta1 on ex vivo differentiation and in vivo marrow repopulating ability of cord blood cells.* Blood 106, 2693-2699.

Ding, X., Lin, Q., Ensenat-Waser, R., Rose-John, S. & Zenke, M. (2011). *Polycomb Group Protein Bmi1 Promotes Hematopoietic Cell Development from Embryonic Stem Cells.* Stem Cells Dev.

Drake, A. C., Khoury, M., Leskov, I., Iliopoulou, B. P., Fragoso, M., Lodish, H. & Chen, J. (2011). *Human CD34+ CD133+ hematopoietic stem cells cultured with growth factors including Angptl5 efficiently engraft adult NOD-SCID Il2rgamma-/- (NSG) mice.* PLoS One 6, e18382.

Duarte, T. L., Cooke, M. S. & Jones, G. D. (2009). *Gene expression profiling reveals new protective roles for vitamin C in human skin cells.* Free Radic Biol Med 46, 78-87.

Duncan, A. W., Rattis, F. M., DiMascio, L. N., Congdon, K. L., Pazianos, G., Zhao, C., Yoon, K., Cook, J. M., Willert, K., Gaiano, N. & Reya, T. (2005). *Integration of Notch and Wnt signaling in hematopoietic stem cell maintenance.* Nat Immunol 6, 314-322.

Eliasson, P. & Jonsson, J. I. (2010). *The hematopoietic stem cell niche: low in oxygen but a nice place to be.* J Cell Physiol 222, 17-22.

Ernst, P., Fisher, J. K., Avery, W., Wade, S., Foy, D. & Korsmeyer, S. J. (2004). *Definitive hematopoiesis requires the mixed-lineage leukemia gene.* Dev Cell 6, 437-443.

Esteban, M. A., Wang, T., Qin, B., Yang, J., Qin, D., Cai, J., Li, W., Weng, Z., Chen, J., Ni, S., et al. (2010). *Vitamin C enhances the generation of mouse and human induced pluripotent stem cells.* Cell Stem Cell 6, 71-79.

Feng, B., Ng, J. H., Heng, J. C. & Ng, H. H. (2009). *Molecules that promote or enhance reprogramming of somatic cells to induced pluripotent stem cells.* Cell Stem Cell 4, 301-312.

Fournier, M., Lebert-Ghali, C. E., Krosl, G. & Bijl, J. J. (2011). *HOXA4 Induces Expansion of Hematopoietic Stem Cells In Vitro and Confers Enhancement of Pro-B-Cells In Vivo.* Stem Cells Dev.

Frisch, B. J., Porter, R. L., Gigliotti, B. J., Olm-Shipman, A. J., Weber, J. M., O'Keefe, R. J., Jordan, C. T. & Calvi, L. M. (2009). *In vivo prostaglandin E2 treatment alters the bone marrow microenvironment and preferentially expands short-term hematopoietic stem cells.* Blood 114, 4054-4063.

Gao, J., Graves, S., Koch, U., Liu, S., Jankovic, V., Buonamici, S., El Andaloussi, A., Nimer, S. D., Kee, B. L., Taichman, R., et al. (2009). *Hedgehog signaling is dispensable for adult hematopoietic stem cell function.* Cell Stem Cell 4, 548-558.

Giampaolo, A., Pelosi, E., Valtieri, M., Montesoro, E., Sterpetti, P., Samoggia, P., Camagna, A., Mastroberardino, G., Gabbianelli, M., Testa, U. & et al. (1995). *HOXB gene expression and function in differentiating purified hematopoietic progenitors.* Stem Cells 13 Suppl 1, 90-105.

Goessling, W., Allen, R. S., Guan, X., Jin, P., Uchida, N., Dovey, M., Harris, J. M., Metzger, M. E., Bonifacino, A. C., Stroncek, D., et al. (2011). *Prostaglandin E2 enhances human cord blood stem cell xenotransplants and shows long-term safety in preclinical nonhuman primate transplant models.* Cell Stem Cell 8, 445-458.

Goey, H., Keller, J. R., Back, T., Longo, D. L., Ruscetti, F. W. & Wiltrout, R. H. (1989). *Inhibition of early murine hemopoietic progenitor cell proliferation after in vivo locoregional administration of transforming growth factor-beta 1.* J Immunol 143, 877-880.

Gupta, R., Karpatkin, S. & Basch, R. S. (2006). *Hematopoiesis and stem cell renewal in long-term bone marrow cultures containing catalase.* Blood 107, 1837-1846.

Han, H., Tanigaki, K., Yamamoto, N., Kuroda, K., Yoshimoto, M., Nakahata, T., Ikuta, K. & Honjo, T. (2002). *Inducible gene knockout of transcription factor recombination signal binding protein-J reveals its essential role in T versus B lineage decision.* Int Immunol 14, 637-645.

Hanna, J., Wernig, M., Markoulaki, S., Sun, C. W., Meissner, A., Cassady, J. P., Beard, C., Brambrink, T., Wu, L. C., Townes, T. M. & Jaenisch, R. (2007). *Treatment of sickle cell anemia mouse model with iPS cells generated from autologous skin.* Science 318, 1920-1923.

Hao, Y., Cheng, D., Ma, Y., Zhou, W. & Wang, Y. (2011). *Antioxidant intervention: a new method for improving hematopoietic reconstitution capacity of peripheral blood stem cells.* Med Hypotheses 76, 421-423.

Hatzfeld, J., Li, M. L., Brown, E. L., Sookdeo, H., Levesque, J. P., O'Toole, T., Gurney, C., Clark, S. C. & Hatzfeld, A. (1991). *Release of early human hematopoietic progenitors from quiescence by antisense transforming growth factor beta 1 or Rb oligonucleotides.* J Exp Med 174, 925-929.

Hermitte, F., Brunet de la Grange, P., Belloc, F., Praloran, V. & Ivanovic, Z. (2006). *Very low O2 concentration (0.1%) favors G0 return of dividing CD34+ cells.* Stem Cells 24, 65-73.

Himburg, H. A., Muramoto, G. G., Daher, P., Meadows, S. K., Russell, J. L., Doan, P., Chi, J. T., Salter, A. B., Lento, W. E., Reya, T., et al. (2010). *Pleiotrophin regulates the expansion and regeneration of hematopoietic stem cells.* Nat Med 16, 475-482.

Hochedlinger, K. & Jaenisch, R. (2006). *Nuclear reprogramming and pluripotency.* Nature 441, 1061-1067.

Hofmann, I., Stover, E. H., Cullen, D. E., Mao, J., Morgan, K. J., Lee, B. H., Kharas, M. G., Miller, P. G., Cornejo, M. G., Okabe, R., et al. (2009). *Hedgehog signaling is dispensable for adult murine hematopoietic stem cell function and hematopoiesis.* Cell Stem Cell 4, 559-567.

Hoggatt, J., Singh, P., Sampath, J. & Pelus, L. M. (2009). *Prostaglandin E2 enhances hematopoietic stem cell homing, survival, & proliferation.* Blood 113, 5444-5455.

Hong, H., Takahashi, K., Ichisaka, T., Aoi, T., Kanagawa, O., Nakagawa, M., Okita, K. & Yamanaka, S. (2009). *Suppression of induced pluripotent stem cell generation by the p53-p21 pathway.* Nature 460, 1132-1135.

Huang, R., Southall, N., Wang, Y., Yasgar, A., Shinn, P., Jadhav, A., Nguyen, D. T. & Austin, C. P. (2011). *The NCGC pharmaceutical collection: a comprehensive resource of clinically approved drugs enabling repurposing and chemical genomics.* Sci Transl Med 3, 80ps16.

Huangfu, D., Maehr, R., Guo, W., Eijkelenboom, A., Snitow, M., Chen, A. E. & Melton, D. A. (2008a). *Induction of pluripotent stem cells by defined factors is greatly improved by small-molecule compounds.* Nat Biotechnol 26, 795-797.

Huangfu, D., Osafune, K., Maehr, R., Guo, W., Eijkelenboom, A., Chen, S., Muhlestein, W. & Melton, D. A. (2008b). *Induction of pluripotent stem cells from primary human fibroblasts with only Oct4 and Sox2.* Nat Biotechnol 26, 1269-1275.

Ichida, J. K., Blanchard, J., Lam, K., Son, E. Y., Chung, J. E., Egli, D., Loh, K. M., Carter, A. C., Di Giorgio, F. P., Koszka, K., et al. (2009). *A small-molecule inhibitor of tgf-Beta signaling replaces sox2 in reprogramming by inducing nanog.* Cell Stem Cell 5, 491-503.

Iiyama, M., Kakihana, K., Kurosu, T. & Miura, O. (2006). *Reactive oxygen species generated by hematopoietic cytokines play roles in activation of receptor-mediated signaling and in cell cycle progression.* Cell Signal 18, 174-182.

Ito, K., Hirao, A., Arai, F., Takubo, K., Matsuoka, S., Miyamoto, K., Ohmura, M., Naka, K., Hosokawa, K., Ikeda, Y. & Suda, T. (2006). *Reactive oxygen species act through p38 MAPK to limit the lifespan of hematopoietic stem cells.* Nat Med 12, 446-451.

Itoh, F., Itoh, S., Goumans, M. J., Valdimarsdottir, G., Iso, T., Dotto, G. P., Hamamori, Y., Kedes, L., Kato, M. & ten Dijke Pt, P. (2004). *Synergy and antagonism between Notch and BMP receptor signaling pathways in endothelial cells.* Embo J 23, 541-551.

Iwama, A., Oguro, H., Negishi, M., Kato, Y., Morita, Y., Tsukui, H., Ema, H., Kamijo, T., Katoh-Fukui, Y., Koseki, H., et al. (2004). *Enhanced self-renewal of hematopoietic stem cells mediated by the polycomb gene product Bmi-1.* Immunity 21, 843-851.

Jaenisch, R. & Young, R. (2008). *Stem cells, the molecular circuitry of pluripotency and nuclear reprogramming.* Cell 132, 567-582.

Jaleco, A. C., Neves, H., Hooijberg, E., Gameiro, P., Clode, N., Haury, M., Henrique, D. & Parreira, L. (2001). *Differential effects of Notch ligands Delta-1 and Jagged-1 in human lymphoid differentiation.* J Exp Med 194, 991-1002.

Jang, Y. Y., Collector, M. I., Baylin, S. B., Diehl, A. M. & Sharkis, S. J. (2004). *Hematopoietic stem cells convert into liver cells within days without fusion.* Nat Cell Biol 6, 532-539.

Jang, Y. Y. & Sharkis, S. J. (2005). *Stem cell plasticity: a rare cell, not a rare event.* Stem Cell Rev 1, 45-51.

Jang, Y. Y. & Sharkis, S. J. (2007). *A low level of reactive oxygen species selects for primitive hematopoietic stem cells that may reside in the low-oxygenic niche.* Blood 110, 3056-3063.

Kaivo-Oja, N., Bondestam, J., Kamarainen, M., Koskimies, J., Vitt, U., Cranfield, M., Vuojolainen, K., Kallio, J. P., Olkkonen, V. M., Hayashi, M., et al. (2003). *Growth differentiation factor-9 induces Smad2 activation and inhibin B production in cultured human granulosa-luteal cells.* J Clin Endocrinol Metab 88, 755-762.

Kambal, A., Mitchell, G., Cary, W., Gruenloh, W., Jung, Y., Kalomoiris, S., Nacey, C., McGee, J., Lindsey, M., Fury, B., et al. (2011). *Generation of HIV-1 resistant and functional macrophages from hematopoietic stem cell-derived induced pluripotent stem cells.* Mol Ther 19, 584-593.

Karanu, F. N., Murdoch, B., Gallacher, L., Wu, D. M., Koremoto, M., Sakano, S. & Bhatia, M. (2000). *The notch ligand jagged-1 represents a novel growth factor of human hematopoietic stem cells.* J Exp Med 192, 1365-1372.

Karanu, F. N., Murdoch, B., Miyabayashi, T., Ohno, M., Koremoto, M., Gallacher, L., Wu, D., Itoh, A., Sakano, S. & Bhatia, M. (2001). *Human homologues of Delta-1 and Delta-4 function as mitogenic regulators of primitive human hematopoietic cells.* Blood 97, 1960-1967.

Karlsson, G., Blank, U., Moody, J. L., Ehinger, M., Singbrant, S., Deng, C. X. & Karlsson, S. (2007). *Smad4 is critical for self-renewal of hematopoietic stem cells.* J Exp Med 204, 467-474.

Kasper, M., Jaks, V., Fiaschi, M. & Toftgard, R. (2009). *Hedgehog signaling in breast cancer.* Carcinogenesis 30, 903-911.

Kirstetter, P., Anderson, K., Porse, B. T., Jacobsen, S. E. & Nerlov, C. (2006). *Activation of the canonical Wnt pathway leads to loss of hematopoietic stem cell repopulation and multilineage differentiation block.* Nat Immunol 7, 1048-1056.

Klump, H., Schiedlmeier, B. & Baum, C. (2005). *Control of self-renewal and differentiation of hematopoietic stem cells: HOXB4 on the threshold.* Ann N Y Acad Sci 1044, 6-15.

Kobune, M., Ito, Y., Kawano, Y., Sasaki, K., Uchida, H., Nakamura, K., Dehari, H., Chiba, H., Takimoto, R., Matsunaga, T., et al. (2004). *Indian hedgehog gene transfer augments hematopoietic support of human stromal cells including NOD/SCID-beta2m-/-repopulating cells.* Blood 104, 1002-1009.

Krivtsov, A. V., Twomey, D., Feng, Z., Stubbs, M. C., Wang, Y., Faber, J., Levine, J. E., Wang, J., Hahn, W. C., Gilliland, D. G., et al. (2006). *Transformation from committed progenitor to leukaemia stem cell initiated by MLL-AF9.* Nature 442, 818-822.

Kroon, E., Krosl, J., Thorsteinsdottir, U., Baban, S., Buchberg, A. M. & Sauvageau, G. (1998). *Hoxa9 transforms primary bone marrow cells through specific collaboration with Meis1a but not Pbx1b.* Embo J 17, 3714-3725.

Krosl, J., Austin, P., Beslu, N., Kroon, E., Humphries, R. K. & Sauvageau, G. (2003). *In vitro expansion of hematopoietic stem cells by recombinant TAT-HOXB4 protein.* Nat Med 9, 1428-1432.

Kugawa, F., Watanabe, M. & Tamanoi, F. (2007). *Chemical Biology/Chemical genetics/chemical genomics: importance of chemical library.* Chem-Bio Informatics Journal 7, 49-68.

Labbe, E., Letamendia, A. & Attisano, L. (2000). *Association of Smads with lymphoid enhancer binding factor 1/T cell-specific factor mediates cooperative signaling by the transforming growth factor-beta and wnt pathways.* Proc Natl Acad Sci U S A 97, 8358-8363.

Larsson, J., Blank, U., Klintman, J., Magnusson, M. & Karlsson, S. (2005). *Quiescence of hematopoietic stem cells and maintenance of the stem cell pool is not dependent on TGF-beta signaling in vivo.* Exp Hematol 33, 592-596.

Lauret, E., Catelain, C., Titeux, M., Poirault, S., Dando, J. S., Dorsch, M., Villeval, J. L., Groseil, A., Vainchenker, W., Sainteny, F. & Bennaceur-Griscelli, A. (2004). *Membrane-bound delta-4 notch ligand reduces the proliferative activity of primitive human hematopoietic CD34+CD38low cells while maintaining their LTC-IC potential.* Leukemia 18, 788-797.

Lengerke, C., Grauer, M., Niebuhr, N. I., Riedt, T., Kanz, L., Park, I. H. & Daley, G. Q. (2009). *Hematopoietic development from human induced pluripotent stem cells.* Ann N Y Acad Sci 1176, 219-227.

Li, W. & Ding, S. (2009). *Small molecules that modulate embryonic stem cell fate and somatic cell reprogramming.* Trends Pharmacol Sci.

Louis, I., Heinonen, K. M., Chagraoui, J., Vainio, S., Sauvageau, G. & Perreault, C. (2008). *The signaling protein Wnt4 enhances thymopoiesis and expands multipotent hematopoietic progenitors through beta-catenin-independent signaling.* Immunity 29, 57-67.

Luis, T. C., Weerkamp, F., Naber, B. A., Baert, M. R., de Haas, E. F., Nikolic, T., Heuvelmans, S., De Krijger, R. R., van Dongen, J. J. & Staal, F. J. (2009). *Wnt3a deficiency irreversibly impairs hematopoietic stem cell self-renewal and leads to defects in progenitor cell differentiation.* Blood 113, 546-554.

Lukaszewicz, A. I., McMillan, M. K. & Kahn, M. (2010). *Small molecules and stem cells. Potency and lineage commitment: the new quest for the fountain of youth.* J Med Chem 53, 3439-3453.

Lyssiotis, C. A., Lairson, L. L., Boitano, A. E., Wurdak, H., Zhu, S. & Schultz, P. G. (2011). *Chemical control of stem cell fate and developmental potential.* Angew Chem Int Ed Engl 50, 200-242.

Matsuno, K., Diederich, R. J., Go, M. J., Blaumueller, C. M. & Artavanis-Tsakonas, S. (1995). *Deltex acts as a positive regulator of Notch signaling through interactions with the Notch ankyrin repeats.* Development 121, 2633-2644.

Melichar, H., Li, O., Ross, J., Haber, H., Cado, D., Nolla, H., Robey, E. A. & Winoto, A. (2011). *Comparative study of hematopoietic differentiation between human embryonic stem cell lines.* PLoS One 6, e19854.

Merchant, A., Joseph, G., Wang, Q., Brennan, S. & Matsui, W. (2010). *Gli1 regulates the proliferation and differentiation of HSCs and myeloid progenitors.* Blood 115, 2391-2396.

Mezey, E., Chandross, K. J., Harta, G., Maki, R. A. & McKercher, S. R. (2000). *Turning blood into brain: cells bearing neuronal antigens generated in vivo from bone marrow.* Science 290, 1779-1782.

Milner, L. A., Kopan, R., Martin, D. I. & Bernstein, I. D. (1994). *A human homologue of the Drosophila developmental gene, Notch, is expressed in CD34+ hematopoietic precursors.* Blood 83, 2057-2062.

Moon, R. T., Kohn, A. D., De Ferrari, G. V. & Kaykas, A. (2004). *WNT and beta-catenin signaling: diseases and therapies.* Nat Rev Genet 5, 691-701.

Murdoch, B., Chadwick, K., Martin, M., Shojaei, F., Shah, K. V., Gallacher, L., Moon, R. T. & Bhatia, M. (2003). *Wnt-5A augments repopulating capacity and primitive hematopoietic development of human blood stem cells in vivo.* Proc Natl Acad Sci U S A 100, 3422-3427.

Nakagawa, M., Koyanagi, M., Tanabe, K., Takahashi, K., Ichisaka, T., Aoi, T., Okita, K., Mochiduki, Y., Takizawa, N. & Yamanaka, S. (2008). *Generation of induced pluripotent stem cells without Myc from mouse and human fibroblasts.* Nat Biotechnol 26, 101-106.

Narayan, A. D., Chase, J. L., Lewis, R. L., Tian, X., Kaufman, D. S., Thomson, J. A. & Zanjani, E. D. (2006). *Human embryonic stem cell-derived hematopoietic cells are capable of engrafting primary as well as secondary fetal sheep recipients.* Blood 107, 2180-2183.

Nemeth, M. J., Topol, L., Anderson, S. M., Yang, Y. & Bodine, D. M. (2007). *Wnt5a inhibits canonical Wnt signaling in hematopoietic stem cells and enhances repopulation.* Proc Natl Acad Sci U S A 104, 15436-15441.

Nishino, T., Miyaji, K., Ishiwata, N., Arai, K., Yui, M., Asai, Y., Nakauchi, H. & Iwama, A. (2009). *Ex vivo expansion of human hematopoietic stem cells by a small-molecule agonist of c-MPL.* Exp Hematol 37, 1364-1377 e1364.

Niwa, A., Umeda, K., Chang, H., Saito, M., Okita, K., Takahashi, K., Nakagawa, M., Yamanaka, S., Nakahata, T. & Heike, T. (2009). *Orderly hematopoietic development of induced pluripotent stem cells via Flk-1(+) hemoangiogenic progenitors.* J Cell Physiol 221, 367-377.

North, T. E., Goessling, W., Walkley, C. R., Lengerke, C., Kopani, K. R., Lord, A. M., Weber, G. J., Bowman, T. V., Jang, I. H., Grosser, T., et al. (2007). *Prostaglandin E2 regulates vertebrate haematopoietic stem cell homeostasis.* Nature 447, 1007-1011.

Ogawa, M., Larue, A. C., Watson, P. M. & Watson, D. K. (2010). *Hematopoietic stem cell origin of connective tissues.* Exp Hematol 38, 540-547.

Ohishi, K., Katayama, N., Shiku, H., Varnum-Finney, B. & Bernstein, I. D. (2003). *Notch signaling in hematopoiesis.* Semin Cell Dev Biol 14, 143-150.

Ohishi, K., Varnum-Finney, B. & Bernstein, I. D. (2002). *Delta-1 enhances marrow and thymus repopulating ability of human CD34(+)CD38(-) cord blood cells.* J Clin Invest 110, 1165-1174.

Ohmizono, Y., Sakabe, H., Kimura, T., Tanimukai, S., Matsumura, T., Miyazaki, H., Lyman, S. D. & Sonoda, Y. (1997). *Thrombopoietin augments ex vivo expansion of human cord blood-derived hematopoietic progenitors in combination with stem cell factor and flt3 ligand.* Leukemia *11*, 524-530.

Ohta, H., Sekulovic, S., Bakovic, S., Eaves, C. J., Pineault, N., Gasparetto, M., Smith, C., Sauvageau, G. & Humphries, R. K. (2007). *Near-maximal expansions of hematopoietic stem cells in culture using NUP98-HOX fusions.* Exp Hematol *35*, 817-830.

Pan, G. & Thomson, J. A. (2007). *Nanog and transcriptional networks in embryonic stem cell pluripotency.* Cell Res *17*, 42-49.

Park, I. K., Qian, D., Kiel, M., Becker, M. W., Pihalja, M., Weissman, I. L., Morrison, S. J. & Clarke, M. F. (2003). *Bmi-1 is required for maintenance of adult self-renewing haematopoietic stem cells.* Nature *423*, 302-305.

Parmar, K., Mauch, P., Vergilio, J. A., Sackstein, R. & Down, J. D. (2007). *Distribution of hematopoietic stem cells in the bone marrow according to regional hypoxia.* Proc Natl Acad Sci U S A *104*, 5431-5436.

Parrinello, S., Samper, E., Krtolica, A., Goldstein, J., Melov, S. & Campisi, J. (2003). *Oxygen sensitivity severely limits the replicative lifespan of murine fibroblasts.* Nat Cell Biol *5*, 741-747.

Peled, T., Glukhman, E., Hasson, N., Adi, S., Assor, H., Yudin, D., Landor, C., Mandel, J., Landau, E., Prus, E., et al. (2005). *Chelatable cellular copper modulates differentiation and self-renewal of cord blood-derived hematopoietic progenitor cells.* Exp Hematol *33*, 1092-1100.

Peled, T., Landau, E., Mandel, J., Glukhman, E., Goudsmid, N. R., Nagler, A. & Fibach, E. (2004a). *Linear polyamine copper chelator tetraethylenepentamine augments long-term ex vivo expansion of cord blood-derived CD34+ cells and increases their engraftment potential in NOD/SCID mice.* Exp Hematol *32*, 547-555.

Peled, T., Landau, E., Prus, E., Treves, A. J., Nagler, A. & Fibach, E. (2002). *Cellular copper content modulates differentiation and self-renewal in cultures of cord blood-derived CD34+ cells.* Br J Haematol *116*, 655-661.

Peled, T., Mandel, J., Goudsmid, R. N., Landor, C., Hasson, N., Harati, D., Austin, M., Hasson, A., Fibach, E., Shpall, E. J. & Nagler, A. (2004b). *Pre-clinical development of cord blood-derived progenitor cell graft expanded ex vivo with cytokines and the polyamine copper chelator tetraethylenepentamine.* Cytotherapy *6*, 344-355.

Pervaiz, S., Taneja, R. & Ghaffari, S. (2009). *Oxidative stress regulation of stem and progenitor cells.* Antioxid Redox Signal *11*, 2777-2789.

Pineault, N., Abramovich, C. & Humphries, R. K. (2005). *Transplantable cell lines generated with NUP98-Hox fusion genes undergo leukemic progression by Meis1 independent of its binding to DNA.* Leukemia *19*, 636-643.

Pineault, N., Abramovich, C., Ohta, H. & Humphries, R. K. (2004). *Differential and common leukemogenic potentials of multiple NUP98-Hox fusion proteins alone or with Meis1.* Mol Cell Biol *24*, 1907-1917.

Pineault, N., Cortin, V., Boyer, L., Garnier, A., Robert, A., Therien, C. & Roy, D. C. (2010). *Individual and synergistic cytokine effects controlling the expansion of cord blood CD34(+) cells and megakaryocyte progenitors in culture.* Cytotherapy *13*, 467-480.

Pineault, N., Helgason, C. D., Lawrence, H. J. & Humphries, R. K. (2002). *Differential expression of Hox, Meis1, & Pbx1 genes in primitive cells throughout murine hematopoietic ontogeny.* Exp Hematol 30, 49-57.

Portela, A. & Esteller, M. (2010). *Epigenetic modifications and human disease.* Nat Biotechnol 28, 1057-1068.

Quesenberry, P. J., Dooner, M. S. & Aliotta, J. M. (2010). *Stem cell plasticity revisited: the continuum marrow model and phenotypic changes mediated by microvesicles.* Exp Hematol 38, 581-592.

Radtke, F., Wilson, A., Stark, G., Bauer, M., van Meerwijk, J., MacDonald, H. R. & Aguet, M. (1999). *Deficient T cell fate specification in mice with an induced inactivation of Notch1.* Immunity 10, 547-558.

Raya, A., Rodriguez-Piza, I., Guenechea, G., Vassena, R., Navarro, S., Barrero, M. J., Consiglio, A., Castella, M., Rio, P., Sleep, E., et al. (2009). *Disease-corrected haematopoietic progenitors from Fanconi anaemia induced pluripotent stem cells.* Nature 460, 53-59.

Rizo, A., Dontje, B., Vellenga, E., de Haan, G. & Schuringa, J. J. (2008). *Long-term maintenance of human hematopoietic stem/progenitor cells by expression of BMI1.* Blood 111, 2621-2630.

Sakamoto, H., Tsuji-Tamura, K. & Ogawa, M. (2010). *Hematopoiesis from pluripotent stem cell lines.* Int J Hematol 91, 384-391.

Salvagiotto, G., Burton, S., Daigh, C. A., Rajesh, D., Slukvin, II, & Seay, N. J. (2011). *A defined, feeder-free, serum-free system to generate in vitro hematopoietic progenitors and differentiated blood cells from hESCs and hiPSCs.* PLoS One 6, e17829.

Sauvageau, G., Lansdorp, P. M., Eaves, C. J., Hogge, D. E., Dragowska, W. H., Reid, D. S., Largman, C., Lawrence, H. J. & Humphries, R. K. (1994). *Differential expression of homeobox genes in functionally distinct CD34+ subpopulations of human bone marrow cells.* Proc Natl Acad Sci U S A 91, 12223-12227.

Sauvageau, G., Thorsteinsdottir, U., Eaves, C. J., Lawrence, H. J., Largman, C., Lansdorp, P. M. & Humphries, R. K. (1995). *Overexpression of HOXB4 in hematopoietic cells causes the selective expansion of more primitive populations in vitro and in vivo.* Genes Dev 9, 1753-1765.

Scadden, D. T. (2006). *The stem-cell niche as an entity of action.* Nature 441, 1075-1079.

Scheller, M., Huelsken, J., Rosenbauer, F., Taketo, M. M., Birchmeier, W., Tenen, D. G. & Leutz, A. (2006). *Hematopoietic stem cell and multilineage defects generated by constitutive beta-catenin activation.* Nat Immunol 7, 1037-1047.

Schiedlmeier, B., Klump, H., Will, E., Arman-Kalcek, G., Li, Z., Wang, Z., Rimek, A., Friel, J., Baum, C. & Ostertag, W. (2003). *High-level ectopic HOXB4 expression confers a profound in vivo competitive growth advantage on human cord blood CD34+ cells, but impairs lymphomyeloid differentiation.* Blood 101, 1759-1768.

Schuringa, J. J., Wu, K., Morrone, G. & Moore, M. A. (2004). *Enforced activation of STAT5A facilitates the generation of embryonic stem-derived hematopoietic stem cells that contribute to hematopoiesis in vivo.* Stem Cells 22, 1191-1204.

Seet, L. F., Teng, E., Lai, Y. S., Laning, J., Kraus, M., Wnendt, S., Merchav, S. & Chan, S. L. (2009). *Valproic acid enhances the engraftability of human umbilical cord blood hematopoietic stem cells expanded under serum-free conditions.* Eur J Haematol *82,* 124-132.

Shi, Y., Desponts, C., Do, J. T., Hahm, H. S., Scholer, H. R. & Ding, S. (2008). *Induction of pluripotent stem cells from mouse embryonic fibroblasts by Oct4 and Klf4 with small-molecule compounds.* Cell Stem Cell *3,* 568-574.

Shimizu, K., Chiba, S., Saito, T., Kumano, K. & Hirai, H. (2000). *Physical interaction of Delta1, Jagged1, & Jagged2 with Notch1 and Notch3 receptors.* Biochem Biophys Res Commun *276,* 385-389.

Simonnet, A. J., Nehme, J., Vaigot, P., Barroca, V., Leboulch, P. & Tronik-Le Roux, D. (2009). *Phenotypic and functional changes induced in hematopoietic stem/progenitor cells after gamma-ray radiation exposure.* Stem Cells *27,* 1400-1409.

Simsek, T., Kocabas, F., Zheng, J., Deberardinis, R. J., Mahmoud, A. I., Olson, E. N., Schneider, J. W., Zhang, C. C. & Sadek, H. A. (2010). *The distinct metabolic profile of hematopoietic stem cells reflects their location in a hypoxic niche.* Cell Stem Cell *7,* 380-390.

Singh, K. P., Casado, F. L., Opanashuk, L. A. & Gasiewicz, T. A. (2009). *The aryl hydrocarbon receptor has a normal function in the regulation of hematopoietic and other stem/progenitor cell populations.* Biochem Pharmacol *77,* 577-587.

Sitnicka, E., Lin, N., Priestley, G. V., Fox, N., Broudy, V. C., Wolf, N. S. & Kaushansky, K. (1996). *The effect of thrombopoietin on the proliferation and differentiation of murine hematopoietic stem cells.* Blood *87,* 4998-5005.

Smith, L. L., Yeung, J., Zeisig, B. B., Popov, N., Huijbers, I., Barnes, J., Wilson, A. J., Taskesen, E., Delwel, R., Gil, J., et al. (2011). *Functional crosstalk between Bmi1 and MLL/Hoxa9 axis in establishment of normal hematopoietic and leukemic stem cells.* Cell Stem Cell *8,* 649-662.

Tadokoro, Y., Ema, H., Okano, M., Li, E. & Nakauchi, H. (2007). *De novo DNA methyltransferase is essential for self-renewal, but not for differentiation, in hematopoietic stem cells.* J Exp Med *204,* 715-722.

Takahashi, K. & Yamanaka, S. (2006). *Induction of pluripotent stem cells from mouse embryonic and adult fibroblast cultures by defined factors.* Cell *126,* 663-676.

Takubo, K., Goda, N., Yamada, W., Iriuchishima, H., Ikeda, E., Kubota, Y., Shima, H., Johnson, R. S., Hirao, A., Suematsu, M. & Suda, T. (2010). *Regulation of the HIF-1alpha level is essential for hematopoietic stem cells.* Cell Stem Cell *7,* 391-402.

Tang, Y., Chen, J. & Young, N. S. (2009). *Expansion of haematopoietic stem cells from normal donors and bone marrow failure patients by recombinant hoxb4.* Br J Haematol *144,* 603-612.

Theise, N. D. (2010). *Stem cell plasticity: recapping the decade, mapping the future.* Exp Hematol *38,* 529-539.

Tian, X. & Kaufman, D. S. (2008). *Differentiation of embryonic stem cells towards hematopoietic cells: progress and pitfalls.* Curr Opin Hematol *15,* 312-318.

Tolar, J., Park, I. H., Xia, L., Lees, C. J., Peacock, B., Webber, B., McElmurry, R. T., Eide, C. R., Orchard, P. J., Kyba, M., et al. (2011). *Hematopoietic differentiation of induced pluripotent stem cells from patients with mucopolysaccharidosis type I (Hurler syndrome).* Blood *117,* 839-847.

Trowbridge, J. J., Scott, M. P. & Bhatia, M. (2006). *Hedgehog modulates cell cycle regulators in stem cells to control hematopoietic regeneration.* Proc Natl Acad Sci U S A *103*, 14134-14139.

Trowbridge, J. J., Snow, J. W., Kim, J. & Orkin, S. H. (2009). *DNA methyltransferase 1 is essential for and uniquely regulates hematopoietic stem and progenitor cells.* Cell Stem Cell *5*, 442-449.

Van Den Berg, D. J., Sharma, A. K., Bruno, E. & Hoffman, R. (1998). *Role of members of the Wnt gene family in human hematopoiesis.* Blood *92*, 3189-3202.

Varnum-Finney, B., Brashem-Stein, C. & Bernstein, I. D. (2003). *Combined effects of Notch signaling and cytokines induce a multiple log increase in precursors with lymphoid and myeloid reconstituting ability.* Blood *101*, 1784-1789.

Varnum-Finney, B., Halasz, L. M., Sun, M., Gridley, T., Radtke, F. & Bernstein, I. D. (2011). *Notch2 governs the rate of generation of mouse long- and short-term repopulating stem cells.* J Clin Invest *121*, 1207-1216.

Varnum-Finney, B., Xu, L., Brashem-Stein, C., Nourigat, C., Flowers, D., Bakkour, S., Pear, W. S. & Bernstein, I. D. (2000). *Pluripotent, cytokine-dependent, hematopoietic stem cells are immortalized by constitutive Notch1 signaling.* Nat Med *6*, 1278-1281.

Walenda, T., Bokermann, G., Ventura Ferreira, M. S., Piroth, D. M., Hieronymus, T., Neuss, S., Zenke, M., Ho, A. D., Muller, A. M. & Wagner, W. (2011). *Synergistic effects of growth factors and mesenchymal stromal cells for expansion of hematopoietic stem and progenitor cells.* Exp Hematol *39*, 617-628.

Walker, L., Lynch, M., Silverman, S., Fraser, J., Boulter, J., Weinmaster, G. & Gasson, J. C. (1999). *The Notch/Jagged pathway inhibits proliferation of human hematopoietic progenitors in vitro.* Stem Cells *17*, 162-171.

Wang, L., Menendez, P., Shojaei, F., Li, L., Mazurier, F., Dick, J. E., Cerdan, C., Levac, K. & Bhatia, M. (2005a). *Generation of hematopoietic repopulating cells from human embryonic stem cells independent of ectopic HOXB4 expression.* J Exp Med *201*, 1603-1614.

Wang, N., Kim, H. G., Cotta, C. V., Wan, M., Tang, Y., Klug, C. A. & Cao, X. (2006). *TGFbeta/BMP inhibits the bone marrow transformation capability of Hoxa9 by repressing its DNA-binding ability.* Embo J *25*, 1469-1480.

Wang, Y. & Nakayama, N. (2009). *WNT and BMP signaling are both required for hematopoietic cell development from human ES cells.* Stem Cell Res *3*, 113-125.

Wang, Y., Umeda, K. & Nakayama, N. (2010). *Collaboration between WNT and BMP signaling promotes hemoangiogenic cell development from human fibroblast-derived iPS cells.* Stem Cell Res *4*, 223-231.

Wang, Y., Yates, F., Naveiras, O., Ernst, P. & Daley, G. Q. (2005b). *Embryonic stem cell-derived hematopoietic stem cells.* Proc Natl Acad Sci U S A *102*, 19081-19086.

Watts, K., Zhang, X., Beard, B., Chiu, S. Y., Trobridge, G. D., Humphries, R. K. & Kiem, H. P. (2011). *Differential Effects of HOXB4 and NUP98-HOXA10hd on Hematopoietic Repopulating Cells in a Nonhuman Primate Model.* Hum Gene Ther.

Weinreich, M. A., Lintmaer, I., Wang, L., Liggitt, H. D., Harkey, M. A. & Blau, C. A. (2006). *Growth factor receptors as regulators of hematopoiesis.* Blood *108*, 3713-3721.

Wernig, M., Lengner, C. J., Hanna, J., Lodato, M. A., Steine, E., Foreman, R., Staerk, J., Markoulaki, S. & Jaenisch, R. (2008). *A drug-inducible transgenic system for direct reprogramming of multiple somatic cell types.* Nat Biotechnol 26, 916-924.

Wiles, M. V. & Keller, G. (1991). *Multiple hematopoietic lineages develop from embryonic stem (ES) cells in culture.* Development 111, 259-267.

Willert, K., Brown, J. D., Danenberg, E., Duncan, A. W., Weissman, I. L., Reya, T., Yates, J. R., 3rd, & Nusse, R. (2003). *Wnt proteins are lipid-modified and can act as stem cell growth factors.* Nature 423, 448-452.

Wojcik, M., Burzynska-Pedziwiatr, I. & Wozniak, L. A. (2010). *A review of natural and synthetic antioxidants important for health and longevity.* Curr Med Chem 17, 3262-3288.

Woods, N. B., Parker, A. S., Moraghebi, R., Lutz, M. K., Firth, A. L., Brennand, K. J., Berggren, W. T., Raya, A., Belmonte, J. C., Gage, F. H. & Verma, I. M. (2011). *Brief report: efficient generation of hematopoietic precursors and progenitors from human pluripotent stem cell lines.* Stem Cells 29, 1158-1164.

Wu, Q., Chen, X., Zhang, J., Loh, Y. H., Low, T. Y., Zhang, W., Zhang, W., Sze, S. K., Lim, B. & Ng, H. H. (2006). *Sall4 interacts with Nanog and co-occupies Nanog genomic sites in embryonic stem cells.* J Biol Chem 281, 24090-24094.

Xu, D., Alipio, Z., Fink, L. M., Adcock, D. M., Yang, J., Ward, D. C. & Ma, Y. (2009). *Phenotypic correction of murine hemophilia A using an iPS cell-based therapy.* Proc Natl Acad Sci U S A 106, 808-813.

Yamazaki, S., Iwama, A., Takayanagi, S., Eto, K., Ema, H. & Nakauchi, H. (2009). *TGF-beta as a candidate bone marrow niche signal to induce hematopoietic stem cell hibernation.* Blood 113, 1250-1256.

Yang, J., Gao, C., Chai, L. & Ma, Y. (2010). *A novel SALL4/OCT4 transcriptional feedback network for pluripotency of embryonic stem cells.* PLoS One 5, e10766.

Yeoh, J. S., van Os, R., Weersing, E., Ausema, A., Dontje, B., Vellenga, E. & de Haan, G. (2006). *Fibroblast growth factor-1 and -2 preserve long-term repopulating ability of hematopoietic stem cells in serum-free cultures.* Stem Cells 24, 1564-1572.

Yoshida, Y., Takahashi, K., Okita, K., Ichisaka, T. & Yamanaka, S. (2009). *Hypoxia enhances the generation of induced pluripotent stem cells.* Cell Stem Cell 5, 237-241.

Young, J. C., Wu, S., Hansteen, G., Du, C., Sambucetti, L., Remiszewski, S., O'Farrell, A. M., Hill, B., Lavau, C. & Murray, L. J. (2004). *Inhibitors of histone deacetylases promote hematopoietic stem cell self-renewal.* Cytotherapy 6, 328-336.

Yu, J., Vodyanik, M. A., Smuga-Otto, K., Antosiewicz-Bourget, J., Frane, J. L., Tian, S., Nie, J., Jonsdottir, G. A., Ruotti, V., Stewart, R., et al. (2007). *Induced pluripotent stem cell lines derived from human somatic cells.* Science 318, 1917-1920.

Zhang, C. C., Kaba, M., Iizuka, S., Huynh, H. & Lodish, H. F. (2008a). *Angiopoietin-like 5 and IGFBP2 stimulate ex vivo expansion of human cord blood hematopoietic stem cells as assayed by NOD/SCID transplantation.* Blood 111, 3415-3423.

Zhang, C. C. & Lodish, H. F. (2005). *Murine hematopoietic stem cells change their surface phenotype during ex vivo expansion.* Blood 105, 4314-4320.

Zhang, X. B., Beard, B. C., Beebe, K., Storer, B., Humphries, R. K. & Kiem, H. P. (2006). *Differential effects of HOXB4 on nonhuman primate short- and long-term repopulating cells.* PLoS Med 3, e173.

Zhang, X. B., Beard, B. C., Trobridge, G. D., Wood, B. L., Sale, G. E., Sud, R., Humphries, R. K. & Kiem, H. P. (2008b). *High incidence of leukemia in large animals after stem cell gene therapy with a HOXB4-expressing retroviral vector.* J Clin Invest *118*, 1502-1510.

Zhao, C., Blum, J., Chen, A., Kwon, H. Y., Jung, S. H., Cook, J. M., Lagoo, A. & Reya, T. (2007). *Loss of beta-catenin impairs the renewal of normal and CML stem cells in vivo.* Cancer Cell *12*, 528-541.

Permissions

The contributors of this book come from diverse backgrounds, making this book a truly international effort. This book will bring forth new frontiers with its revolutionizing research information and detailed analysis of the nascent developments around the world.

We would like to thank Rosana Pelayo, for lending her expertise to make the book truly unique. She has played a crucial role in the development of this book. Without her invaluable contribution this book wouldn't have been possible. She has made vital efforts to compile up to date information on the varied aspects of this subject to make this book a valuable addition to the collection of many professionals and students.

This book was conceptualized with the vision of imparting up-to-date information and advanced data in this field. To ensure the same, a matchless editorial board was set up. Every individual on the board went through rigorous rounds of assessment to prove their worth. After which they invested a large part of their time researching and compiling the most relevant data for our readers. Conferences and sessions were held from time to time between the editorial board and the contributing authors to present the data in the most comprehensible form. The editorial team has worked tirelessly to provide valuable and valid information to help people across the globe.

Every chapter published in this book has been scrutinized by our experts. Their significance has been extensively debated. The topics covered herein carry significant findings which will fuel the growth of the discipline. They may even be implemented as practical applications or may be referred to as a beginning point for another development. Chapters in this book were first published by InTech; hereby published with permission under the Creative Commons Attribution License or equivalent.

The editorial board has been involved in producing this book since its inception. They have spent rigorous hours researching and exploring the diverse topics which have resulted in the successful publishing of this book. They have passed on their knowledge of decades through this book. To expedite this challenging task, the publisher supported the team at every step. A small team of assistant editors was also appointed to further simplify the editing procedure and attain best results for the readers.

Our editorial team has been hand-picked from every corner of the world. Their multi-ethnicity adds dynamic inputs to the discussions which result in innovative outcomes. These outcomes are then further discussed with the researchers and contributors who give their valuable feedback and opinion regarding the same. The feedback is then collaborated with the researches and they are edited in a comprehensive manner to aid the understanding of the subject.

Apart from the editorial board, the designing team has also invested a significant amount of their time in understanding the subject and creating the most relevant covers. They scrutinized every image to scout for the most suitable representation of the subject and create an appropriate cover for the book.

The publishing team has been involved in this book since its early stages. They were actively engaged in every process, be it collecting the data, connecting with the contributors or procuring relevant information. The team has been an ardent support to the editorial, designing and production team. Their endless efforts to recruit the best for this project, has resulted in the accomplishment of this book. They are a veteran in the field of academics and their pool of knowledge is as vast as their experience in printing. Their expertise and guidance has proved useful at every step. Their uncompromising quality standards have made this book an exceptional effort. Their encouragement from time to time has been an inspiration for everyone.

The publisher and the editorial board hope that this book will prove to be a valuable piece of knowledge for researchers, students, practitioners and scholars across the globe.

List of Contributors

Takafumi Yokota, Kenji Oritani and Yuzuru Kanakura
Department of Hematology and Oncology, Osaka University Graduate School of Medicine, Suita, Japan

Stefan Butz, Stephan Ewers and Dietmar Vestweber
Department of Vascular Cell Biology, Max-Planck-Institute for Molecular Biomedicine, Münster, Germany

Rasmus Freter
Ludwig Institute for Cancer Research, University of Oxford, United Kingdom

Eliana Abdelhay, Luciana Pizzatti and Renata Binato
Instituto Nacional de Câncer, Rio de Janeiro, Brazil

Yasushi Kubota
Division of Hematology, Respiratory Medicine and Oncology, Department of Internal Medicine, Faculty of Medicine, Saga University, Japan
Department of Transfusion Medicine, Saga University Hospital, Japan

Shinya Kimura
Division of Hematology, Respiratory Medicine and Oncology, Department of Internal Medicine, Faculty of Medicine, Saga University, Japan

Atsuko Masumi
Department of Safety Research on Blood and Biological Products, National Institute of Infectious Diseases, Tokyo, Japan

Shoichiro Miyatake
Laboratory of Self Defense Gene Regulation, Tokyo Metropolitan Institute of Medical Science, Tokyo, Japan

Tomoko Kohno and Toshifumi Matsuyama
Department of Molecular Microbiology and Immunology, Nagasaki University Graduate School of Biomedical Sciences, Nagasaki, Japan

Keiyo Takubo
Department of Cell Differentiation, The Sakaguchi Laboratory of Developmental Biology, Keio University School of Medicine, Tokyo, Japan

Mayumi Naramura
University of Nebraska Medical Center, USA

Elizabeth Sweeney and Olena Jacenko
University of Pennsylvania, USA

Aysegul Ocal Sahin and Miranda Buitenhuis
Department of Hematology and Erasmus MC Stem Cell Institute for Regenerative Medicine, Erasmus MC, Rotterdam, The Netherlands

Jeanne Grosselin, Karine Sii-Felice and Diana Tronik-Le Roux
CEA, Institute of Emerging Diseases and Innovative Therapies (iMETI), Fontenay-aux-Roses, France
Inserm U962 and University Paris 11, CEA-iMETI, Fontenay-aux-Roses, France

Philippe Leboulch
CEA, Institute of Emerging Diseases and Innovative Therapies (iMETI), Fontenay-aux-Roses, France
Inserm U962 and University Paris 11, CEA-iMETI, Fontenay-aux-Roses, France
Harvard Medical School and Genetics Division, Brigham & Women's Hospital, Boston, USA

Printed in the USA
CPSIA information can be obtained
at www.ICGtesting.com
JSHW011436221024
72173JS00004B/823

9 781632 412492